€55-00

TL2451

D1355303

Textbook of Disaster Psychiatry

This is the first textbook to focus specifically on disaster psychiatry. It brings together international experts to provide a comprehensive review of the psychological, biological, and social responses to disaster, describing evidence-based clinical and service-led interventions to meet mental health needs and foster resilience and recovery. Chapters address the epidemiology of disaster response, the neurobiology of disaster exposure, socio-cultural issues, early intervention and consultation-liaison care, the role of non-governmental organizations, workplace policies, and implications for public health planning at the level of the individual and the community. This book is essential reading for all those involved in preparing for traumatic events and their clinical and social outcomes for public health planning.

ROBERT J. URSANO is Professor of Psychiatry and Neuroscience and Chairman of the Department of Psychiatry at the Uniformed Services University of the Health Sciences, Bethesda, Maryland. He is also Director of the Center for the Study of Traumatic Stress.

CAROL S. FULLERTON is Research Professor in the Department of Psychiatry at the Uniformed Services University of the Health Sciences, Bethesda, Maryland. She is also the Scientific Director of the Center for the Study of Traumatic Stress.

LARS WEISAETH is Professor of Psychiatry and Director of Research in the Division of Disaster Psychiatry at the Norwegian Centre for Violence and Traumatic Stress Studies, University of Oslo, Norway.

BEVERLEY RAPHAEL is Professor of Population Mental Health and Disasters and Director of the Centre for Disasters and Terrorism at the University of Western Sydney. She is Emeritus Professor of Psychiatry, at the University of Queensland and holds professorial appointments at the Universities of Sydney, New South Wales, and Newcastle.

Textbook of Disaster Psychiatry

Edited by

Robert J. Ursano
Carol S. Fullerton
Uniformed Services University of the Health Sciences

Lars Weisaeth
University of Oslo

Beverley Raphael
University of Western Sydney

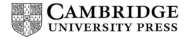
CAMBRIDGE
UNIVERSITY PRESS

CAMBRIDGE UNIVERSITY PRESS
Cambridge, New York, Melbourne, Madrid, Cape Town, Singapore, São Paulo

Cambridge University Press
The Edinburgh Building, Cambridge CB2 8RU, UK

Published in the United States of America by Cambridge University Press, New York

www.cambridge.org
Information on this title: www.cambridge.org/9780521852357

© Cambridge University Press 2007

First published 2007

Printed in the United Kingdom at the University Press, Cambridge

A catalogue record for this publication is available from the British Library

ISBN 978-0-521-85235-7 hardback

Contents

Contributors

David M. Benedek, M.D.
Associate Professor
Department of Psychiatry
Center for the Study of Traumatic Stress
Uniformed Services University of the
  Health Sciences
4301 Jones Bridge Road
Bethesda, MD 20814
USA

Melissa J. Brymer, Psy.D.
Director, Terrorism and Disaster Programs
National Center for Child Traumatic Stress
University of California, Los Angeles
11150 W. Olympic Boulevard, Suite 650
Los Angeles, CA 90064
USA

Dennis S. Charney, M.D.
Professor and Dean, Psychiatry
Mount Sinai School of Medicine
One Gustave L. Levy Place, Box 1217
New York, NY 10029
USA

Zelde Espinel, M.D., MA, MPH
Center for Disaster and Extreme Event
Preparedness (DEEP Center)
University of Miami Miller
School of Medicine
1120 NW 14th St. Suite 1043
Miami, FL
USA

Brian W. Flynn, Ed.D.
Adjunct Psychiatry Professor
Department of Psychiatry
Center for the Study of Traumatic Stress
Uniformed Services University of the
    Health Sciences
P.O. Box 1205
Severna Park, MD 21146
USA

Carol S. Fullerton, Ph.D.
Research Professor
Department of Psychiatry
Center for the Study of Traumatic Stress
Uniformed Services University of the
    Health Sciences
4301 Jones Bridge Road
Bethesda, MD 20814
USA

Sandro Galea, M.D., Dr P.H., MPH
Associate Professor
Center for Social Epidemiology and
    Population Health
School of Public Health
The University of Michigan
1214 S. University
Ann Arbor, MI 48104-2548
USA

Robert K. Gifford, Ph.D.
Senior Scientist
Department of Psychiatry
Center for the Study of Traumatic Stress
Uniformed Services University of the
    Health Sciences
4301 Jones Bridge Road
Bethesda, MD 20814
USA

Harry C. Holloway, M.D.
Professor
Department of Psychiatry
Center for the Study of Traumatic Stress
Uniformed Services University of the
    Health Sciences

4301 Jones Bridge Road
Bethesda, MD 20814
USA

Joop de Jong, M.D.
Director of Public Health & Research
Transcultural Psychosocial Organization
Keizersgracht 329
1016EE Amsterdam
The Netherlands

Craig L. Katz, M.D.
Assistant Clinical Professor, Psychiatry
Mount Sinai School of Medicine
One Gustave L. Levy Place, Box 1217
New York, NY 10029
USA

James E. McCarroll, M.D., MPH
Research Professor
Department of Psychiatry
Center for the Study of Traumatic Stress
Uniformed Services University of the
    Health Sciences
4301 Jones Bridge Road
Bethesda, MD 20814
USA

Carol S. North, M.D.
Professor of Psychiatry
Nancy and Ray L. Hunt Chair in Crisis Psychiatry
Southwestern Medical Center
The University of Texas
Department of Psychiatry
6363 Forest Park Road
Dallas, TX 75390-8828
USA

Ann E. Norwood, M.D.
Senior Advisor for Public Health
Risk Communications
HHS/OS/OASPHEP
200 Independence Avenue, S.W. Room 636G
Washington, DC 20201
USA

Robert S. Pynoos, M.D., MPH
Center Director
Professor of Psychiatry
National Center for Child Traumatic Stress
UCLA
11150 W. Olympic Boulevard
Suite 650
Los Angeles, CA 90064
USA

Beverley Raphael, AM, MBBS, M.D.
Professor of Population Mental Health and Disasters
University of Western Sydney
Penrith South
NSW DC 1797
Australia

Dori B. Reissman, M.D., MPH
Capt. U.S.
Public Health Service
Senior Medical Advisor, Office of the Director
National Institute for Occupational
Safety and Health
395 E Street SW
Patriots Plaza I,
Suite 9200
Washington, DC 20201
USA

James R. Rundell, M.D.
Professor of Psychiatry
Mayo Clinic College of Medicine
200 First Street, SW, West 11
Rochester, MN 55905
USA

James M. Shultz, MS, Ph.D.
Director, Center for Disaster and Extreme Event
Preparedness (DEEP Center)
University of Miami Miller School of Medicine
1120 NW 14th St.
Suite 1043
Miami, FL
USA

Rebecca P. Smith, M.D.
World Trade Center Worker and Volunteer Mental
Health Screening, Monitoring and Interventions
Programs
Assistant Clinical Professor of Psychiatry
Mount Sinai School of Medicine
1212 5th Avenue, 3rd Floor
New York, NY 10029
USA

Steven M. Southwick, M.D.
Section of Child Study Center
Yale University
Department of Psychiatry
300 George Street
New Haven, CT 06511
USA

Alan M. Steinberg, Ph.D.
Associate Director
The National Child
Traumatic Stress Network
University of California, Los Angeles
11150 W. Olympic Boulevard
Suite 650
Los Angeles, CA 90064
USA

Robert J. Ursano, M.D.
Professor and Chairman
Department of Psychiatry
Director, Center for the Study of Traumatic Stress
Uniformed Services University of the
Health Sciences
4301 Jones Bridge Road
Bethesda, MD 20814
USA

Nancy T. Vineburgh, MA
Assistant Professor
Department of Psychiatry
Center for the Study of Traumatic Stress
Uniformed Services University of the
Health Sciences

4301 Jones Bridge Road
Bethesda, MD 20814
USA

Patricia J. Watson, Ph.D.
National Center for PTSD
VA Medical and Regional office
White River Junction, VT 05009
USA

Lars Weisaeth, MD
Professor, Division of Disaster Psychiatry
University of Oslo/The Military Medical Competence
Center, Building 20
Sognsvannsveien 21, 0320 Oslo
Norway

Douglas Zatzick, M.D.
Department of Psychiatry
University of Washington School of Medicine
325 Ninth Avenue, Box 359911
Seattle, WA 98104
USA

Preface

Disasters are a prominent part of our history and will be a part of our future. From gene to protein, cell to organ, and individual to group, the complexity of human responses to disaster trauma is profound. Understanding both individual and community mental health responses to disasters is critical to developing and planning for postdisaster interventions across the biological, psychological, and sociocultural levels.

Disaster planning begins with individual, family, community, and workplace preparedness prior to a disaster. Effective interventions are dependent on rapid, effective, and sustained mobilization of resources. Evidence-based interventions at multiple levels strengthen clinical care and community responses and facilitate resilience and recovery. Knowing the psychiatric and behavioral responses to disaster enables medical experts and community leaders to communicate to the public, deliver evidence-based care, promote resilience, foster adherence to recommendations, encourage behaviors which can facilitate recovery, and sustain the social fabric of the disaster communities and nations.

This textbook, the first specifically on disaster psychiatry, brings together international experts to provide a comprehensive view of the psychological, biological, and social processes of response to, and intervention for, disaster mental health needs. The chapters present cutting-edge scientific knowledge with implications for clinical care and interventions, services and public health policy development. The volume is organized to provide scientific information about psychiatric illness, disaster-related stress and health risk behaviors, as well as the treatment and public health services that are needed for disaster mental health care for individuals and communities in countries throughout the world. We believe that the comprehensive examination of disaster and its impact gives this textbook broad clinical and public health relevance.

The textbook is organized from basic concepts to care delivery and public health concerns. The information spans from the epidemiology of disaster response and disaster ecology to the neurobiology of disaster exposure; from early intervention to consultation-liaison care for injured disaster victims; from nongovernmental organizations and disaster care to workplace trauma and healthcare systems. The volume as a whole and each chapter have broad public health planning implications for individual and community mental healthcare following disasters and terrorism.

We hope that the knowledge in this volume of how mental health is altered by the experience of disaster trauma will lead to more effective approaches to treatment, intervention and recovery to inform both the mental health practitioner and the public health planner.

PART I

Introduction

Individual and community responses to disasters

Robert J. Ursano, Carol S. Fullerton, Lars Weisaeth,
& Beverley Raphael

While most of our work force returned to work soon after the hurricanes many were walking wounded. They were unfocused, spacey, not performing at their usual levels, and performance was inconsistent. I noticed this in other people before I realized that it was happening to me. The feelings and changes lingered longer than I would have thought – for months. The change in the environment – the loss of trees, "blue tarp" roofs, boarded-up houses that stayed boarded-up long after the threat of storms – and living in a dark cluttered home, all seemed to add to my deep sense of lethargy. It all weighed heavily on myself, my family, friends, and co-workers ... We didn't do any of the usual summer social get-togethers. The storms didn't just affect us when the wind blew, but changed the landscape of our lives ... I remember thinking that my neighborhood looked like an abandoned ghost town. The only neighbors I saw day to day were those who were out walking their dogs. Things are back to normal now, but there is still an edginess to us all I think. I guess now that the repairs are done it's time again to "board-up" and wait for this year's storms.

(Public Health Worker 9 months after five hurricanes had struck Florida in the summer of 2004)

In 2005, an estimated 162 million people worldwide were affected by disaster (i.e., natural disasters, industrial and other accidents, and epidemics). Over 105 000 people died and damages totaled over $176 million (World Health Organization, 2006). Concern for weather-related disasters – hurricanes and tsunamis – has increased over the past decade as has the concern for pandemic flu, which raises special issues of health protective behaviors such as adherence with medical recommendations, quarantine and travel restrictions. Terrorism and wars are human-made disasters. From the World Trade Center attacks of 2001, anthrax attacks in the United States, the 2004 train bombings in Madrid, the London tube attacks of 2005, to the ongoing terrorist attacks in the Middle East, terrorism has new prominence in disaster mental health planning for individuals, communities, and nations. In addition, there are at least 23 ongoing wars (http://en.wikipedia.org/wiki/Ongoing_wars) – with mass casualties, famine, and community devastation involving an estimated 40 countries (www.globalsecurity.org). Worldwide in the year 2000, over 300 000 people died from war (World Health Organization, 2001). Every disaster, natural or human-made, places extreme demands on health care and mental health care in particular across federal, state and local agencies, communities, and workplaces.

Disasters affect large and diverse populations. How the psychological response to a disaster is managed may be the defining factor in the ability of a community to recover (Holloway *et al.*, 1997). Interventions require rapid, effective, and sustained mobilization of resources (Ursano & Friedman, 2006). Sustaining the social fabric of the community and facilitating recovery depend on leadership's

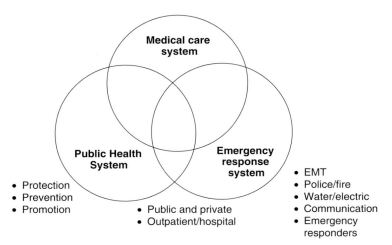

Figure 1.1 Coordinated systems approach

knowledge of a community's resilience and vulnerabilities as well as an understanding of the distress, disorder, and health risk behavioral responses to the event (Institute of Medicine, 2003; Raphael & Wooding, 2004). A coordinated systems approach across the medical care system, public health system, and emergency response system is necessary to meet the mental health care needs of a disaster region (see Figure 1.1).

Over time, the resilience of individuals and communities is the expected response to a disaster. But for some the effects can be severe and lasting. Experiencing an altered sense of safety, increased fear and arousal, and concern for the future affect not only those who may develop mental health problems but also those who continue to work and care for their families and loved ones. Consequence management for mental health – fostering resilience, decreasing and treating disorders and responding to health risk behaviors – requires preparing for, responding to, and focusing on the mitigation of disaster effects and recovery. For those directly exposed and those indirectly affected, the additional burdens of lost supports and increased demands are an ongoing part of disaster recovery. Importantly, in the aftermath of large-scale disasters, such as the Asian tsunami of 2004 which affected

thousands, early identification of individuals at risk for developing psychiatric disorders from those experiencing transient distress is key to delivering effective treatment (Bryant & Njenga, 2006).

The nature of disaster

A disaster is the result of exposure to a hazard that threatens personal safety, disrupts community and family structures, and results in personal and societal loss creating demands that exceed existing resources. Disasters are grouped into two major types: natural and human-made. Human-made disasters include technological accidents resulting from human error and intentional human acts such as terrorism. In general, human-made disasters have been shown to cause more frequent and more persistent psychiatric symptoms and distress (for review see Norris *et al.*, 2002). However, this distinction is increasingly difficult to make. The etiology and consequences of natural disasters often are the result of human beings. For example, the damage and loss of life caused by an earthquake can be magnified by poor construction practices and high-density occupancy. Similarly, humans may cause or contribute to natural disasters through poor land-management practices that increase the probability of floods. Interpersonal violence between individuals (assault) or groups (war, terrorism) is perhaps the most disturbing traumatic experience. Technological disasters may also bring specific fears about usually normal life events – for example, fear of flying after a plane crash or claustrophobia after a mine accident. Each of these may require public education or individual evaluation and intervention to assist population-level concerns or treat a persistent specific phobia and limit generalization to other areas of life (e.g., "I cannot cook anymore because the boiling water reminds me of the explosion"). Mass violence is the most disturbing of disasters. A review of over 60 000 disaster victims found 67% of those exposed to mass violence were severely impaired compared to 39% of those exposed to technological disasters and 34% of those exposed to natural disasters (Norris et al., 2002).

Psychiatric morbidity is associated with specific aspects of disasters. The risk of psychiatric morbidity is greatest for those with high perceived threat to life, low controllability, lack of predictability, high loss, injury, the possibility that the disaster will recur, and exposure to the dead and the grotesque (Boudreaux et al., 1998; Epstein et al., 1997; Green et al., 1985; North et al., 1999; Schuster et al., 2001; Wain et al., 2006; Zatzick et al., 2001). Disasters with a high degree of community destruction and those in developing countries are associated with worse outcomes (for review, see Davidson & McFarlane, 2006). Terrorism can be distinguished from other natural and human-made disasters by the characteristic extensive fear, loss of confidence in institutions, unpredictability and pervasive experience of loss of safety (Fullerton et al., 2003). In New York City after the terrorist attacks of September 11, 2001, 7.5% of southern Manhatten had probable posttraumatic stress disorder (PTSD; Galea et al., 2002). Nearly one-third of people with the highest levels of exposure (e.g., 37% of those in the building or 30% of the injured) had PTSD. Rates of PTSD decreased to 0.6% 6 months later.

In addition the effects of terrorism can echo through a nation. In a longitudinal national study of the reactions to the September 11 disaster, 64.6% of the United States outside of New York City reported fear of future terrorism at 2 months and 37.5% at 6 months (Silver et al., 2002). In addition, 59.5% reported fear of harm to family at 2 months and 40.6% at 6 months. In the weeks following the bombings in London, 31% of Londoners reported substantial stress and 32% reported that they intended to travel less (Rubin et al., 2005). Those reporting greater stress were 3.8 times more likely to have thought they could have been injured or killed and 1.7 times more likely to report having difficulty contacting friends or family by mobile phone. Four to seven months after Hurricane Katrina in the United States, in the highest impact area (the city of New Orleans), 49.6% reported nightmares and 8% reported these nightmares were occurring nearly every night (Kessler et al., 2006). Similarly, 58.2% reported being more jumpy or easily startled, and 79.4% reported being more irritable or angry. Findings following the Madrid March 11 train bombings again indicate that the magnitude of a terrorist attack is one of the primary determinants of the prevalence of PTSD (Miguel-Tobal et al., 2006). Terrorism is one of the most powerful and pervasive generators of psychiatric illness, distress and disrupted community and social functioning (Holloway et al., 1997; North et al., 1999).

Community response to disaster

Disasters overwhelm local resources and threaten the function and safety of the community. With the advent of instantaneous communication and media coverage, word of a disaster is disseminated quickly, and often is witnessed in real time around the globe. The disaster community is soon flooded with outsiders: people offering assistance, curiosity seekers, and the media. This sudden influx of strangers affects the community in many ways. The presence of large numbers of media representatives can be experienced as intrusive and insensitive. Hotel rooms have no vacancies, restaurants are crowded with unfamiliar faces, and the normal

Table 1.1 Generic and unique challenges in natural disaster, technological disaster, and terrorism

Dimension	Natural disaster[a]	Technological disaster[b]	Terrorism[c]
Altered sense of safety	+++	+++	+++
Intentional			+++
Unpredictable	++	+++	+++
Localized geographically	+++	++	
Local fear	+++	+++	++
National fear			+++
National bereavement	+	+	+++
Consequences spread over time	++	++	+++
Loss of confidence in institutions	+	+++	+++
Community disruption	+++	+++	+++
Target basic societal infrastructure			+++
Overwhelm health care systems	+++	++	+
Hoaxes/copycats			+++

[a] Natural disaster, e.g., hurricanes, tornados, earthquakes.
[b] Technological disasters, e.g., nuclear leaks, toxic spills.
[c] Terrorism, e.g., bombings, hostage taking.

routine of the community is altered. In the face of disaster, communities tend to pull together often with outside assistance, such as the financial and humanitarian aid seen following the Asian tsunami (Ghodse & Galea, 2006). At a time when, traditionally, communities turn inward to grieve and assist affected families, the normal social supports are strained and disrupted by outsiders.

Disruption of the community and workplace increases distress, health risk behaviors and risk of post-traumatic stress disorders. In the immediate aftermath of a disaster or terrorist attack, individuals and communities may respond in adaptive, effective ways or they may make fear-based decisions, resulting in unhelpful behaviors. Psychiatric disease and psychological function, including the subthreshold distress of individuals, depend upon the rapid, effective, and sustained mobilization of health care resources as well as community-level responses and resources. Knowledge of an individual's and community's resilience and vulnerability before a disaster or terrorist event as well as an understanding of the psychiatric and psychological responses to such an event enables leaders and

medical experts to talk to the public, in order to promote resilient healthy behaviors, sustain the social fabric of the community, and facilitate recovery (Institute of Medicine, 2003; Ursano et al., 2003b). The adaptive capacities of individuals and groups within a community are variable and need to be understood before a crisis in order to target needs effectively after a disaster. For example, community embeddedness – the degree to which one belongs to and is connected in one's neighborhood and community – may be both a risk factor and a protective factor after community-level disasters (see Fullerton et al., 1999; Sampson, 2003; Sampson et al., 1997).

The community and workplace also serve as important physical and emotional support systems. The larger the scale of the disaster, the greater the potential disruption of the community and workplace. It is helpful to compare the generic and unique challenges facing survivors of an airplane crash as well as those confronting victims of disasters such as tornados, earthquakes, or terrorist attacks (see Table 1.1). If family members are involved in the same airplane crash, the plane crash survivor can return home to family, friends, and coworkers. They will most likely go back to a structurally intact house, to a community unaffected by the accident, and to the same job with the same financial security. In contrast, a tornado involves additional factors that amplify the traumatic event itself. Although the tornado survivor may experience and witness comparably gruesome sights, the recovery environment is markedly different. Home and work site may have been destroyed, job lost, schools closed, food and water scarce, relatives and friends moved or perished, and coworkers may be dead, injured, or displaced. Thus, psychiatric morbidity is affected by both the degree of the disaster's impact on the community and its effects on the recovery environment (Gerrity & Steinglass, 1994; Hobfoll & Jackson, 1991; Steinglass & Gerrity, 1990; Noji, 1997).

The economic impacts of disasters are substantial. Loss of a job is a major post event predictor of negative psychiatric outcome (Galea *et al.*, 2002; Nandi *et al.*, 2004). These effects can be seen at the macro level; for example, a dip in consumer confidence was seen during and after the sniper attacks in the Washington, D.C. area in October 2002. Since terrorism targets the social capital of the nation – a nation's cohesion, values, and ability to function – economic behavioral changes may be substantial. Counterterrorism and national continuity are crucially dependent upon our having effective interventions to sustain the psychological, behavioral, and social function of the nation and its citizens. The psychological and behavioral consequences of disasters are a complex interaction between the disaster impact (e.g., destruction and death), the consequences of the response (e.g., economic loss, disruption, etc.), and the impact of subsequent preparedness or counterterrorism strategies themselves (e.g., behavioral and social ramifications of new security procedures).

Certain economic behaviors and decisions are affected by both the characteristics of disaster or terrorist attack and the psychological and behavioral responses to that disaster. For example, after Hurricane Katrina in the United States or the terrorist attacks seen on cities around the world, decisions and behaviors related to travel, home purchase, food consumption, and medical care visits were altered by changes in availability (Weisler *et al.*, 2006), and also by changes in perceived safety, and optimism about the future. Terrorism also can affect economic behavior through threats and hoaxes. These also carry with them economic costs and consequences. The local or national economy may see altered savings, insurance and investment, as well as changes in work attendance and productivity, and broader national or industry-specific consequences such as altered financial and insurance markets or disrupted transportation, communication, and energy networks.

Early after disaster there is often a sense of cohesion and a "honeymoon" of working together (see Figure 1.2). Later, disillusionment, mistrust, and anger are common. Inevitably, after any major disaster, there are also rumors circulated within the community about the circumstances leading up to the event and the government response. Sometimes there is a heightened state of fear. For example, a study of a school shooting in Illinois noted that a high level of anxiety continued for a week after the event, even after it was known that the perpetrator had committed suicide (Schwarz & Kowalski, 1991). Similarly after the Hurricane Katrina in the United States, rumors and expectations of looting, and shootings by police changed trust in law enforcement and in the community. After the London bombings and the regrettable shooting of a fleeing individual by police, the community had to recover and understand.

Over time, anger often emerges in communities. Typically, there is a focus on accountability, a search for someone who was responsible for a lack of preparation or inadequate response. Mayors, police and fire chiefs, and other community leaders are often targets of these strong feelings. Scapegoating can be an especially destructive process when leveled at those who already hold themselves responsible, even if, in reality, there was nothing they could have done to prevent adverse outcomes. In addition, nations and communities experience

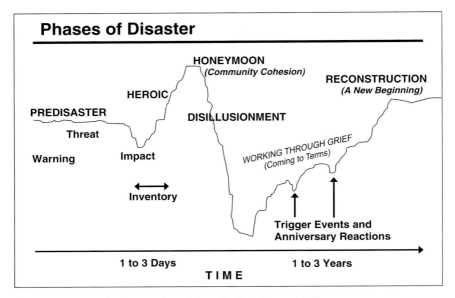

Figure 1.2 Phases of Disaster (adapted from Zunih & Myers, 2000)

ongoing hypervigilance and a sense of lost safety while trying to establish normality in their lives.

There are many milestones of a disaster which both affect the community and may offer opportunities for recovery. Outpourings of sympathy for the injured, dead, and their friends and families are common and expected. There are the normal rituals associated with burying the dead. Later, energy is poured into creating appropriate memorials. Memorialization carries the potential to cause harm as well as to do good. There can be heated disagreement about what the monument should look like and where it should be located. Special thought must be given to the placement of memorials: if it is situated too prominently so that community members cannot avoid encountering it, the memorial may heighten intrusive recollections and interfere with the resolution of grief reactions. Impromptu memorials of flowers, photographs, and memorabilia are frequently erected. It is important to distinguish between this type of spontaneous memorialization, e.g., candles and photos after 9/11, and more formalized and planned memorials. Churches and synagogues play an important role in assisting communities in their search for meaning

from such tragedy and in assisting in the grief process. Anniversaries of the disaster (e.g., 1 year) often stimulate renewed grief.

Disorder, distress and health risk behaviors

The majority of people exposed to disasters do well; however, some individuals develop psychiatric disorders, distress, or health risk behaviors such as an increase in alcohol or tobacco use (see Figure 1.3). The effects of disaster may be rekindled by new experiences that remind the person of the past traumatic event (Holloway & Ursano, 1984). At times, disasters may also have unexpected beneficial effects by serving as organizing events and providing a sense of purpose and an opportunity for positive growth experiences (Foa *et al.*, 2000; Ursano, 1987).

Exposure to a traumatic event, the essential element for development of acute stress disorder (ASD) or post-traumatic stress disorder (PTSD), is a relatively common experience. Approximately 50%–70% of the United States population is exposed to a traumatic event sometime during their lifetime;

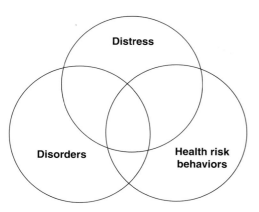

Figure 1.3 Disaster responses

Table 1.2 Trauma-related disorders

Psychiatric diagnoses

- Post-traumatic stress disorder
- Acute stress disorder
- Major depression
- Substance use disorders
- Generalized anxiety disorder
- Adjustment disorder
- Organic mental disorders secondary to head injury, toxic exposure, illness, and dehydration
- Somatization
- Psychological factors affecting physical disease (in the injured)

however, only 5%–12% develop PTSD. In a nationally representative study of 5 877 people aged 15–45 in the United States, the National Comorbidity Study (NCS) (Kessler *et al.*, 1995) found the lifetime prevalence of exposure to trauma to be 60.7% in men and 51.2% in women. In a nationally representative sample of women in the United States, the National Women's Study (NWS) (Resnick *et al.*, 1993) found that 69.0% of women were exposed to a traumatic event at some time in their lives. Over a lifetime, any given individual is very likely to be exposed to a traumatic event.

Disorder

Post-traumatic stress disorder has been widely studied following both natural and human-made disasters (for review, see Fullerton & Ursano 1997; Saigh & Bremner, 1999; Breslau *et al.*, 2005). Post-traumatic stress disorder is not uncommon following many traumatic events, from terrorism to motor vehicle accidents to industrial explosions. In its acute form, PTSD may be more like the common cold, experienced at some time in one's life by nearly all. However, when it persists, it can be debilitating and require psychotherapeutic and/or pharmacological intervention.

The NCS found rates of PTSD to be 7.8%, while the NWS found rates of PTSD to be 12.3%. In an epidemiological study of people belonging to an urban health maintenance organization in the United States, Breslau *et al.* (1991) found the lifetime prevalence of PTSD to be 9.2% for adults.

Post-traumatic stress disorder is not, however, the only trauma related disorder, nor perhaps the most common (Fullerton & Ursano, 1997; Norris *et al.*, 2002; North *et al.*, 1999) (see Table 1.2). People exposed to disaster are at increased risk for depression (e.g., Miguel-Tobal *et al.*, 2006), generalized anxiety disorder, panic disorder, and increased substance use (Breslau *et al.*, 1991; Kessler *et al.*, 1995; North *et al.*, 1999, 2002; Vlahov *et al.*, 2002). Nearly 40.5% of disaster workers following a plane crash met criteria for at least one diagnosis (i.e., acute stress disorder, PTSD, or depression) in a 13-month longitudinal study (Fullerton *et al.*, 2004). Exposed disaster workers with acute stress disorder were 7.33 times more likely to meet PTSD criteria at 13 months. Forty-five percent of survivors of the Oklahoma City bombing had a postdisaster psychiatric disorder. Of these 34.3% had PTSD and 22.5% had major depression (North *et al.*, 1999). Nearly 40% of those with PTSD or depression had no previous history of psychiatric illness (North *et al.*, 1999).

After a disaster or terrorist event, the contribution of the psychological factors to medical illness can also be pervasive – from heart disease (Leor *et al.*, 1996) to diabetes (Jacobson, 1996). Injured survivors often have psychological factors affecting their physical condition (Benedek *et al.*, 2002;

Kulka *et al.*, 1990; North *et al.*, 1999; Shore *et al.*, 1989; Smith *et al.*, 1990; Zatzick *et al.*, 2001).

Acute stress disorder was introduced into the diagnostic nomenclature in DSM-IV (American Psychiatric Association, 1994). Acute stress disorder is a constellation of symptoms very similar to PTSD but persists for a minimum of 2 days and a maximum of 4 weeks and occurs within 4 weeks of the trauma (see Bryant & Harvey, 2000). The only difference in symptom requirements between the two diagnoses is that dissociative symptoms must be present in order to diagnose ASD. The dissociative symptoms can occur during the traumatic event itself or after it. A common early response to traumatic exposure appears to be a disturbance in our sense of time, our internal time clock, resulting in time distortion – time feeling speeded up or slowed down (Ursano & Fullerton, 2000). Along with other dissociative symptoms this time distortion indicates an over four times greater risk for chronic PTSD and may also be an accompaniment of depressive symptoms. Acute stress disorder is diagnosed in 15%–20% of survivors of civilian trauma (Brewin *et al.*, 1999). As many as 80% of persons with ASD will develop PTSD at 6 months. However, it is also true that not everyone who develops PTSD had ASD in the first month. A recent review suggests that although acute dissociation is an important factor in early response to trauma, many people develop PTSD in the absence of dissociative symptoms (Bryant, 2005).

Major depression, generalized anxiety disorder, substance abuse, and adjustment disorders in disaster victims have been less often studied than ASD and PTSD, but available data suggest that these disorders also occur at higher than average rates (Galea *et al.*, 2002; Kessler *et al.*, 1999; Miguel-Tobal *et al.*, 2006). Major depression, substance abuse, and adjustment disorders (anxiety and depression) may be relatively common in the 6–12 months after a disaster and may reflect survivors' reactions to their injuries, to feelings stimulated by the disaster, and/or to their attributions of symptoms to the disaster. The occurrence of these psychiatric disorders is also mediated by secondary stressors following a disaster (Epstein *et al.*, 1998; Vlahov *et al.*, 2002). These include the problems of disaster recovery, such as negotiations with insurance companies for reimbursement, or unemployment secondary to destroyed businesses. Major depression and substance abuse (drugs, alcohol, and tobacco) are frequently comorbid with PTSD and warrant further study (Davidson & Fairbank, 1992; Rundell *et al.*, 1989; Shalev *et al.*, 1990). Increased substance use (without abuse) is also seen and affects morbidity and mortality through potential risk behaviors such as motor vehicle accidents, risky sexual behaviors, and family violence (Fullerton *et al.*, 2004; Galea *et al.*, 2002).

Grief reactions are common after all disasters, however little is known about complex grief as a disaster-specific outcome. Available studies of grief reactions following trauma do not greatly aid our understanding of who is at risk for persistent depression. Single parents may be at high risk for developing psychiatric disorders since they often have fewer resources to begin with, and they lose some of their social supports after a disaster (Solomon & Smith, 1994).

Distress and health risk behaviors

Distress and health risk behaviors include non-specific distress (for review, see Norris *et al.*, 2002), stress-related psychological and psychosomatic symptoms (Ford, 1997; McCarroll *et al.*, 2002), sleep disturbance, increased alcohol, caffeine, and cigarette use (Shalev *et al.*, 1990; Vlahov *et al.*, 2002) as well as family conflict and family violence (see Tables 1.3 and 1.4). Following the 7 July, 2005 bombings in London, 31% of Londoners reported substantial distress and 32% of Londoners reported behavioral changes, i.e., the intent to travel less (Rubin *et al.*, 2005). Anger, disbelief, sadness, anxiety, fear, and irritability are expected responses following trauma. Anxiety and family conflict can accompany the distress and fear of recurrence of a traumatic event, the ongoing threat of terrorism and the economic impact of lost jobs and companies closing or moving as a result of a disaster.

Table 1.3 Post-traumatic distress

- Grief reactions and other normal responses to an abnormal event
- Altered interpersonal interactions (withdrawal, aggression, violence, family conflict, family violence)
- Decreased work functioning (ability to do work, concentration, absenteeism, quitting, effectiveness on the job)
- Change in safety/travel
- Sleep disturbance
- Loss of concentration

Table 1.4 Health risk behaviors

- Change in smoking
- Change in alcohol
- Balancing home and work
- Disaster behaviors
  - Evacuation
  - Overdedication
  - Adherence to medical recommendations

After September 11, substantial numbers of people wished to stay home and might well have met the diagnosis of separation anxiety.

Somatic symptoms can also be an indicator of disaster-related distress. Assessing exposure to disaster events may be overlooked by overburdened primary care physicians after a disaster. Somatization is common after a disaster and must be managed both in the community at large and in individual patients (Rundell & Ursano, 1996). Disaster and rescue workers also report increased somatic symptoms after disaster exposure (McCarroll *et al.*, 2002). Somatization is a frequent presentation of anxiety and depression in patients seeking care in medical clinics. Recognizing these symptoms as an indicator of distress can help in the appropriate diagnosis and treatment and minimize inappropriate medical treatments. Medical evaluation, which includes inquiring about family conflict, can provide reassurance as well as begin a discussion for referral, and be a primary preventive intervention for children whose first experience of a disaster or terrorist

attack is mediated through their parents. Sleep disturbances following trauma are common clinical problems that present to clinicians for treatment. Sleep difficulties can be due to grief, anxiety related to recurrent disaster events (e.g., aftershocks), or the ongoing threat of terrorist attacks, or to underlying psychiatric disease such as depression or PTSD (Mellman *et al.*, 1995). Post-traumatic distress must be considered in the differential diagnosis and appropriate treatments initiated.

Hostility with its accompanying social disruption, feelings of frustration, and perception of chaos are also common following disaster (Forster, 1992; Ursano *et al.*, 1995). Although in some cases it is helpful for individuals to recognize that the return of anger can be a sign of a return to normal (i.e., it is again safe to be angry and express one's losses, disappointments, and needs), in others hostility should remind the care provider to assess the risk of family violence and substance abuse.

Disaster behavior, how one acts at the time of impact of a disaster, also affects morbidity and at times mortality. Studies of evacuation from the World Trade Center towers in 1993 after a terrorist truck bomb showed that those evacuating in groups greater than 20 took more than 6 min longer to decide to evacuate (Aguirre *et al.*, 1998). In addition, the more people knew each other in the group, the longer the group took to initiate evacuation. After the 9/11 attacks, rather than leave the disaster area, victims from the twin towers tended to congregate at the site (Gershon *et al.*, 2004). Overdedication to one's group can also lead firefighters, police, and other first responders to needlessly risk their lives. In pandemics, or after a bioterrorism attack, adherence to medical recommendations is a lifesaving behavior.

Bereavement and grief

Increasingly, traumatic loss and the bereavement and grief associated with the traumatic loss are recognized as posing special challenges to survivors of disasters and other traumatic events (Fullerton *et al.*, 1999; Prigerson *et al.*, 1999, 2000; Raphael *et al.*, 2004; Raphael & Minkov, 1999; Raphael & Wooding, 2004; Shear *et al.*, 2001, 2005). While the death of loved ones is always painful, an unexpected and violent death is most difficult. Even when not directly witnessing the death, family members may develop intrusive images based on information gleaned from authorities or the media. In children, traumatic play, a phenomenon similar to intrusive symptoms in adults, is both a sign of distress and an effort at mastery (Terr, 1981). Effective leadership after disasters includes "grief leadership," an important aspect of giving permission to grieve, and teaching and showing people how to grieve (Ursano & Fullerton, 1990).

Risk factors and vulnerable populations

We are only beginning to understand why some people exposed to disasters develop post-traumatic psychopathology and some people do not (for two recent meta-analyses of risk factors for PTSD, see Brewin *et al.*, 2000; Ozer *et al.*, 2003). Protecting vulnerable individuals and communities against disaster is a critical component of disaster preparedness and response (Norris *et al.*, 2002; Somasundaram & van de Put, 2006). Special populations such as women, children and adolescents, individuals with pre-existing health problems, and the poor are at increased risk for psychological morbidity following disasters (for review, see Somasundaram & van de Put, 2006). Trauma severity, lack of social support, and life stress have a greater effect on the development of PTSD than pre-existing factors such as demographics, pre-existing psychiatric illness, and family psychiatric history (Brewin *et al.*, 2000).

Post-traumatic psychiatric disorders are most often seen in the primary victims, those directly exposed to the threat to life and the horror of a disaster. The greater the "dose" of traumatic stressors, the more likely an individual or group is to develop high rates of psychiatric morbidity. In addition, those who have significant attachments with the primary victims, first responders, and

Table 1.5 High-risk groups

- Directly exposed to life threat
- Injured
- First responders
- Bereaved
- Single parents
- Children
- Elderly
- Women
- Individuals with:
  - Prior post-traumatic stress disorder
  - Prior exposure to trauma
  - Prior or current psychiatric or medical illness
  - Lack of supportive relationships

support providers are all at risk (Wright & Bartone, 1994) (see Table 1.5). Adults, children, and the elderly in particular who were in physical danger and who directly witnessed the events are at risk. Those who were psychologically vulnerable before exposure to a disaster are also buffeted by the fears and realities of job loss, untenably longer commutes or eroded interpersonal and community support systems overtaxed now by increased demands (Norris *et al.*, 2002).

Persons who are injured are at high risk, reflecting both their high level of exposure to life threat and the added persistent reminders and additional stress burden accompanying an ongoing injury and necessary rehabilitation. The Epidemiologic Catchment Area study of Vietnam veterans documented a higher rate of PTSD in wounded than in nonwounded veterans (Helzer *et al.*, 1987). Similar findings were noted in the Veterans Affairs study (Kulka *et al.*, 1990, 1991). Co-occurring psychiatric symptoms are frequently seen in injured survivors who may be dealing with the stress of their injury (Brandt *et al.*, 1997; Goenjian, 1993; Kulka *et al.*, 1990; North *et al.*, 1999; North *et al.*, 1989; Shore *et al.*, 1989; Zatzick *et al.*, 2001). Since studies indicate a high rate of psychiatric disorder in the physically injured, a proactive psychiatric consultation and liaison approach is a necessary part of a hospital emergency response plan.

Police, paramedics and other first responders who assist the injured and evacuate them to medical care, and hospital personnel who care for the injured need opportunities to process what happened to them in disaster events, education on normal responses, and information on when to seek further help. Those who are charged with cleaning up the site of a tragedy – and are exposed to death and the dead, as well as extended demanding work schedules – are also vulnerable to persistent symptoms. Overidentification with the victims (e.g., "It could have been me") and their pain and grief can perpetuate the fear response (Ursano et al., 1999). This normally health and growth promoting mechanism of identification with victims and heroes can turn against us in this setting like an autoimmune disorder. Inevitably, each disaster situation will also contain individuals who are "silent" victims and often overlooked. By paying close attention to the patterns and types of exposure, these individuals can be identified and receive proper care.

Pre-existing psychiatric illness

Pre-existing psychiatric illness or symptoms are not necessary for psychiatric morbidity after a disaster, nor are they sufficient to account for it (Goldberg et al., 1990; McFarlane, 1989; Ursano, 1981; Ursano et al., 1981). However, people with pre-existing psychiatric illness are especially likely to experience psychiatric illness after a disaster (Bromet et al., 1982; McFarlane, 1989; North et al., 1989, 1994, 1999; Ramsay, 1990; Smith et al., 1990; Weisaeth, 1985). Similarly, pre-existing personality features have been shown to predict the occurrence of postdisaster psychopathology including PTSD (Chen et al., 2001; Liao et al., 2002; Maes et al., 2001; McFarlane, 1989; Roy, 1982; Southwick et al., 1993).

Importantly, nearly 40% of survivors of the Oklahoma City bombing with PTSD or depression had no previous history of psychiatric illness (North et al., 1999). Therefore, those needing treatment after a disaster will not all have the usually expected accompanying risk factors and coping strategies of the usual mental health populations, which has a much higher frequency of past psychiatric problems and altered coping and functioning. The less severe the disaster, the more important predisaster variables such as neuroticism or a history of psychiatric disorder appear to be (Fullerton et al., 1999; McFarlane, 1986, 1988a, 1988b). The more severe the stressor, the less pre-existing psychiatric disorders predict outcome.

Demographic risk factors

Women are at greater risk for PTSD and major depression, and men are at greater risk for substance abuse after disasters (Kasl et al., 1981a, 1981b; Lopez-Ibor et al., 1985; Maes et al., 1998; North et al., 1999, 2002; Robins et al., 1984; Steinglass & Gerrity, 1990; Weisaeth, 1985). However, for war stressors some data show no differences in female soldiers compared to male soldiers (Hoge et al., 2004). This may reflect the importance of training and previous experience with traumatic events as protective factors for PTSD. Of the other demographic factors tested in the literature – including age, race, and socioeconomic status – either the findings have been mixed or the evidence has been insufficient to conclude that they have consistent associations with postdisaster outcome.

The role of race/ethnicity in the development of adverse mental health consequences in the aftermath of disasters remains unclear. Some studies have found racial/ethnic differences in the incidence of PTSD, depression, and anxiety after individual trauma and disasters (Kulka et al., 1990; Ortega & Rosenheck, 2000; Penk et al., 1989; Pole et al., 2001; Ruef et al., 2000) while others have not (Bromet et al., 1998; Kessler et al., 1995). Two recent meta-analyses of the risk factors for PTSD in trauma-exposed adults suggested that race/ethnicity was a predictor of PTSD in some populations, but not in others (Brewin et al., 2000; Ozer et al., 2003). A number of studies conducted among military populations have found an increased risk of PTSD symptoms among ethnic minorities, compared to Whites (Kang et al., 2003; Orcutt et al., 2004;

Ruef *et al.*, 2000; Sutker *et al.*, 1995), though it is unclear if these differences remain when accounting for differing combat exposure and other factors (Frueh *et al.*, 1998). Recent studies of New York City residents following the 2001 World Trade Center terrorist attacks show diversity in outcome as well as in utilization of mental health services among populations. In a large-scale epidemiologic study, one of the predictors of PTSD was Hispanic ethnicity (Galea *et al.*, 2002). African-American and Hispanic respondents were also less likely than White respondents to either use services or take medications. Asian Americans were less likely to seek emotional help from mental health specialists than White Americans. The authors attributed this to various cultural aspects, including cultural values of self-reliance, reservation, and passiveness to self-expression.

Few studies have explored the empirical link from ethnicity to preparedness for disasters (for review see, Peacock *et al.*, 1997). The frequency, intensity, and form of social interaction among members of ethnic groups are prime suspects in how disaster information is passed along, made acceptable, and integrated into appropriate disaster preparedness behaviors (Kirschenbaum, 2004). These networks create the social structural conditions for heightened interaction, increased trust and accepted lines for information dissemination. Ethnicity may be a catalyst for stimulating groups or individuals with similar cultural backgrounds, languages, values, and norms through emergent social networks to become sensitive to potential disasters and prepare for them. This sensitivity will then have a direct impact on how well prepared they are for a disaster and whether they may evacuate when asked, comply with quarantine or trust leadership and community interventions. In the face of Hurricane Katrina, Blacks across the disaster region were less inclined than Whites to evacuate before the storm because they did not believe the hurricane would be as devastating as it was (Elliott & Pais, 2006). Following the London bombings, being Muslim was associated with a greater presence of substantial stress (odds ratio 4.0) (Rubin *et al.*,

2005). After Hurricane Katrina in the United States, 40.6% of the disaster-exposed region reported experiencing five or more significant stressors (e.g., significant financial loss, had to be rescued, housing loss) (Kessler *et al.*, 2006). All of these stressors were more commonly reported by socially disadvantaged people (e.g., poor, minorities, low education). Of those in the lowest quartile of income, 47.6% experienced five or more stressors compared to 23% in the highest quartile of income.

Children are also vulnerable after disasters (see Bromet *et al.*, 2000; Cohen *et al.*, 2006; Pfefferbaum, 2005; Pynoos *et al.*, 1996; Shaw *et al.*, 1995, 1996; Shaw 2003; Chapter 3). The prevalence rates of PTSD symptoms 2 months following the Asian tsunami in children aged 7–14 years were 13% for children living in camps, 11% among children from affected villages, and 6% among children from unaffected villages (Thienkrua *et al.*, 2006). Delayed evacuation, feeling that you or a family member's life was in danger, and having felt extreme panic or fear were associated with PTSD symptoms. These rates did not decrease 9 months after the tsunami. Following 9/11 parents of children with greater levels of distress spent more time talking with their children, potentially trying to reassure them (Schuster *et al.*, 2001). However, in a situation in which parents as well as children may feel threatened, more information is needed regarding such parent–child conversations before such a conclusion can be reached. It is also possible that such parent–child conversations actually heighten children's worries and psychological reactions, particularly in those families whose parents caution children to avoid public places and take precautions against anthrax. Six months following 9/11, of children in grades 4–12 in the New York City public schools, 28.6% had one or more of six probable anxiety/depressive disorders (Hoven *et al.*, 2005). The most prevalent probable diagnoses were agoraphobia (14.8%), separation anxiety (12.3%), and PTSD (10.6%).

In studies in Israel of children with continuing exposure to terrorism, many children experienced insecurity, concerns with safety, and a readiness to expect the worst (Shaw, 2003). Worries about being a victim of terrorism remained common in children several months after September 11 (Schuster et al., 2001). Efforts are needed to monitor whether such changes in children's view of their safety might occur as a result of repeated warnings or threats about terrorism in the absence of actual terrorist events. Children's parents play a substantial role in moderating how children respond to terrorism, and in few other types of traumatic events are the potential threat to both parent and child comparable (see Bromet et al., 2000; Shaw, 2000). Further research examining how parent–child dyads and family units respond to and are affected by terrorism will begin to build an evidence base that will allow more informed recommendations to parents about how to help their child cope with terrorism (see Cohen et al., 2006; Schuster et al., 2001).

The nature of homelessness requires people to live in a constant, crisis level of coping and adaptation in order to meet basic needs. Despite the high number of people who are homeless living in densely populated urban areas around the globe and in developed countries, few studies have examined the homeless during times of heightened crisis. Many surveys which employ phone and internet-based approaches typically exclude people who are homeless, unless they are done in cooperation with nonprofit social service agencies (Ahern et al., 2004; Schlenger et al., 2002). Consequently, little is known about this population's reactions to disaster and terrorism.

Social support and resources

Social support is linked to mental health outcomes (Bland et al., 1997; Norris et al., 2002; Regehr et al., 2001). There is substantial evidence that the perceived availability of social support buffers the effect of stress on distress and psychological symptoms including depression and anxiety (see Cohen & Wills, 1985; Kawachi & Berkman, 2001; Norris et al., 2002). Greater social supports are in general associated with lower stress symptoms (Ursano

et al., 2003). Although social support appears to strengthen the psychosocial adjustment of men, there is evidence that social networks may be more of a burden than a support for women (Solomon et al., 1987). Social support, however, may be the result of an individual's psychosocial strength as well as a mediator. Those with good social support networks tend to be better adjusted regardless of disaster exposure. A longitudinal study of social support mobilization and deterioration after Mexico's 1999 flood showed lower social support in those who had experienced mass casualties and displacement, among women and persons with lower education (Norris et al., 2005). These disparities grew larger as time passed, suggesting the importance of social as well as psychological functioning in the aftermath and in the long-term following disaster.

From a resource perspective, a critical goal of interventions postdisaster is to replace valued resources as quickly as possible (Hobfoll & Lilly, 1993). Loss can occur on multiple ecological levels such as family, organization, and community (Hobfoll & Jackson, 1991). The Conservation of Resources (COR) theory posits that people strive to obtain and protect resources (Hobfoll, 1989). These resources can include personal or material resources and life conditions. In the aftermath of disasters the losses incurred are related to one's survival, and the losses tend to be numerous and profound, resulting in high levels of stress. For example, in the case of natural disasters, people often lose their homes, job, and social network. In a recent large-scale study of terrorism in Israel, psychosocial resources and psychosocial resource loss and gain were significantly related to exposure to terrorism, greater PTSD, and depressive symptoms (Hobfoll et al., 2006).

Organizations such as schools, churches, employee assistance programs, and employers who already have relationships with large and specific segments of the community play important roles after terrorism in particular (Institute of Medicine, 2003). These organizations are also well positioned to provide information and support to individuals with specific concerns or in need of additional support, thus greatly enhancing the effectiveness of the overall response (Stein *et al.*, 2004a, 2004b). With prior education and planning, citizens are in a better position to utilize their existing infrastructures by shielding within their own communities rather than engaging in spontaneous evacuations to more vulnerable environments (Saathoff & Everly, 2002; Pilch, 2004).

Treatment, intervention, and recovery

The normal process of recovery includes talking with others about the disaster and available resources for recovery, learning new coping strategies, and seeking help. Effective treatments for post-traumatic disorder, acute stress disorder, depression and other post-traumatic disorders are available (see Ursano *et al.*, 2004). These include psychological and pharmacologic interventions (see Chapters 6–9) (for reviews, see Foa, 2006; Foa *et al.*, 2000; Ritchie *et al.*, 2006; Yehuda, 2002).

Importantly, treatment effectiveness depends on the cultural sensitivity of assessment and treatment tools (Bryant & Njenga, 2006). Early psychiatric interventions after disaster are directed to minimizing exposure to additional traumatic stressors and educating about normal responses to trauma and disasters (see National Institute of Mental Health, 2002; Chapter 6). Consultations with other health care professionals, who will see individuals seeking medical care for injuries, and with community leaders, who need assistance in identifying at-risk groups and understanding the phases of recovery, are also important early on. More traditional health care services such as advising people on when to seek professional treatment, assisting in the resolution of acute symptomatology occurring in the days and weeks after the initial exposure, identifying those who are at higher risk for the development of psychiatric disorders and engaging them in treatment and support are important to the health of the community. Educating patients and their families can also help them to identify worsening or persistent symptoms. Anxiety and family conflict can be triggered by the fear of new threats or by the economic impact of the loss of a job after a traumatic event.

Early symptoms usually respond to a number of approaches, such as helping patients and their families identify the cause of the stress and limiting further exposure (e.g., by avoiding excessive news coverage of the traumatic event) and advising patients to get enough rest and maintain their biologic rhythms (e.g., going to sleep at the same time each night, eating at the same times each day). Key components of early intervention can be provided by mental health professionals and by other health care providers (National Institute of Mental Health, 2002).

Psychological First Aid (PFA) is an evidence-informed approach designed to reduce the initial distress in the immediate aftermath of traumatic events and to foster adaptive functioning in children, adolescents, adults, and families (National Child Traumatic Stress Network and National Center for PTSD, 2005). The primary principles of early PFA for individual care are safety, calming, connectedness, efficacy (ability and belief that one can cope/respond), and optimism. Application of these principles is the present state of the art for early intervention.

Psychological First Aid applied across all domains involves meeting basic needs for physical safety, food, protection from the elements, connectedness, survival, and security (see Chapter 6; Young, 2006). It involves early assessment of needs, monitoring the rescue and recovery environment, outreach and information dissemination, technical assistance, consultation and training, fostering resilience/recovery, triage, and early treatment. The principles and techniques of PFA are: (1) consistent with evidenced-based research on risk and resilience following disaster; (2) applicable in field settings; (3) age appropriate for developmental levels across the lifespan; and (4) culturally informed and adaptable across cultures (National Child Traumatic Stress Network and National Center for PTSD, 2005).

One of the goals of psychiatric care is to facilitate the treatment of the injured by removing individuals who do not require emergency medical care from the patient flow. Designation of a location near the hospital but separate from the chaos is important for initial treatment and triage. Hospitals or other institutions serving as entry points for care can act as locations where persons with psychologic symptoms can receive respite (Benedek et al., 2002).

Interpersonal withdrawal and social isolation are particularly difficult symptoms and often bode a complex trauma response. Social withdrawal tends to limit the normal recovery mechanisms, e.g., the "natural debriefing process" (Ursano et al., 2000), talking with others, active coping, and help seeking. Depression may be a primary contribution to withdrawal and requires evaluation and treatment.

Increased somatic symptoms have been frequently reported after disasters, particularly toxic exposures (Engel & Katon, 1999) and exposure to the dead (McCarroll et al., 2002), and can be an expression of anxiety or depression. In these individuals, conservative medical management with education and reassurance are the core of medical treatment. Discussion of specific worries and fears can decrease symptoms, initiate the normal metabolism and digestion of stress symptoms, and identify any need for further specific treatment.

Risk and protective factors: resilience and response trajectories

Resilience and post-traumatic growth

Although the psychiatric consequences of disasters have been associated with debility that can persist for decades, the effects of traumatic events are not exclusively bad. Understanding the range of trajectories of response – e.g., resilience, distress, illness, recovery – is an important longitudinal perspective on disaster-exposed individuals and communities. In recent years there has been increased interest in the role of resilience in response to disaster (e.g., see Bonanno et al., 2006; Connor, 2006; Wessely, 2005) and post-traumatic growth (for reviews see Linley &

Joseph, 2004; Zoellner & Maercker, 2006). Resilience has been defined as having either no PTSD symptoms or one symptom (Bonnano et al., 2006) and also as a measure of coping and personal qualities that allow individuals and communities to grow in the face of adversity (Connor & Davidson, 2003; Luthar et al., 2000; Richardson, 2002). For some people trauma and loss can facilitate a move toward health (Card, 1983; Tedeschi et al., 1998; Ursano, 1981).

Resilience and recovery need to be differentiated. Bonanno (2004) defined resilience as "the ability of adults *in otherwise normal circumstances* who are exposed to an isolated and potentially highly disruptive event such as the death of a close relation or a violent or life-threatening situation to maintain relatively stable, healthy levels of psychological and physical functioning . . . as well as the capacity for generative experiences and positive emotions" (pp. 20–21). Key to this definition is the distinction between resilience and recovery. Whereas recovering individuals often experience subthreshold symptom levels, resilient individuals are hypothesized to experience transient perturbations in normal functioning (e.g., several weeks of sporadic preoccupation or restless sleep), but generally exhibit a stable trajectory of healthy functioning across time. A growing body of evidence has been garnered in support of this definition (for reviews see Bonanno, 2004; Bonanno & Kaltman, 2001), including a recent study examining the resilient trajectory among a high-exposure group of people who had been in or near the World Trade Center on September 11 when the first plane struck the towers (Bonanno, 2004). In addition to being in physical danger, most of these individuals had also witnessed death and injury to others. Not only did the majority fail to meet criteria for either depression or PTSD, the most common outcome trajectory was a resilient pattern of stable low symptom levels. This study also provided important validity data by showing a high concordance between the resilience trajectory and ratings of resilience provided independently by participants' close friends and relatives.

A traumatic experience can become the center around which a victim reorganizes a previously disorganized life, reorienting values and goals (Ursano, 1981, 1987). Traumatic events may function as psychic organizers by linking event-related feelings, thoughts, and behaviors that are later accessed en bloc following symbolic, environmental, or biological stimuli (Holloway & Ursano, 1984). Many survivors of the 1974 tornado in Xenia, Ohio experienced psychological distress, but the majority described positive outcomes: they learned that they could handle crises effectively (84%) and believed that they were better off for having met this type of challenge (69%) (Quarentelli, 1985; Taylor, 1977). This "benefited response" is also reported in the combat trauma literature. Sledge et al. (1980) found that approximately one-third of United States Air Force Vietnam-era prisoners of war reported having benefited from their prisoner of war experience; they believed that they had developed an important reprioritization of their life goals, placing new emphasis on the importance of family and country. The individuals reporting these benefits tended to be the ones who had suffered the most traumatic experiences. More recently, after Hurricane Katrina in the United States, 88.5% of the disaster-impacted population reported that their experiences with the hurricane helped them develop a deeper sense of meaning or purpose in life (Kessler et al., 2006). The vast majority (89.3%) and 81% of the highest impacted area, the City of New Orleans, reported they would be better able to cope with future life stressors.

Meaning and cognitive appraisal of disaster events

Clinical studies and treatment interventions suggest that the psychiatric consequences following disasters are influenced by the meaning (i.e., cognitive appraisal) of the traumatic event (Bryant, 2006; Dollinger, 1986; Green et al., 1985; Holloway & Ursano, 1984). Beliefs about the cause of the disaster and the ramifications of these beliefs (such as self-blame, the shattering of assumptions about human nature, and rage at "those responsible" when the event is viewed as preventable) should be assessed in psychiatric evaluation and represent potential areas for intervention. Chronic PTSD may be particularly related to the meaning of a disaster experience. Therapists can assist patients in modifying distorted attributions (e.g., "It's all my fault; if only I had insisted that we not go away for the weekend, we wouldn't have been caught in the tornado and my wife would still be alive"). Cognitive models of responses to traumatic events indicate that the appraisal of the traumatic event and its consequences is critical to levels of stress and disorder after the event (Ehlers & Clark, 2000). Catastrophic appraisals in particular increase the experience of threat (Resick & Schnicke, 1993). Maladaptive appraisals appear related to altered beliefs in the safety of our world or our own sense of efficacy versus helplessness (Bryant & Guthrie, 2005; Foa & Rothbaum, 1998).

Some events are more likely than others to shatter one's faith in a just and safe world (Holloway & Fullerton, 1994). Consider the implications of the following scenarios: an individual has survived an airplane crash in which many people were injured and killed. Various explanations for the crash exist; each would stimulate a different meaning and emotional response. The plane may have crashed because of sudden and unexpected wind shears, because of uncomplicated pilot error, or because of "complicated" pilot error (e.g., the pilot was under the influence of drugs or alcohol). At the far end of this continuum would be a crash caused by an act of terrorism or greed in which the plane was destroyed to further the interests of a group or an individual.

The construction of meaning is an active process that affects the outcome of the disaster experience and recovery (Ursano & Fullerton, 1990; Ursano et al., 1992). The meaning of a disaster to any one person results from the interaction of his or her past history, present context, and physiological state. The ascribed meaning will then direct individual behaviors of what to do, what to fix, and whom or what to blame. Meaning is dynamic, not static: it changes over time as the individual's psychosocial context changes. Such alterations can aid or inhibit recovery. For example, immediately following the crash of an Air Force C-141 cargo plane, the remaining members of the squadron were convinced that the accident was caused by aircraft failure. However, this belief was modified as the date grew nearer for the squadron members to fly the same type of plane again. By that time, the squadron's belief had changed, and members thought that the crash must have been caused by human error. If it were human error, one could feel safe: "I would never do that."

Leadership is an important aspect of the construction of meaning in the aftermath of disaster and in preparedness for disaster. In the workplace, corporate leaders acknowledge that communicating to employees a recognition of their value to the corporation – of instilling in employees the idea that they "mattered" – was important to preservation of function in times of disaster and crises (Ursano, 2005).

Conclusion

Natural and human-made disasters will continue to be a primary cause of mental health need. Those most directly exposed, those most vulnerable, and the disaster community require individual care and population-level health interventions. Community leadership is critical to fostering recovery, providing treatment and maximizing community restoration.

REFERENCES

Aguirre, B. E., Wenger, D. & Vigo, G. (1998). A test of the emergent norm theory of collective behavior. *Sociological Forum*, **13**, 301–320.

Ahern, J., Galea, S., Resnick, H. & Vlahov, D. (2004). Television images and probable posttraumatic stress disorder after September 11: the role of background characteristics, event exposures, and perievent panic. *Journal of Nervous and Mental Disease*, **192**, 217–226.

American Psychiatric Association (1994). *Diagnostic and Statistical Manual of Mental Disorders*, 4th edn. Washington, D.C.: American Psychiatric Press.

Benedek, D. M., Holloway, H. C. & Becker, S. M. (2002). Emergency mental health management in bioterrorism events. *Emergency Medicine Clinics of North America*, **20**, 393–407.

Bland, S. H., O'Leary, E. S., Farinaro, E. *et al.* (1997). Social network disturbances and psychological distress following earthquake evacuation. *Journal of Nervous and Mental Disease*, **185**, 188–194.

Bonanno, G. A. (2004). Loss, trauma, and human resilience: have we underestimated the human capacity to thrive after extremely aversive events? *The American Psychologist*, **59**, 20–28.

Bonanno, G. A. & Kaltman, S. (2001). The varieties of grief experience. *Clinical Psychology Review*, **21**, 705–734.

Bonanno, G. A., Galea, S., Bucciarelli, A. & Vlahov, D. (2006). Psychological resilience after disaster: New York City in the aftermath of the September 11th terrorist attack. *Psychological Science*, **17**, 181–186.

Boudreaux, E., Kilpatrick, D. G., Resnick, H. S., Best, C. L. & Saunders, B. E. (1998). Criminal victimization, posttraumatic stress disorder, and comorbid psychopathology among a community sample of women. *Journal of Traumatic Stress*, **11**, 665–678.

Brandt, G. T., Norwood, A. E., Ursano, R. J. *et al.* (1997). Psychiatric morbidity in medical and surgical patients evacuated from the Persian Gulf War. *Psychiatric Services*, **48**, 102–104.

Breslau, N., Davis, G. C., Andreski, P. & Peterson E. (1991). Traumatic events and posttraumatic stress disorder in an urban population of young adults. *Archives of General Psychiatry*, **48**, 216–222.

Breslau, N., Reboussin, B. A., Anthony, J. C. & Storr, C. L. (2005). The structure of posttraumatic stress disorder. Latent class analysis in 2 community samples. *Archives of General Psychiatry*, **62**, 1343–1351.

Brewin, C. R., Andrews, B., Rose, S. & Kirk, M. (1999). Acute stress disorder and posttraumatic stress disorder in victims of violent crime. *American Journal of Psychiatry*, **156**, 360–366.

Brewin, C. R., Andrews, B. & Valentine, J. D. (2000). Meta-analysis of risk factors for posttraumatic stress disorder in trauma-exposed adults. *Journal of Consulting and Clinical Psychology*, **68**, 746–766.

Bromet, E., Schulberg, H. C. & Dunn, L. (1982). Reactions of psychiatric patients to the Three Mile Island nuclear accident. *Archives of General Psychiatry*, **39**, 725–730.

Bromet, E., Sonnega, A. & Kessler, R. C. (1998). Risk factors for DSM-III-R posttraumatic stress disorder: findings from the national comorbidity survey. *American Journal of Epidemiology*, **147**, 353–361.

Bromet, E. J., Goldgaber, D., Carlson, G. *et al.* (2000). Children's well-being 11 years after the Chernobyl catastrophe. *Archives of General Psychiatry*, **57**, 563–571.

Bryant, R. (2006). Early intervention and treatment of acute stress disorder. Presented at conference, "Early psychological intervention following mass trauma: the present and future directions." Valhalla, New York: New York Medical College, School of Public Health.

Bryant, R. A. (2005). Predicting posttraumatic stress disorder from acute reactions. *Journal of Trauma Dissociation*, **6**(2), 5–15.

Bryant, R. A. & Guthrie, R. M. (2005). Maladaptive appraisals as a risk factor for posttraumatic stress. A study of trainee firefighters. *Psychological Science*, **16**, 749–752.

Bryant, R. A. & Harvey, A. G. (2000). *Acute Stress Disorder: A Handbook of Theory, Assessment, and Treatment.* Washington, D.C.: American Psychological Association.

Bryant, R. A. & Njenga, F. G. (2006). Cultural sensitivity: making trauma assessment and treatment plans culturally relevant. *Journal of Clinical Psychiatry*, **67** (Suppl 2), 74–79.

Card, J. J. (1983). *Lives after Viet Nam.* Lexington: Lexington Books.

Chen, C. C., Yeh, T. L., Yang, Y. K. *et al.* (2001). Psychiatric morbidity and post-traumatic symptoms among survivors in the early stage following the 1999 earthquake in Taiwan. *Psychiatry Research*, **105**, 13–22.

Cohen, J. P., Mannarino, A. P., Gibson, L. E. *et al.* (2006). Interventions for children and adolescents following disasters. In *Interventions Following Mass Violence and Disasters*, eds. E. C. Ritchie, P. J. Watson & M. J. Friedman, pp. 227–256. Strategies for Mental Health Practice, New York: Guilford Press.

Cohen, S. & Wills, T. A. (1985). Stress, social support, and the buffering hypothesis. *Psychological Bulletin*, **98**, 310–357.

Connor, K. M. (2006). Assessment of resilience in the aftermath of trauma. *Journal of Clinical Psychiatry*, **67** (Suppl 2), 46–49.

Connor, K. M. & Davidson, J. R.T. (2003). Development of a new resilience scale: the Connor-Davidson Resilience Scale (CD-RISC). *Depression and Anxiety*, **18**, 76–82.

Davidson, J. R.T. & Fairbank, J. A. (1992). The epidemiology of posttraumatic stress disorder. In *Posttraumatic Stress Disorder: DSM-IV and Beyond*, eds. J. R.T. Davidson &

E. B. Foa, pp. 147–169. Washington, D.C.: American Psychiatric Press.

Davidson, J. R. & McFarlane, A. C. (2006). The extent and impact of mental health problems after disaster. *Journal of Clinical Psychiatry*, **67** (Suppl 2), 9–14.

Dollinger, S. J. (1986). The need for meaning following disaster: attributions and emotional upset. *Personality and Social Psychology Bulletin*, **12**, 300–310.

Ehlers, A. & Clark, D. M. (2000). A cognitive model of posttraumatic stress disorder. *Behaviour Research and Therapy*, **38**, 319–345.

Elliott, J. R. & Pais, J. (2006). Race, class and Hurricane Katrina: social differences in human responses to disaster. *Social Science Research*, **35**, 295–321.

Engel, C. C. & Katon, W. J. (1999). Population and need-based prevention of unexplained physical symptoms in the community (Appendix A). In *Strategies to Protect the Health of Deployed US Forces*, eds. L. M. Jollenbeck, P. K. Russell & S. B. Guze, pp. 173–212. Washington, D.C.: National Academy Press.

Epstein, J. N., Saunders, B. E. & Kilpatrick, D. G. (1997). Predicting PTSD in women with a history of childhood rape. *Journal of Traumatic Stress*, **10**, 573–588.

Epstein, R. S., Fullerton, C. S. & Ursano, R. J. (1998). Posttraumatic stress disorder following an air disaster: a prospective study. *American Journal of Psychiatry*, **155**, 934–938.

Foa, E. B. (2006). Psychosocial therapy for posttraumatic stress disorder. *Journal of Clinical Psychiatry*, **67** (Suppl 2), 40–45.

Foa, E. B. & Rothbaum, B. O. (1998). *Treating the Trauma of Rape: Cognitive-Behavioral Therapy for PTSD.* New York: Guilford.

Foa, E. B., Keane, T. M. & Friedman, M. J. (2000). *Effective Treatments for PTSD.* New York: Guilford Press.

Ford, C. V. (1997). Somatic symptoms, somatization, and traumatic stress: an overview. *Nordic Journal of Psychiatry*, **51**, 5–13.

Forster, P. (1992). Nature and treatment of acute stress reactions. In *Responding to Disaster: A Guide for Mental Health Professionals*, ed. L. S. Austin, pp. 25–51. Washington, D.C.: American Psychiatric Press.

Frueh, B. C., Brady, K. L. & de Arellano, M. A. (1998). Racial differences in combat-related PTSD: empirical findings and conceptual issues. *Clinical Psychology Review*, **18**, 287–305.

Fullerton, C. S. & Ursano, R. J. (eds.) (1997). *Posttraumatic Stress Disorder: Acute and Long Term Responses to*

Trauma and Disaster. Washington, D.C.: American Psychiatric Press.

Fullerton, C. S., Ursano, R. J., Kao, T. C. & Bharitya, V. R. (1999). Disaster-related bereavement: acute symptoms and subsequent depression. *Aviation, Space, and Environmental Medicine*, **70**, 902–909.

Fullerton, C. S., Ursano, R. J., Norwood, A. E. & Holloway, H. C. (2003). Trauma, terrorism, and disaster. In *Terrorism and Disaster. Individual and Community Mental Health Interventions*, eds. R. J. Ursano, C. S. Fullerton & A. E. Norwood, pp. 1–20. Cambridge: Cambridge University Press.

Fullerton, C. S., Ursano, R. J. & Wang, L. (2004). Acute stress disorder, posttraumatic stress disorder, and depression in disaster or rescue workers. *American Journal of Psychiatry*, **161**, 1370–1376.

Galea, S., Ahern, J., Resnick, H. *et al.* (2002). Psychological sequelae of the September 11 terrorist attacks in New York City. *New England Journal of Medicine*, **346**, 982–987.

Gerrity, E. T. & Steinglass, P. (1994). Relocation stress following natural disasters. In *Individual and Community Responses to Trauma and Disaster*, eds. R. J. Ursano, B. G. McCaughey & C. S. Fullerton, pp. 220–247. Cambridge: Cambridge University Press.

Gershon, R., Hogan, E., Qureshi, K. A. & Doll, L. (2004). Preliminary results from the world trade center evacuation study – New York City. *MMWR: Morbidity and Mortality Weekly Reports*, **53**, 815–817.

Ghodse, H. & Galea, S. (2006). Tsunami: understanding mental health consequences and the unprecedented response. *International Review of Psychiatry*, **18**, 289–297.

Goenjian, A. (1993). A mental health relief program in Armenia after the 1988 earthquake: implementation and clinical observations. *British Journal of Psychiatry*, **163**, 230–239.

Goldberg, J., True, W. R., Eisen, S. A. & Henderson, W. G. (1990). A twin study of the effects of the Vietnam War on posttraumatic stress disorder. *Journal of the American Mental Association*, **263**, 1227–1232.

Green, B. L., Wilson, J. P. & Lindy, J. D. (1985). Conceptualizing post-traumatic stress disorder: a psychosocial framework. In *Trauma and its Wake* (Vol. 1). *The Study and Treatment of Post-Traumatic Stress Disorder*, ed. C. R. Figley, pp. 53–69. New York: Brunner/Mazel.

Helzer, J. E., Robins, L. N. & McEvoy, L. (1987). Post-traumatic stress disorder in the general population. *New England Journal of Medicine*, **317**, 1630–1634.

Hobfoll, S. E. (1989). Conservation of resources. A new attempt at conceptualizing stress. *American Psychologist*, **44**, 513–524.

Hobfoll, S. E. & Jackson, A. P. (1991). Conservation of resources in community intervention. *American Journal of Community Psychology*, **19**, 111–121.

Hobfoll, S. & Lilly, R. (1993). Resource conservation as a strategy for community psychology. *Journal of Community Psychology*, **21**, 128–148.

Hobfoll, S. E., Canetti-Nisim, D. & Johnson, R. J. (2006). Exposure to terrorism, stress-related mental health symptoms, and defensive coping among Jews and Arabs in Israel. *Journal of Consulting and Clinical Psychology*, **74**, 207–218.

Hoge, C. W., Castro, C. A., Messer, S. C. *et al.* (2004). Combat duty in Iraq and Afghanistan, mental health problems, and barriers to care. *New England Journal of Medicine*, **351**, 13–22.

Holloway, H. C. & Fullerton, C. S. (1994). The psychology of terror and its aftermath. In *Individual and Community Responses to Trauma and Disaster*, eds. R. J. Ursano, B. G. McCaughey & C. S. Fullerton, pp. 31–45. Cambridge: Cambridge University Press.

Holloway, H. C. & Ursano, R. J. (1984). The Vietnam veteran: memory, social context, and metaphor. *Psychiatry*, **47**, 103–108.

Holloway, H. C., Norwood, A. E., Fullerton, C. S., Engel, C. C. & Ursano, R. J. (1997). The threat of biological weapons: prophylaxis and mitigation of psychological and social consequences. *Journal of the American Mental Association*, **278**, 425–427.

Hoven, C. W., Duarte, C. S., Lucas, C. P. *et al.* (2005). Psychopathology among New York city public school children 6 months after September 11. *Archives of General Psychiatry*, **62**, 545–552.

Institute of Medicine (IOM) (2003). *Preparing for the Psychological Consequences of Terrorism: A Public Health Strategy*. Washington, D.C.: National Academies of Science, National Academies Press.

Jacobson, A. M. (1996). The psychological care of patients with insulin-dependent diabetes mellitus. *New England Journal of Medicine*, **334**, 1249–1253.

Kang, H. K., Natelson, B. H., Mahan, C. M., Lee, K. Y. & Murphy, F. M. (2003). Post-traumatic stress disorder and chronic fatigue syndrome-like illness among gulf war veterans: a population-based survey of 30,000 veterans. *American Journal of Epidemiology*, **157**, 141–148.

Kasl, S. V., Chisholm, R. F. & Eskenazi, B. (1981a). The impact of the accident at the Three Mile Island on the behavior and well-being of nuclear workers. Part I: Perceptions and evaluations, behavioral responses, and work-related attitudes and feelings. *American Journal of Public Health*, **71**, 472–483.

Kasl, S. V., Chisholm, R. F. & Eskenazi, B. (1981b). The impact of the accident at the Three Mile Island on the behavior and well-being of nuclear workers. Part II: Job tension, psychophysiological symptoms, and indices of distress. *American Journal of Public Health*, **71**, 484–495.

Kawachi, I. & Berkman, L. F. (2001). Social ties and mental health. *Journal of Urban Health*, **78**, 458–467.

Kessler, R., Brewin, C., Galea, S. *et al.* (2006). Overview of baseline survey results: Hurricane Katrina community advisory group. Available at: http://hurricanekatrina. med.harvard.edu/pdf/baseline_report%208-25-06.pdf.

Kessler, R. C., Sonnega, A., Bromet, E., Hughes, M. & Nelson, C. B. (1995). Posttraumatic stress disorder in the National Comorbidity Survey. *Archives of General Psychiatry*, **52**, 1048–1060.

Kessler, R. C., Barber, C., Birnbaum, H. G. *et al.* (1999). Depression in the workplace: effects of short-term disability. *Health Affairs*, **18**, 163–171.

Kirschenbaum, A. (2004). *Chaos, Organization and Disaster Management*. New York: Marcel Dekker, Inc.

Kulka, R. A., Schlenger, W. E., Fairbank, J. A. *et al.* (1990). *Trauma and the Vietnam War Generation*. New York: Brunner/Mazel.

Kulka, R. A., Schlenger, W. E., Fairbank, J. A. *et al.* (1991). Assessment of posttraumatic stress disorder in the community: prospects and pitfalls from recent studies of Vietnam veterans. *Psychological Assessment*, **3**, 547–560.

Leor, J., Poole, W. K. & Kloner, R. A. (1996). Sudden cardiac death triggered by an earthquake. *New England Journal of Medicine*, **334**, 413–419.

Liao, S. C., Lee, M. B., Lee, Y. J. *et al.* (2002). Association of psychological distress with psychological factors in rescue workers within two months after a major earthquake. *Journal of the Formososan Medical Association*, **101**, 169–176.

Linley, P. A. & Joseph, S. (2004). Positive change following trauma and adversity: a review. *Journal of Traumatic Stress*, **17**, 11–21.

Lopez-Ibor, J. J., Jr., Soria, J., Canas, F. & Rodriguez-Gamazo, M. (1985). Psychopathological aspects of the toxic oil syndrome catastrophe. *British Journal of Psychiatry*, **147**, 352–365.

Luthar, S. S., Cicchetti, D. & Becker, B. (2000). The construct of resilience: a critical evaluation and guidelines for future work. *Child Development*, **71**, 543–562.

Maes, M., Delmeire, L., Schotte, C. *et al.* (1998). Epidemiologic and phenomenological aspects of post-traumatic stress disorder: DSM-III-R diagnosis and diagnostic criteria not validated. *Psychiatry Research*, **81**, 179–193.

Maes, M., Mylle, J., Delmeire, L. & Janca, A. (2001). Pre- and post-disaster negative life events in relation to the incidence and severity of post-traumatic stress disorder. *Psychiatry Research*, **105**, 1–12.

McCarroll, J. E., Ursano, R. J., Fullerton, C. S., Liu, X. & Lundy, A. (2002). Somatic symptoms in Gulf War mortuary workers. *Psychosomatic Medicine*, **64**, 29–33.

McFarlane, A. C. (1986). Posttraumatic morbidity of a disaster: a study of cases presenting for psychiatric treatment. *Journal of Nervous and Mental Disease*, **174**, 4–14.

McFarlane, A. C. (1988a). The longitudinal course of posttraumatic morbidity: the range of outcomes and their predictors. *Journal of Nervous and Mental Disease*, **176**, 30–39.

McFarlane, A. C. (1988b). The phenomenology of posttraumatic stress disorders following a natural disaster. *Journal of Nervous and Mental Disease*, **176**, 22–29.

McFarlane, A. C. (1989). The aetiology of post-traumatic morbidity: predisposing, precipitating and perpetuating factors. *British Journal of Psychiatry*, **154**, 221–228.

Mellman, T. A., Kulick-Bell, R., Ashlock, L. E. & Nolan, B. (1995). Sleep events among veterans with combat-related posttraumatic stress disorder. *American Journal of Psychiatry*, **52**, 110–115.

Miguel-Tobal, J. J., Cano-Vindel, A., Gonzalez-Ordi, H. *et al.* (2006). PTSD and depression after the Madrid March 11 train bombings. *Journal of Traumatic Stress*, **19**, 69–80.

Nandi, A., Galea, S., Tracy, M. *et al.* (2004). Job loss, unemployment, work stress, job satisfaction, and the persistence of posttraumatic stress disorder one year after the September 11 attacks. *Journal of Occupational and Environmental Medicine*, **46**, 1057–1064.

National Child Traumatic Stress Network and National Center for PTSD. (2005). Psychological first aid: field operations guide. Available at: www.NCTSN.org and www.NCPTSD.va.gov.

National Institute of Mental Health (2002). Mental health and mass violence: evidence-based early psychological intervention for victims/survivors of mass violence: a workshop to reach consensus on best practices, NIH Publication No. 02–5138. Washington, D.C.: US Government Printing Office.

Noji, E. K. (ed.) (1997). *The Public Health Consequences of Disasters*. New York: Oxford University Press.

Norris, F. H., Friedman, M. J., Watson, P. J. *et al.* (2002). 60,000 disaster victims speak, Part I. An empirical review of the empirical literature: 1981–2001. *Psychiatry*, **65**, 207–239.

Norris, F. H., Baker, C. K., Murphy, A. D. & Kaniasty, K. (2005). Social support mobilization and deterioration after Mexico's 1999 flood: effects of context, gender, and time. *American Journal of Community Psychology*, **36**, 15–28.

North, C. S., Smith, E. M., McCool, R. E. & Lightcap, P. E. (1989). Acute post-disaster coping and adjustment. *Journal of Traumatic Stress*, **2**, 353–360.

North, C. S., Smith, E. M. & Spitznagel, E. L. (1994). Post-traumatic stress disorder in survivors of a mass shooting. *American Journal of Psychiatry*, **151**, 82–88.

North, C. S., Nixon, S. J., Shariat, S. *et al.* (1999). Psychiatric disorders among survivors of the Oklahoma City bombing. *Journal of the American Medical Association*, **282**, 755–762.

North, C. S., Tivis, L., McMillen, J. C. *et al.* (2002). Psychiatric disorders in rescue workers after the Oklahoma City bombing. *American Journal of Psychiatry*, **159**, 857–859.

Orcutt, H. K., Erickson, D. J. & Wolfe, J. (2004). The course of PTSD symptoms among gulf war veterans: a growth mixture modeling approach. *Journal of Traumatic Stress*, **17**, 195–202.

Ortega, A. N. & Rosenheck, R. (2000). Posttraumatic stress disorder among Hispanic Vietnam veterans. *American Journal of Psychiatry*, **157**, 615–619.

Ozer, E. J., Best, S. R., Lipsey, T. L. & Weiss, D. S. (2003). Predictors of posttraumatic stress disorder and symptoms in adults: a meta-analysis. *Psychological Bulletin*, **129**, 52–73.

Peacock, W. G., Morrow, B. H. & Gladwin, H. (1997). *Hurricane Andrew: Ethnicity, Gender and the Sociology of Disasters*. New York: Routledge.

Penk, W. E., Robinowitz, R., Black, J. *et al.* (1989). Ethnicity: post-traumatic stress disorder (PTSD) differences among black, white, and Hispanic veterans who differ in degrees of exposure to combat in Vietnam. *Journal of Clinical Psychology*, **45**, 729–735.

Pfefferbaum, B. J. (2005). Aspects of exposure in childhood trauma: the stressor criterion. *Journal of Trauma Dissociation*, **6**, 17–26.

Pilch F. (2004). The worried well: strategies for installation commanders. USAF Institute for National Security Studies. Colorado Springs, CO: USAF Academy.

Pole, N., Best, S. R., Weiss, D. S. *et al.* (2001). Effects of gender and ethnicity on duty-related posttraumatic stress symptoms among urban police officers. *The Journal of Nervous and Mental Disease*, **189**, 442–448.

Prigerson, H. G., Shear, M. K., Jacobs, S. C. *et al.* (1999). Consensus criteria for traumatic grief: a preliminary empirical test. *British Journal of Psychiatry*, **174**, 67–73.

Prigerson, H. G., Shear, M. K., Jacobs, S. *et al.* (2000). Grief and its relationship to posttraumatic stress disorder. In *Posttraumatic Stress Disorders: Diagnosis, Management and Treatment*, eds. D. Nutt, J. R. Davidson & J. Zohar, pp. 163–177. New York: Martin Dunitz Publishers.

Pynoos, R. S., Steinberg, A. M. & Goenjian, A. (1996). Traumatic stress in childhood and adolescence: recent developments and current controversies. In: *Traumatic Stress: The Effect of Overwhelming Experience on Mind, Body, and Society*, eds. B. A. vanderKolk, A. C. McFarlane & L. Weisaeth, pp. 331–358. New York: Guilford Press.

Quarentelli, E. L. (1985). An assessment of conflicting views on mental health: the consequences of traumatic events. In *Trauma and its Wake*, ed. C. R. Figley, pp. 173–215. New York: Brunner/Mazel.

Ramsay, R. (1990). Invited review: post-traumatic stress disorder; a new clinical entity? *Journal of Psychosomatic Research*, **34**, 355–365.

Raphael, B. & Minkov, C. (1999). Abnormal grief. *Current Opinion in Psychiatry*, **12**, 99–102.

Raphael, B. & Wooding, S. (2004). Early mental health interventions for traumatic loss in adults. In *Early Intervention for Trauma and Traumatic Loss*, ed. B. T. Litz, pp. 147–178. New York: Guilford Press.

Raphael, B., Martinek, N. & Wooding, S. (2004). Assessing traumatic bereavement. In *Assessing Psychological Trauma and PTSD*, 2nd edn., eds. J. P. Wilson & T. M. Keane, pp. 492–510. New York: Guilford Press.

Regehr, C., Hemsworth, D. & Hill, J. (2001). Individual predictors of posttraumatic distress: a structural equation model. *Canadian Journal of Psychiatry*, **46**, 156–161.

Resick, P. A. & Schnicke, M. K. (1993). *Cognitive Processing Therapy for Rape Victims: A Treatment Manual*. London: Sage.

Resnick, H. S., Kilpatrick, D. G., Dansky, B. S., Saunders, B. E. & Best, C. L. (1993). Prevalence of civilian trauma and posttraumatic stress disorder in a representative national sample of women. *Journal of Consulting Clinical Psychology*, **61**, 984–991.

Richardson, G. E. (2002). The metatheory of resilience and resiliency. *Journal Clinical Psychology*, **58**, 307–321.

Robins, L. N., Helzer, J. E., Weissman, M. M. *et al.* (1984). Lifetime prevalence of specific psychiatric disorders in three sites. *Archives of General Psychiatry*, **41**, 949–958.

Roy, W. (1982). Risk factors for suicide in psychiatric patients. *Archives of General Psychiatry*, **39**, 1089–1095.

Rubin, G. J., Brewin, C. R., Greenberg, N., Simpson, J. & Wessely, S. (2005). Psychological and behavioural reactions to the bombings in London on 7 July 2005: cross sectional survey of a representative sample of Londoners. *British Medical Journal*, **331**, 606.

Ruef, A. M., Litz, B. T. & Schlenger, W. E. (2000). Hispanic ethnicity and risk for combat-related posttraumatic stress disorder. *Cultural Diversity and Ethnic Minority Psychology*, **6**, 235–251.

Rundell, J. R. & Ursano, R. J. (1996). Psychiatric responses to trauma. In *Emotional Aftermath of the Persian Gulf War: Veterans, Communities, and Nations*, eds. R. J. Ursano & A. E. Norwood, pp. 43–81. Washington, D.C.: American Psychiatric Press.

Rundell, J. R., Ursano, R. J., Holloway, H. C. & Silberman, E. K. (1989). Psychiatric responses to trauma. *Hospital and Community Psychiatry*, **40**, 68–74.

Saathoff, G. & Everly, G. S. Jr. (2002). Psychological challenges of bioterror: containing contagion. *International Journal of Emergency Mental Health*, **4**, 245–252.

Saigh, P. A. & Bremner, J. D. (eds.) (1999). *Posttraumatic Stress Disorder: A Comprehensive Text*. Boston, MA: Allyn & Bacon.

Sampson, R. J. (2003). The neighborhood context of well-being. *Perspectives in Biology and Medicine*, **46**, S53–S64.

Sampson, R. J., Raudenbush, S. W. & Earls, F. (1997). Neighborhoods and violent crime: a multilevel study of collective efficacy. *Science*, **277**, 918–924.

Schlenger, W. E., Caddell, J. M., Ebert, L. *et al.* (2002). Psychological reactions to terrorist attacks: findings from the National Study of Americans' Reactions to September 11. *Journal of the American Medical Association*, **288**, 581–588.

Schuster, M. A., Stein, B. D., Jaycox, L. H. *et al.* (2001). A national survey of stress reactions after the September 11, 2001, terrorist attack. *New England Journal of Medicine*, **345**, 1507–1512.

Schwarz, E. D. & Kowalski, J. M. (1991). Malignant memories: PTSD in children and adults after a school shooting. *Journal of the American Academy of Child and Adolescent Psychiatry*, **30**, 936–944.

Shalev, A., Bleich, A. & Ursano, R. J. (1990). Posttraumatic stress disorder: somatic comorbidity and effort tolerance. *Psychosomatics*, **31**, 197–203.

Shaw, J. A. (2000). Children, adolescents and trauma. *Psychiatric Quarterly*, **71**, 227–243.

Shaw, J. A. (2003). Children exposed to war/terrorism. *Clinical Child and Family Psychology Review*, **6**, 237–246.

Shaw, J. A., Applegate, B., Tanner, S. *et al.* (1995). Psychological effects of Hurricane Andrew on an elementary school population. *Journal of the American Academy of Child and Adolescent Psychiatry*, **34**, 1185–1192.

Shaw, J. A., Applegate, B. & Schorr, C. (1996). Twenty-one month follow-up study of school-age children exposed to Hurricane Andrew. *Journal of the American Academy of Child and Adolescent Psychiatry*, **35**, 359–364.

Shear, K., Frank, E., Houck, P. R. & Reynolds, C. F. (2005). Treatment of complicated grief. A randomized controlled trial. *Journal of the American Medical Association*, **293**, 2601–2608.

Shear, M. K., Frank, E., Foa, E. *et al.* (2001). Traumatic grief treatment: a pilot study. *American Journal of Psychiatry*, **158**, 1506–1508.

Shore, J. H., Vollmer, W. M. & Tatum, E. L. (1989). Community patterns of posttraumatic stress disorders. *Journal of Nervous and Mental Disease*, **177**, 681–685.

Silver, R. C., Holman, E. A., McIntosh, D. N., Poulin, M. & Gil-Rivas, V. (2002). Nationwide longitudinal study of psychological responses to September 11. *Journal of the American Medical Association*, **288**, 1235–1244.

Sledge, W. H., Boydstun, J. A. & Rahe, A. J. (1980). Self-concept changes related to war captivity. *Archives of General Psychiatry*, **37**, 430–443.

Smith, E. M., North, C. S., McCool, R. E. & Shea, J. M. (1990). Acute postdisaster psychiatric disorders: identification of those at risk. *American Journal of Psychiatry*, **147**, 202–206.

Solomon, S. D. & Smith, E. M. (1994). Social support and perceived control as moderators of responses to dioxin and flood exposure. In *Individual and Community Responses to Trauma and Disaster*, eds. R. J. Ursano, B. G. McCaughey & C. S. Fullerton, pp. 179–200. Cambridge: Cambridge University Press.

Solomon, S. D., Smith, E. M., Robins, L. N. & Fischbach, R. L. (1987). Social involvement as a mediator of disaster-induced stress. *Journal of Applied and Social Psychology*, **17**, 1092–1112.

Somasundaram, D. J & van de Put, W. (2006). Management of trauma in special populations after a disaster. *Journal of Clinical Psychiatry*, **67** (Suppl 2), 64–73.

Southwick, S. M., Morgan, A., Nagy, L. M. *et al.* (1993). Trauma-related symptoms in veterans of operation desert storm: a preliminary report. *The American Journal of Psychiatry*, **150**, 1524–1528.

Stein, B. D., Elliott, M. N., Jajcox, L. H. *et al.* (2004a). A national longitudinal study of the psychological consequences of the September 11, 2001 terrorist attacks: reactions, impairment, and help-seeking. *Psychiatry*, **67**, 105–117.

Stein, B. D., Tanielian, T. L., Eisenman, D. P. *et al.* (2004b). Emotional and behavioral consequences of bioterrorism: planning a public health response. *The Milbank Quarterly*, **82**, 413–455.

Steinglass, P. & Gerrity, E. (1990). Natural disasters and post-traumatic stress disorder: short-term versus long-term recovery in two disaster-affected communities. *Journal of Applied Social Psychology*, **20**, 1746–1765.

Sutker, P. B., Davis, J. M., Uddo, M. & Ditta, S. R. (1995). Assessment of psychological distress in persian gulf troops: ethnicity and gender comparisons. *Journal of Personality Assessment*, **64**, 415–427.

Taylor, V. (1977). Good news about disaster. *Psychology Today*, **11**, 93–94, 124–126.

Tedeschi, R. G., Park, C. L. & Calhoun, L. G. (1998). *Posttraumatic Growth: Positive Changes in the Aftermath of Crisis*. Mahwah: Lawrence Erlbaum.

Terr, L. C. (1981). "Forbidden games": post-traumatic child's play. *Journal of the American Academy of Child Psychiatry*, **20**, 741–760.

Thienkrua, W., Cardozo, B. L., Chakkraband, M. L. *et al.* (2006). Symptoms of posttraumatic stress disorder and depression among children in tsunami-affected areas in southern Thailand. *Journal of the American Medical Association*, **296**, 549–559.

Ursano, R. J. (1981). The Vietnam era prisoner of war: precaptivity personality and development of psychiatric illness. *American Journal of Psychiatry*, **138**, 315–318.

Ursano, R. J. (1987). Commentary. Posttraumatic stress disorder: the stressor criterion. *Journal of Nervous and Mental Disease*, **175**, 273–275.

Ursano, R. J. (2005). Workplace preparedness for terrorism: report of findings to Alfred P. Sloan Foundation. Available at: www.usuhs.mil/psy/WorkplacePreparednessTerrorism.pdf.

Ursano, R. J. & Friedman, M. J. (2006). Mental health and behavioral interventions for victims of disasters and mass violence: systems, caring, planning, and needs. In *Interventions Following Mass Violence and Disasters: Strategies for Mental Health Practice*, eds. E. C. Ritchie, P. J. Watson & M. J. Friedman, pp. 405–414. New York, NY: Guilford Press.

Ursano, R. J. & Fullerton, C. S. (1990). Cognitive and behavioral responses to trauma. *Journal of Applied Psychology*, **20**, 1766–1775.

Ursano, R. J. & Fullerton, C. S. (2000). Posttraumatic stress disorder: cerebellar regulation of psychological, interpersonal and biological responses to trauma? *Psychiatry*, **62**, 325–328.

Ursano, R. J., Boydstun, J. A. & Wheatley, R. D. (1981). Psychiatric illness in US Air Force Vietnam prisoners of war: a five-year follow-up. *American Journal of Psychiatry*, **138**, 310–314.

Ursano, R. J., Kao, T. C. & Fullerton, C. S. (1992). Posttraumatic stress disorder and meaning: structuring human chaos. *Journal of Nervous and Mental Disease*, **180**, 756–759.

Ursano, R. J., Fullerton, C. S., Bhartiya, V. & Kao, T. C. (1995). Longitudinal assessment of posttraumatic stress disorder and depression after exposure to traumatic death. *Journal of Nervous and Mental Disease*, **183**, 36–42.

Ursano, R. J., Fullerton, C. S., Vance, K. & Wang, L. (2000). Debriefing: its role in the spectrum of prevention and acute management of psychological trauma. In *Psychological Debriefing: Theory, Practice, and Evidence*, eds. B. Raphael & J. P. Wilson, pp. 32–42. Cambridge: Cambridge University Press.

Ursano, R. J., Norwood, A. E., Fullerton, C. S., Holloway, H. C. & Hall, M. (2003). Terrorism with weapons of mass destruction: chemical, biological, nuclear, radiological, and explosive agents. In *Trauma and Disaster: Responses and Management*, eds. R. J. Ursano & A. E. Norwood, pp. 125–154. Arlington, Va.: American Psychiatric Press.

Vlahov, D., Galea, S., Resnick, H. *et al.* (2002). Increased use of cigarettes, alcohol, and marijuana among Manhattan, New York, residents after the September 11 terrorist attacks. *American Journal of Epidemiology*, **155**, 988–996.

Wain, H. J., Grammer, G. G., Stasinos, J. & DeBoer, C. M. (2006). Psychiatric intervention for medical and surgical patients following traumatic injuries. In *Interventions Following Mass Violence and Disasters: Strategies for Mental Health Practice*, eds. E. C. Ritchie, P. J. Watson & M. J. Friedman, pp. 278–299. New York: Guilford Press.

Weisaeth, L. (1985). Post-traumatic stress disorder after an industrial disaster. In *Psychiatry – the State of the Art*, eds. P. Pichot, P. Berner, R. Wolf *et al.*, pp. 299–307. New York: Plenum.

Weisler, R. H., Barbee, J. G. & Townsend, M. H. (2006). Mental health and recovery in the Gulf Coast after Hurricanes Katrina and Rita. *Journal of the American Medical Association*, **296**, 585–588.

Wessely, S. (2005). Victimhood and resilience. *New England Journal of Medicine*, **353**, 548–550.

World Health Organization (2001). *World Health Report 2001*. Geneva: World Health Organization.

World Health Organization (2006). Collaborating Centre for Research on the Epidemiology of Disasters. EM-DAT: The OFDA/CRED International Disaster Database. Available at: www.em-dat.net/.

Wright, K. M. & Bartone, P. T. (1994). Community responses to disaster: the Gander plane crash. In *Individual and Community Responses to Trauma and Disaster: The Structure of Human Chaos*, eds. R. J. Ursano, B. G. McCaughey & C. S. Fullerton, pp. 267–284. Cambridge: Cambridge University Press.

Yehuda, R. (2002). Post-traumatic stress disorder. *New England Journal of Medicine*, **346**, 108–114.

Young, B. H. (2006). The immediate response to disaster: guidelines for adult psychological first aid. In *Interventions Following Mass Violence and Disasters*, eds. E. C. Ritchie, P. J. Watson & M. J. Friedman, pp. 134–154. New York: Guilford Press.

Zatzick, D. F., Kang, S. M., Hinton, L. *et al.* (2001). Post-traumatic concerns: a patient-centered approach to outcome assessment after traumatic physical injury. *Medical Care*, **39**, 327–339.

Zoellner, T. & Maercker, A. (2006). Posttraumatic growth in clinical psychology – a critical review and introduction of a two component model. *Clinical Psychology Review*, **26**, 626–653.

Zunih, L. M. & Myers, D. (2000). *Training Manual for Human Service Workers in Major Disasters*, 2nd edn. Washington, D. C.: Department of Health and Human Services, Substance Abuse and Mental Health Services Administration, Center for Mental Health Services, DHHS Publication no. ADM 90–538.

PART II

Foundations of disaster psychiatry

Epidemiology of disaster mental health

Carol S. North

Introduction

Psychiatric epidemiology provides a broad foundation for general understanding of the mental health effects of extreme trauma and secondarily helps to inform the field of mental health response to less extreme stress. Disaster mental health has considerable relevance in today's world, with disasters and terrorism increasingly occupying concerns of communities internationally.

The study of the mental health effects of traumatic events suffers from inherent methodological limitations. Studies of personal traumatic events endemic to community settings (such as motor vehicle accidents, gunshot wounds, and violent assault) suffer from confounding resulting from the nonrandom nature of their occurrence.

Pre-existing characteristics of individuals may be associated with risk for exposure to traumatic events (Breslau *et al.*, 1998), such as drug abuse, other psychopathology, high novelty-seeking and low harm-avoidance characteristics of personality, and low socioeconomic status (Breslau *et al.*, 1991). Risk for exposure to traumatic events in community settings is thus confounded with the mental health consequences of them. Studies of trauma in community settings may therefore be unable to determine what part of post-trauma effects is due to the traumatic experience, and what is pre-existing in individuals predisposed to such exposure. Because pre-existing characteristics

of individuals exposed to trauma in individual incidents in communities determine their status after the event, findings from studies of other kinds of traumatic events may not apply to populations affected by disasters. Adding further layers of bias to research on psychological trauma, many studies sample from treatment populations (such as posttraumatic stress disorder (PTSD) clinics), where virtually all individuals studied have psychiatric illness.

Disaster studies have the potential to sidestep many of these problems. Disasters strike more random cross-sections of the population, or groups without special characteristics other than, for example, having shown up for work on the day of a workplace disaster. Therefore, disasters provide opportunities to study mental health effects of extreme trauma in the most pure form, generally unencumbered by biases of characteristics conferring vulnerability to traumatic events. A noteworthy exception to the "equal opportunity" style of selection in disasters, however, is Midwestern flooding, which preferentially affects lower socioeconomic status populations that are attracted to live on the inexpensive land on flood plains. Lower socioeconomic status is associated with elevated population base rates of psychiatric illness (Koppel & McGuffin, 1999; Rutter, 2003) and therefore this characteristic, more than the effects of the flood itself, may be a major source of mental health problems after the flood.

Despite the importance of disaster research in understanding general mental health effects of community-wide catastrophes, conducting this research is difficult. Obstacles to disaster research include lack of timely funding for rapid deployment of research initiatives, barriers to affected populations created by lack of appreciation for research and unsubstantiated concerns about effects on study samples, and difficulties initiating research in postdisaster settings where chaos is proportional to the scope and magnitude of the event.

The majority of available information on mental health effects of traumatic events has accumulated from studies of nondisaster trauma such as military combat (Brewin *et al.*, 2000) and individual traumatic experiences in communities (motor vehicle accidents, assaults, childhood sexual abuse). Experience from nondisaster events may not necessarily apply to postdisaster mental health work. Studies focused on disaster mental health are therefore critical to understanding post-traumatic mental health outcomes specific to disasters.

This chapter will provide an overview of epidemiologic research on the mental health effects of major disasters. It will begin by examining disaster typology and then proceed to examine various outcomes of disasters, and predictors such as pre-existing characteristics, exposure status, and time frame. The chapter will also critically review other predictors of potential relevance for postdisaster settings, and finally will synthesize from this information relevant implications for disaster intervention policy and practice.

Disaster typology

Characteristics of disaster agents may contribute to the occurrence and course of ensuing mental health problems. The generally accepted typology of disasters divides disaster agents into: (1) natural disasters, such as earthquakes, floods, tornados, and volcanoes – sometimes referred to as "acts of God"; (2) technological accidents, such as mass transportation accidents, structural collapses, and

Table 2.1 Disaster typology

- Natural disasters
- Technological accidents
- Willful human-induced incidents

explosions, involving human error rather than intent; and (3) willful human-induced incidents, including mass murders in workplaces and domestic or international terrorism (see Table 2.1). Of the various disaster types, natural disasters are thought to be associated with the mildest mental health consequences (Baum *et al.*, 1983), although this assertion is not uniformly accepted (Rubonis & Bickman, 1991). Technological accidents involving human error may generate greater psychopathology. Acts of terrorism with their willful human origins may be associated with the most severe mental health sequelae (Baum *et al.*, 1983; Beigel & Berren, 1985; Frederick, 1980; Gleser *et al.*, 1981; Norris *et al.*, 2002b; Shalev *et al.*, 2004).

Determining the relative severity of different types of disasters constitutes a challenge, because other characteristics of disasters that also affect outcomes, such as scope and magnitude of the event (reflected in numbers of fatalities and injuries, size of the geographic area involved, and amount of property destruction), terror (fear for one's life), horror (contact with the grotesque), duration, and repetition and recurrence, are inextricably tied to specific events. This thwarts dissection of disaster typology from the associated characteristics of individual disasters.

Untangling the effects of other characteristics of disasters from effects attributable to the type of disaster will require comparisons of mental health outcomes of many disasters of different types controlling for variation in other disaster agent characteristics. This task is further complicated by the lack of uniformity of study methods from one disaster study to the next, especially inconsistencies in outcomes measured, measurement tools, timing of assessment, and sampling strategies. For example, studies of the September 11 terrorist attacks differed in timing of data collection from days to months later, and sampled groups with different exposure levels varying from being in the World Trade Center at the time the towers were attacked to random samples of the surrounding areas. The studies differed in instruments of measure and outcomes examined often deviating from critical elements of accepted diagnostic criteria. Inconsistency in research methodology among studies defies meaningful comparison of the estimates of post September 11 PTSD prevalence between populations in Manhattan and other parts of the country (Breslau, 2001).

Further complicating disaster typology, catastrophic events do not necessarily fall neatly into one category (World Health Organization, 1991). For example, a commercial airplane crash landing during a severe storm in Little Rock, Arkansas in 1999 was not just a technological accident, but it also involved elements of natural catastrophe, with the central role played by the weather in causing the accident. When the Mississippi and Missouri Rivers overflowed their banks in the Great Midwestern Floods of 1993, people blamed the Army Corps of Engineers for contributing to the catastrophe by its practices of containment and diversion of river water.

Catastrophes resulting from deliberate human acts can be subdivided into ordinary criminal acts such as mass murders, and terrorist acts. Terrorist acts are intended "...to intimidate or coerce a government, the civilian population, or any segment thereof, in furtherance of political or social objectives" (U.S. Code of Federal Regulations, 28 C.F.R. Section 0.85). Terrorist acts most often involve conventional explosives in the form of bombings. Use of biological, chemical, and radiological agents (sometimes referred to as Weapons of Mass Destruction) in terrorist attacks is classified as bioterrorism.

The goals of terrorism are to create widespread fear and demoralization, disrupt society, and erode trust in government and authorities (Alexander & Klein, 2003). The intent is to affect far greater numbers of people than those in direct contact with the damaging agent and intimidate members of

Table 2.2 Characteristics of bioterrorism

- Exposure not perceptible
- Uncertainty about exposure
- Misinterpretation of symptoms
- Behavior directed by perception of exposure, not actual exposure

communities or societies (Pfefferbaum et al., 2002, 2005). Assessment of mental health effects and the scope of mental health interventions will therefore need to encompass a population far wider than the circumscribed number of individuals in direct contact with the disaster agent, and to measure mental health effects outside the confines of PTSD and other psychiatric disorders.

Bioterrorism has unique features not observed in conventional terrorism. In bioterrorism, exposure may not be perceptible (see Table 2.2). This characteristic has earned the term "stealth terrorism" (Lamberg, 2005). Damaging effects of bioterrorism may not be apparent immediately, declaring themselves only days, weeks or even years later. Facing uncertainty about exposure, people may be influenced by their own perceptions and contagion from rumors, speculation, and their own imaginations. People may misinterpret their own physiological fear responses as symptoms of biological exposures, seeking treatment in large numbers and overwhelming the health care system's ability to attend to patients with serious injuries and illness (Norwood et al., 2001). Psychiatric responses to bioterrorism may become disarticulated from their level of exposure or injury. People's *perceptions* of their exposure, regardless of their *actual* exposures, may direct their behavior after bioterrorism.

Little research has been carried out on bioterrorist incidents, therefore studies of "mass hysteria," also known as "mass sociogenic illness," following actual or perceived exposures to biologic or toxic agents may be relevant to bioterrorism (Bartholomew & Wessely, 2002; Doyle et al., 2004; Jones, 2000; Pastel, 2001). Psychological responses to toxic contamination accidents and natural epidemics such as severe acute respiratory syndrome

(SARS) may also be applicable to understanding mental health effects of bioterrorist incidents (Arata *et al.*, 2000; Bowler *et al.*, 1994a, 1994b; Lopez-Ibor *et al.*, 1985). Risk communication is a critical public health response from leadership to help the public react safely and appropriately (Covello *et al.*, 2001; Marks, 1993; Moscrop, 2001; National Research Council, 1999; Norwood *et al.*, 2001).

Mental health outcomes of disasters

A fundamental principle in contemplating mental health interventions after disasters is to fit the response to the population, its exposure, and the needs of the individual. Psychiatric sequelae may not only differ from one individual to the next, but also from disaster to disaster and population to population.

Post-traumatic stress disorder (PTSD) is the signature diagnosis of disaster, and mental health responses to disasters typically focus on it. Unlike most psychiatric diagnoses, PTSD incorporates an etiology in its definition. Diagnosis of PTSD requires "direct personal experience of an event that involves actual or threatened death or serious injury" (American Psychiatric Association, 1994) (p. 424). Additional potentially qualifying experiences for the diagnosis may include vicarious exposure through directly witnessing others in such an event and learning that a loved one was involved in such an event. Symptoms in three categories (intrusive re-experience, avoidance and numbing, and hyperarousal) are required for the diagnosis of PTSD once a qualifying exposure has been established.

Intrusion and hyperarousal are nearly universal experiences after intense exposure to a severe trauma. Among directly exposed survivors of the Oklahoma City bombing, 96% described at least one post-traumatic symptom (North *et al.*, 1999), and four out of five had the required number of symptoms in the intrusion and hyperarousal categories to diagnose PTSD. The most commonly reported symptoms were intrusive recollections (intrusion),

trouble concentrating (hyperarousal), sleep disturbance (hyperarousal), and jumpiness (hyperarousal). The avoidance and numbing symptom profile was less common, described by just one-third, and 94% of Oklahoma City bombing survivors who reported three or more avoidance/numbing symptoms (the minimum number required for diagnosis) met full criteria for PTSD, yielding a 94% specificity and 100% sensitivity for PTSD. The avoidance and numbing symptoms were further associated with problems functioning, treatment-seeking, psychiatric comorbidity, and drinking alcohol to cope. Intrusion and hyperarousal symptoms in the absence of avoidance and numbing were not associated with these variables. It appears, therefore, that intrusion and hyperarousal symptoms are common and themselves nonpathological, and that avoidance/numbing responses are the pathological part of PTSD (McMillen *et al.*, 2000).

One does not have to be directly exposed to a traumatic event to develop PTSD. Witnessing an event with exposure to grotesque and horrifying images may lead to PTSD. Additionally, exposure to a traumatic event only through learning that a loved one was in a traumatic event may also provide a sufficient stimulus for the development of PTSD.

Post-traumatic symptoms do not count toward a diagnosis of PTSD unless they are new after the event, interfere with functioning or are very disturbing, continue for at least one month, and are not better accounted for by another disorder. This is to differentiate from clinically nonsignificant responses, brief psychological upset experienced by most people after severely traumatic events, chronic symptoms unrelated to the event, and symptoms of other disorders from post-traumatic illness. Most measures of PTSD, however, do not take into account the individual's actual exposure to a traumatic event, specificity of symptoms for the event, effects of the symptoms on the person's life, duration of symptoms, or other potential medical explanations for the symptoms. These measures may inflate population estimates of PTSD and overdiagnose individual cases.

Table 2.3 Disaster psychiatric responses

- PTSD
- Major depression
- Panic disorder
- Phobic disorder
- Substance use
- Medically unexplained symptoms
- Distress
- Resilience

For people who become symptomatic in the first two days after a traumatic event, before a diagnosis of PTSD can be established, the diagnosis of acute stress disorder may be applied. This diagnosis requires any PTSD symptom plus one or more dissociative symptoms. After four weeks, acute stress disorder is no longer a consideration, and the diagnosis is dropped, or else upgraded to PTSD if all the criteria for the diagnosis of PTSD are met.

The prevalence of PTSD described in association with disasters ranges widely. Only 2%–4% of survivors of natural disasters such as tornados (North *et al.*, 1989), mudslides (Canino *et al.*, 1990), and volcanoes (Shore *et al.*, 1986b) were found to develop PTSD. Post-traumatic stress disorder was reported in association with dioxin contamination among only 4%–8% of people exposed to it (Smith *et al.*, 1986). Other disaster studies have documented far higher rates of PTSD, including 44% associated with a dam break and flood (Green *et al.*, 1990), 53% following bushfires, 54% after an airplane crash landing (Sloan, 1988), and 50%–100% exposed to a plane crash into a shopping mall (Newman & Foreman, 1987).

Post-traumatic stress disorder is not the only important mental health consequence of disasters (see Table 2.3). Whether following individual traumatic events or disaster, PTSD more often than not presents with comorbidity, especially when it presents in mental health treatment settings (North *et al.*, 1994, 1999; Smith *et al.*, 1990). Therefore, once PTSD has been assessed, consideration of other disorders must follow, because other disorders are likely. Post-traumatic stress disorder cases with diagnostic comorbidity tend to have the greatest severity and associated disability (North *et al.*, 1999).

After PTSD, major depression is typically the next most prevalent disorder in most populations directly exposed to disasters (David *et al.*, 1996; Green *et al.*, 1992; McFarlane & Papay, 1992; North *et al.*, 1994, 1999). Individuals with pre-existing major depression are likely to suffer from major depression after disasters (North *et al.*, 1989, 1994, 1999); therefore, disaster-exposed individuals with a history of depression may warrant surveillance for signs of depression. Bereavement following violent death is seen among close family and associates after disasters, and can be confused with major depression, but it is distinct.

Other anxiety disorders besides PTSD, especially panic disorder and phobic disorders, may also be found in disaster-exposed populations (David *et al.*, 1996; Green *et al.*, 1992; McFarlane & Papay, 1992), but are not as prevalent as PTSD or major depression after disasters (David *et al.*, 1996; North *et al.*, 1994, 1999, 2002b).

The prevalence of alcohol and drug use disorders in populations is likely to be reflected in the occurrence of such problems after disasters, especially in men. Nevertheless, substance abuse after disaster is commonly assumed to represent self-medication or efforts to cope with the traumatic event (Jacobsen *et al.*, 2001; Saxon *et al.*, 2001; Zatzick *et al.*, 2001). Because of the prevalence of substance disorders in the population, and especially in certain populations at risk for them, the postdisaster setting may represent an opportunity to identify cases and direct cases to treatment. After disasters, people with pre-existing substance abuse problems may be flushed out of their private dwellings into public settings such as shelters, where their substance abuse may be exposed. In populations studied after disasters, alcohol and drug use disorders identified are almost always pre-existing (David *et al.*, 1996; North *et al.*, 1994, 1999, 2002b).

A number of studies have described increased use of alcohol, tobacco, and other drugs after disasters (Joseph *et al.*, 1993; Marcus 2001; McFarlane 1998; Pfefferbaum & Doughty, 2001; Sims & Sims, 1998;

Smith *et al.*, 1999; Vlahov *et al.*, 2002), although this is not a universal finding (Shimizu *et al.*, 2000). Most reported increases in substance use in disaster studies are observed in individuals with pre-existing substance abuse or other psychiatric difficulties (Joseph *et al.*, 1993; McFarlane, 1998; Pfefferbaum & Doughty, 2001; Sims & Sims, 1998; Smith *et al.*, 1999; Vlahov *et al.*, 2002). Conversely, decreases in alcohol consumption were described following a major earthquake in Japan (Shimizu *et al.*, 2000). Studies reporting such findings have provided little relevant information to demonstrate negative effects of increased substance use on employment, family relations, social and recreational activities, and health and legal status. Individuals seeking out the camaraderie of friends in social settings that involve consuming moderately more alcohol and cigarettes for a circumscribed period after a community-wide catastrophe may not necessarily be demonstrating evidence of a problem requiring a clinical response or intervention.

Patterns of increased *use* of alcohol and other drugs must be differentiated from abuse/dependence *diagnoses*. Any small but statistically significant increases in use of substances after disasters may represent nonpathological and possibly temporary disaster-related alterations in consumption patterns, and/or problematic increases in use among individuals with established abuse or dependence, but reports of changes in use of substances after disasters apparently do not often translate into new alcohol or drug use disorders after the event (David *et al.*, 1996; North *et al.*, 1989, 1994, 1999, 2002b).

Somatization disorder, characterized by a lifelong pattern of endorsing multiple medically unexplained complaints, is not a disorder that emerges after trauma (Breslau, 1998). A large disaster literature, however, has accumulated a repository of medically unexplained complaints, otherwise known as somatization, following traumatic events. Unfortunately, many instruments purporting to measure somatization cannot discern medically unexplained from medically based symptoms (Merskey, 1995; Ramsay *et al.*, 1993; Tennant *et al.*, 1986; Viel *et al.*, 1997), fail to distinguish clinically

significant somatic complaints from minor annoyances, and do not distinguish new symptoms after the disaster from pre-existing symptoms, thus artifactually elevating post-traumatic problems.

In general populations, some individuals report multiple medically unexplained somatic symptoms. Some, often the same, individuals may endorse an array of psychological symptoms without basis in established psychiatric disorders (Lenze *et al.*, 1999). In disaster-exposed populations, pre-existing symptom-reporting tendencies tend to persist afterward, with those reporting the most pre-existing symptoms also reporting more current symptoms. Tools designed to measure somatization may be insensitive to individual symptom-endorsement proclivities, further elevating estimates of post-traumatic problems (Wetzel *et al.*, 2000).

Somatization following disaster exposure was compared with that in unexposed comparison populations in two prospective studies. Following torrential rains and mudslides in Puerto Rico, somatization increased by a clinically small, but statistically significant, amount. The effect on somatization was considered nonspecific and potentially explained by known medical and psychiatric disorders or the unsanitary postdisaster conditions (Bravo *et al.*, 1990). A study of multiple disasters, including dioxin contamination, tornados, floods, and discovery of radioactive well water affecting one geographic area, found no new somatization symptoms and only one case of somatization disorder, occurring in the unexposed comparison group and predating the disaster (Robins *et al.*, 1986). The study concluded that somatization was not a product of the disasters and the affected population was resilient.

The resilience of populations affected by disasters is easily overlooked in the rush to identify psychiatric cases for mental health interventions. Most people do not become psychiatrically ill after disasters, even after exposure to the most catastrophic events (Galea *et al.*, 2002; North *et al.*, 1999; Schlenger *et al.*, 2002; Schuster *et al.*, 2001; Silver *et al.*, 2002). Fewer than one-half of people in the direct path of the blast of the Oklahoma City bombing developed a psychiatric disorder (North *et al.*, 1999). Strong emotional reactions, described by the majority of people affected by severe disasters, are normative and can hardly be considered pathological in these settings. Such strong emotions have been described as "normal responses to abnormal events" and have been termed "subdiagnostic distress" (North & Pfefferbaum, 2002). After the Oklahoma City bombing, 96% of survivors acknowledged one or more post-traumatic symptoms. Emotional reactions occurring outside the context of PTSD consist largely of intrusion and arousal symptoms such as nightmares, insomnia, problems concentrating, and jumpiness without prominent avoidance and numbing (North *et al.*, 1999). These symptoms tend to diminish with the healing processes of time. Outside the context of psychiatric illness, it might be advisable to refer these reactions in nonpathologizing language such as "reactions" or "responses" rather than "symptoms" (North & Pfefferbaum, 2002).

Distinguishing distress from PTSD or other psychiatric illness is pivotal for application of post-disaster interventions appropriate to the needs of affected individuals and populations. For post-disaster mental health intervention, one size does not fit all. Available treatments for psychiatric disorders, including psychopharmacologic agents and psychotherapy, are effective and should be utilized. These measures may not be appropriate for sub-diagnostic distress, for which support, education, and reassurance are more applicable interventions. Just as it is important to avoid pathologizing the distress of individuals affected by disasters, it is also important not to overlook postdisaster psychiatric illness. Post-traumatic stress disorder is a serious medical condition deserving treatment and is not considered a normal response to traumatic events.

Not all mental health outcomes after severe adversity are necessarily negative. Many people are challenged or stimulated to grow or develop in positive ways by cataclysmic life events (Frazier *et al.*, 1995; McMillen, 1999; McMillen *et al.*, 1997). After disasters, most people are able to identify something positive that came about as a result of the experience, such as appreciation of life, or people treating one another better (McMillen, 1999; McMillen *et al.*, 1997). Failure to inquire into positive outcomes may overlook them altogether, in the process painting an especially pessimistic portrait and missing opportunities to appreciate and enhance these positive effects.

Considerations of space and time frames apply to the mental health effects of disasters. Mental health effects differ by physical proximity to a disaster agent as well as in different time frames.

It is intuitive that the degree of an individual's exposure to a disaster agent predisposes to likelihood of development of PTSD in association with it. Studies have demonstrated that those directly exposed to severe incidents are at highest risk for PTSD and other psychiatric sequelae (North *et al.*, 1999), and risk for mental health consequences generally decreases with increasing distance from the disaster agent and decreasing exposure of affected individuals (Shore *et al.*, 1989). The prevalence of PTSD in relation to the Mt. St. Helens volcano eruption was associated with proximity of the individual's home to the volcano (Shore *et al.*, 1986a, 1989). Severity of PTSD was found to decrease with greater distance from an earthquake's epicenter (Abdo *et al.*, 1997). Degree of injury among survivors of the Oklahoma City bombing predicted development of PTSD (North *et al.*, 1999). Even though exposure is required for a diagnosis of PTSD in individuals and is critical for considering mental health effects of disasters on populations, psychopathology should not be automatically assumed in individuals with intense exposure to a severely traumatic event.

In populations, exposure level is a fundamental determinant of the mental health effects of disasters (Abdo *et al.*, 1997; Baum *et al.*, 1983; Beigel & Berren, 1985; Frederick, 1980; Gleser *et al.*, 1981; North *et al.*, 1999; Rubonis & Bickman, 1991; Shore *et al.*. 1986a, 1989). Exposure level is a pivotal factor for conceptualizing different population groups after disasters. People may be indirectly exposed to a disaster's effects in a variety of ways, such as disruption of business, damage to the workplace, financial loss, inconvenience of disrupted electricity and other utilities, and commuting delays caused by detours and damaged throughways or transportation systems. Indirectly exposed groups can be expected to show a lower prevalence of psychiatric problems after disasters compared to those directly exposed, and those less directly exposed who do develop postdisaster psychiatric disorders may have elevated rates of pre-existing psychiatric problems (Breslau & Davis, 1992).

The scope and magnitude of the 1995 Oklahoma City bombing and especially the September 11, 2001 attacks stimulated new thinking about the potential range of disaster mental health effects. People may potentially be affected in places remote to the disasters. With widespread economic consequences following immense disasters such as the September 11 attacks, significant mental health consequences may be anticipated in the population (Bland, 1998). At the farthest extremes of the ripple effects of disasters are people geographically distant, such as people in other parts of the country who may hear about the event indirectly such as through television news coverage.

After the Oklahoma City bombing, the surrounding communities were psychologically affected (Pfefferbaum et al., 1999, 2000; Smith et al., 1999; Sprang, 2001). After the September 11 attacks, psychiatric symptoms spread outward concentrically from Ground Zero in diminishing ripple patterns (Anonymous, 2002; Galea et al., 2002, 2003). The psyche of the entire nation was said to be affected, with evidence of widespread emotional and attitudinal changes (Blanchard et al., 2005; Ford et al., 2003; Linley et al., 2003; Schlenger et al., 2002; Schuster et al., 2001) as well as psychological vulnerability to disaster-related mental health problems (Baker, 2002). After the Oklahoma City bombing and the September 11 attacks, community and household surveys of the surrounding metropolitan areas and more distant populations reported prevalence rates of PTSD, probable PTSD, subthreshold PTSD, PTSD symptoms and symptom levels, symptoms "consistent with" PTSD, and post-traumatic stress disorder components (Galea et al., 2002; Pfefferbaum

et al., 1999, 2000; Schlenger et al., 2002; Schuster et al., 2001).

Remotely affected populations lack sufficient exposure to the traumatic event for its members to be considered candidates for a diagnosis of PTSD in relation to the event (Abdo et al., 1997). By definition, psychiatric effects will be qualitatively different among indirectly exposed and remotely affected groups compared to those of directly exposed groups, based on the dependence of mental health effects on the level of exposure. Members of populations without sufficient exposure to a qualifying traumatic event cannot be considered to be candidates for a diagnosis of PTSD due to the event. Measuring PTSD after disasters becomes problematic among members of large populations affected by disasters of national and international proportions, because most individuals in such populations do not meet trauma exposure criteria, and for them PTSD cannot be meaningfully assessed. Aggregate PTSD data reported from populations with mixed exposures, including large segments distant from the event, therefore become uninterpretable. Such data characterize a nonexistent amorphous average, describing no part of the population. Sampling in studies of large-scale disasters must measure effects in direct and indirect exposure groups independently from one another and from remotely affected populations, reporting findings separately to estimate the population burden of PTSD.

The significance of PTSD symptoms unassociated with an exposure to a qualifying traumatic event is uncertain. In this context, "symptoms" of a disorder that by definition cannot occur are paradoxical. PTSD "symptoms" in this case disembodied from a disorder that cannot occur suggests need for revision of terminology characterizing these experiences as nonpathological responses or reactions, rather than as "symptoms."

After the September 11 terrorist attacks, concerns arose that people might develop post-traumatic mental health problems with exposure only to graphic television images of the incident. Published reports claimed that contact with media coverage of disasters is associated with PTSD symptoms

(Ahern *et al.*, 2002; Associated Press, 2001; Pfeffer-baum *et al.*, 1999, 2003; Schlenger *et al.*, 2002; Schuster *et al.*, 2001). Studies do not always take into account that the experience of observing disaster media coverage does not meet diagnostic criteria for exposure to a significant trauma, and that causal relationships are not necessarily in the anticipated direction between viewing television media coverage of an event and emotional responses to it.

Although the news of the September 11 attacks and the graphic images on television were upsetting to the public viewing the media reports, this stimulus is not in the same league as being directly exposed to the event, and by itself would not lead individuals to develop PTSD. To characterize the distress of viewing media coverage of a disaster as equivalent to an exposure precipitating PTSD unnecessarily pathologizes a population and trivializes the experience of groups with high-intensity exposure (North & Pfefferbaum, 2002). Such responses may represent the norm in such circumstances.

Rescue and recovery workers are a group that may have varying exposures to a disaster and also pre-existing characteristics that shape mental health outcomes. They may be exposed to grotesque and horrific experiences in the aftermath of disaster, and in some disasters, as in the September 11 attacks on the World Trade Center, they may personally encounter danger and sustain injuries, may experience bereavement for fallen colleagues, and they may know direct victims. These types of exposure may translate into different mental health effects. Additionally, self-selection and selection for this type of work, training, and experience in this work may lend resilience to this group (Cardeña, 1994; North *et al.*, 2002a). Among firefighters who served as rescue and recovery workers after the Oklahoma City bombing, PTSD was less prevalent compared to survivors of the bomb blast (North *et al.*, 2002b). The most prevalent disorder among the firefighters was alcohol abuse or dependence, diagnosed in one-quarter of the firefighters after the bombing; nearly all of these cases were pre-existing. A study of firefighters not involved in community-wide

catastrophes reported current alcohol abuse rates of 29% (Boxer & Wild, 1993), suggesting that these high rates of alcohol use disorders may be more a function of the population than a response to trauma work, which has often been assumed (Jacobsen *et al.*, 2001; Saxon *et al.*, 2001; Zatzick *et al.*, 2001).

Differences in potential mental health outcomes determined by exposure status dictate different assessment designs for studying disaster-affected populations by exposure level. For small, highly exposed samples exposed to a severe disaster, which may be expected to have high rates of psychopathology, full diagnostic assessment may be feasible. Larger, less exposed populations, however, may overwhelm potential resources because numbers to be assessed are larger and the expected yield of cases is smaller. Full diagnostic assessment may be too resource-intensive, and screening for high-risk cases may be more feasible (Norris *et al.*, 2002a). Psychiatric screening tools are appropriate and more economical for this task, to identify high-risk cases that warrant full psychiatric evaluation. Screening tools, however, should not be used for diagnosis, to determine treatment decisions, or to estimate population rates of disorders. Screening instruments often fail to assess all DSM-IV criteria for the diagnosis of PTSD, including establishing exposure to a traumatic event, differentiating new from predisaster symptoms, determining duration of symptoms, and demonstrating the clinical or functional significance of the symptoms. Individuals identified as high risk for PTSD using screening tools need follow-up with a full diagnostic assessment to direct treatment decisions and provide accurate estimations of population rates of psychopathology.

Taking into account the many methodological determinants of outcomes, including type and severity of disaster, level of exposure, the type of outcome measured, and instruments of measure, a wide range of outcomes in disaster studies is expected. Even within directly exposed populations, the proportion with PTSD appears to vary markedly from one disaster to the next, ranging from virtually none (North, 2001; Shore *et al.*, 1986b) to essentially all of those exposed (Newman & Foreman, 1987). Among 182 randomly sampled directly exposed survivors of the Oklahoma City bombing, 87% of whom sustained injuries, one-third developed PTSD in association with it as measured by structured diagnostic interviews (North *et al.*, 1999). This can be considered to be a solid benchmark against which other highly disaster-exposed populations can be compared.

Varied mental health consequences may manifest in different postdisaster time frames. After disasters, post-traumatic stress begins quickly, most often within a day (North *et al.*, 1997, 1999). Delayed onset (defined as PTSD beginning six months or more after the event) is rarely observed in disaster survivors, unlike PTSD studied in the context of military combat (Helzer *et al.*, 1987; Prigerson *et al.*, 2001) or childhood abuse (McNally *et al.*, 2000). Occasionally PTSD begins early after a disaster but not quite enough symptoms are present to meet criteria for a diagnosis; later, an emergent symptom may nudge the symptom count over the diagnostic threshold. Such cases should not be mistaken for late-onset PTSD (North *et al.*, 1997), although longitudinal studies typically do not attend to this issue. People may delay in seeking treatment for PTSD after disasters, but this should not be assumed to represent delayed onset (North *et al.*, 1997; Weisaeth, 2001).

The longitudinal course of PTSD tends to be chronic (defined as lasting at least three months) after disasters as well as endemic in general populations (Breslau & Davis, 1992; Kessler *et al.*, 1995; North *et al.*, 1997, 1999). After the Oklahoma City bombing, no cases had recovered by three months (North *et al.*, 2004), and a year later most people with PTSD remained symptomatic (North *et al.*, 2004). A year after a mass murder episode, approximately one-half of PTSD cases had fully recovered (North *et al.*, 1994). Few predictors of recovery from PTSD have been identified (North *et al.*, 1994, 2004).

Post-traumatic symptoms not rising to the level of PTSD are more likely than symptoms of full PTSD to diminish within weeks to months after the event (Galea *et al.*, 2003; Silver *et al.*, 2002). The difference in the time course of symptoms among those with and without PTSD validates an important conceptual difference between symptoms and post-traumatic illness.

Predictors of disaster outcomes

Predicting mental health outcomes of disasters is vital to directing mental health resources that may be scarce in postdisaster settings. Because only some people develop psychiatric disorders, being able to identify the high-risk cases early through effective screening can conserve resources (see Table 2.4). Although prominent avoidance and numbing responses may be a marker for PTSD (McMillen *et al.*, 2000; North *et al.*, 1999) and the onset of PTSD symptoms is known to occur early after disasters, it is not known whether these symptoms are part of the early response or whether they appear later. Prospective study of the timing of onset of specific symptoms is needed to determine how early avoidance and numbing symptoms begin. If they are part of the early symptom response, then avoidance and numbing symptoms may be useful in early identification of people at high risk for PTSD. Regardless, prominent avoidance and numbing symptoms at any time after a disaster signal risk for PTSD not conveyed by intrusion or arousal symptoms alone.

Although the severity of disaster agents and degree of individual or population exposure to the disaster are considered predictors of PTSD (Abdo *et al.*, 1997; Green, 1993; North *et al.*, 1999; Shore *et al.*, 1986a; Shore *et al.*, 1989), disaster severity and exposure are not among the strongest predictors of outcomes (Sungur & Kaya, 2001). Gender is a strong predictor of post-traumatic anxiety and depressive disorders. In the general population, women exhibit twice the prevalence of PTSD, other anxiety disorders, and major depression as men (Blazer *et al.*, 1991; Breslau, 2002; Eaton *et al.*, 1991; Fullerton *et al.*, 2001; Helzer *et al.*, 1987; Kessler *et al.*, 1995; Pincinelli & Wilkinson, 2000; Weissman

Table 2.4 Predictors of disaster outcomes

- Gender
- Pre-existing psychopathology
- Age
- Education
- Socioeconomic status
- Postdisaster adverse life events

et al., 1991), while men are more prone to substance use disorders (Anthony & Helzer, 1991; Brady & Randall, 1999; Bucholz, 1999; Helzer *et al.*, 1991). After disasters, gender is also a robust predictor of PTSD and major depression (Kasl *et al.*, 1981; Lopez-Ibor *et al.*, 1985; Moore & Friedsam, 1959; Rubonis & Bickman, 1991; Steinglass & Gerrity, 1990; Weisaeth, 1985).

A second robust predictor of disaster mental health outcomes in individuals is pre-existing psychopathology (Bromet *et al.*, 1982; Chen *et al.*, 2001; Feinstein & Dolan, 1991; Hocking, 1970; Liao *et al.*, 2002; Maes *et al.*, 2001; McFarlane, 1989; North *et al.*, 1989, 1994, 1999; Ramsay, 1990; Smith *et al.*, 1990; Southwick *et al.*, 1993; Steinglass *et al.*, 1988; Weisaeth, 1985). Pre-existing psychiatric illness, however, is neither necessary nor sufficient to generate PTSD after disasters. Post-traumatic stress disorder may occur in people with no prior psychiatric difficulties; conversely, many people with previous psychiatric illness remain free from psychopathology after disasters (North *et al.*, 1994, 1999; Smith *et al.*, 1990). With exposure to mild events or with minimal exposure to more severe events, previous psychiatric history is an especially strong predictor of PTSD (Breslau & Davis, 1992; Feinstein & Dolan, 1991; Hocking, 1970; Shore *et al.*, 1986b; Smith *et al.*, 1993). With increasing exposure and greater severity of the traumatic event, previous psychiatric history is less predictive, and greater numbers of those with no prior psychiatric history develop PTSD (Hocking, 1970).

Few studies of predisposing psychopathology have examined the predictive potential of personality. Limited research suggests that pre-existing personality disorders predict postdisaster mental health problems (Chen *et al.*, 2001; Liao *et al.*, 2002; Maes *et al.*, 2001; McFarlane, 1989; Roy, 1982; Southwick *et al.*, 1993). A difficulty in conducting this research is differentiating the temporary effects of extreme events on people's patterns of interacting with others and the world from pre-existing personality disorders. This differentiation is addressed by documenting a lifelong pattern of maladaptive behaviors with early origins well before the disaster.

Other, less consistent predictors of PTSD and other psychopathology after disasters include age, education, and socioeconomic status. Apparent associations of some of these variables with psychopathology may lie with their confounding with significantly associated variables. For example, in two studies, lack of education was associated with PTSD only because it was a characteristic of women, who had a significantly higher incidence of PTSD than men (North *et al.*, 1994, 1999).

A well-known predictor of postdisaster mental health problems is the occurrence of other adverse life events in the postdisaster period, including events directly related to the disaster as well as indirectly associated and unrelated events such as being assaulted or loss of an elderly parent to natural causes (Epstein *et al.*, 1998; Maes *et al.*, 2001; North *et al.*, 1999). Disasters intrude into people's lives in the context of their existing situations and problems, and these existing issues are likely to continue to be a powerful predictor of outcomes in disaster settings.

Although social support has been linked to positive mental health outcomes (Bland *et al.*, 1997; Regehr *et al.*, 2001), especially among men (Solomon *et al.*, 1987), causal directionalities are uncertain, and likely to be complex. Social support may be as much a function of an individual's psychosocial strength as a determiner of mental health, because well-adjusted people tend to develop healthy social support networks. The same might be said about uncertainty of causal directionalities in coping as a predictor of mental health outcomes. Ineffective coping strategies, especially avoidant or passive coping rather than active problem-solving strategies (Arata *et al.*, 2000; Gibbs, 1989; North, 1995; North *et al.*, 1994, 2001), predict adverse mental health outcomes. Even though these associations have been demonstrated prospectively, it could be argued that while ineffective coping styles may increase vulnerability to psychiatric problems, those psychiatric problems may impair the individual's ability to cope.

Community response to disaster may affect mental health problems that may be reduced by an outpouring of community support (North *et al.*, 1989) or raised in settings of community conflict (Johnes, 2000). The postdisaster adjustment of rescue workers, whose mission is to serve the community, may be especially influenced by community response (Green & Linday, 1994; Hassling, 2000).

Implications

From the information reviewed in this chapter, practical recommendations can be made for post-disaster intervention policy and practice.

Interventions are needed early after disasters, and the need can be expected to continue through the long term

Based on available research, the acute onset and chronicity of post-traumatic disorders are now well known. Even though psychiatric illness may not be diagnosable for weeks after disasters, the evidence indicates it starts right away, and that considerable chronicity can be expected. After disasters, especially large-scale incidents, when psychopathology and anguish are acute, mental health professionals are moved to want to help. These sentiments sometimes bring so much help in the first few hours and days that the response overwhelms the situation.

In later weeks and months, however, as psychiatric disorders solidify in the affected population, signaling a larger need for formal mental health services, attention to the plight of the exposed population fades. The mental health professionals have returned to their offices and their mental health practices. At this point, mental health resources may be difficult to access by those in need. Mental health professionals are encouraged to save their benevolent urges to help for the long-term needs that are almost certain to manifest later. Even though delayed PTSD is not a generally observed phenomenon after disasters, people may delay in seeking mental health assistance, and many may obtain no help at all (Weisaeth, 2001). Outreach to members of the affected population who may be reluctant to venture outside its usual support network to accept help from strangers may therefore be needed (Lindy *et al.*, 1981; North & Hong, 2000).

Postdisaster populations can be most effectively approached by considering levels of exposure and pre-existing characteristics

Mental health interventions have traditionally focused on the most directly and highly exposed subsets of populations. The far-reaching effects of the September 11 terrorist attacks have necessitated reconsideration of the scope of attention for mental health sequelae. Not all subsets of populations, however, have the same sets of mental health issues and needs. Because groups diverge in post-disaster characteristics according to their level of exposure and pre-existing characteristics that shape outcomes, different approaches are needed to utilize limited mental health resources in post-disaster settings. Large surrounding populations with minimal direct exposure must be screened for the minority who will be at risk for clinically significant mental health problems, while full-scale systematic psychiatric evaluation may be feasible with available resources for responding to mental health outcomes of small, highly exposed groups who are expected to have the highest risk for mental health problems.

Although exposure level has utility for predicting psychopathology in groups or populations, it can be misleading if applied to individuals as an indicator of psychiatric illness. Research suggests that prominent avoidance and numbing responses may indicate high risk for PTSD (McMillen *et al.*, 2000; North *et al.*, 1999, 2002b). A screening tool with demonstrated high sensitivity and specificity is based almost entirely upon assessment of these symptoms (Breslau *et al.*, 1999). Screening instruments do not provide psychiatric diagnoses or a confident basis for determining population rates of psychiatric disorders, however. Psychiatric disorders in individuals must not be assumed based on exposure level or on screening instruments, but must be individually determined according to application of diagnostic criteria.

Differentiating psychiatric illness from distress facilitates treatment of psychiatric disorders without discounting or unnecessarily pathologizing distress

The first task in responding to mental health effects following disasters is to differentiate psychiatric illness from distress, because these two entities generally require different approaches and interventions tailored to their needs (National Academy of Sciences Institute of Medicine, 2003). Most people without psychiatric illness find talking about their traumatic experiences with trusted others to be helpful (North *et al.*, 1999; Smith *et al.*, 1990). Interventions designed to increase social support and sharing may be beneficial for many. Distress that does not merit a psychiatric diagnosis should not be discounted, because appropriately directed interventions may provide benefit for reactions not constituting illness.

People with prominent avoidance and numbing profiles that are central to PTSD may be unable to tolerate the level of exposure to reminders of the disaster required by interventions that force them to come face to face with reminders, which may be retraumatizing for them. Post-traumatic stress disorder and other disorders need psychiatric evaluation and treatment, because effective treatments are available. Special attention should be paid to: individuals with intense exposure to severe disasters, those experiencing additional adverse life events, female gender, those with pre-existing psychopathology, and those with prominent avoidance and numbing symptoms, who are at greatest risk for PTSD. Assessment should not stop with PTSD, because comorbid disorders are usually present, and may be at least as important to the course of recovery and the choice of treatment as the PTSD.

Summary

This chapter has provided an overview of epidemiologic research on mental health effects of major disasters, beginning with disaster typology and proceeding to examine various mental health outcomes and predictors of them. Practical recommendations for mental health policy and practice in disaster settings have been distilled from relevant empirical data from disaster research.

REFERENCES

Abdo, T., al-Dorzi, H., Itani, A. R., Jabr, F. & Zaghloul, N. (1997). Earthquakes: health outcomes and implications in Lebanon. *The Lebanese Medical Journal*, **45**, 197–200.

Ahern, J., Galea, S., Resnick, H. *et al.* (2002). Television images and psychological symptoms after the September 11 terrorist attacks. *Psychiatry*, **65**, 289–300.

Alexander, D. A. & Klein, S. (2003). Biochemical terrorism: too awful to contemplate, too serious to ignore: subjective literature review. *British Journal of Psychiatry*, **183**, 491–497.

American Psychiatric Association (1994). *Diagnostic and Statistical Manual of Mental Disorders*, 4th edn. Washington, D.C.: American Psychiatric Association Press.

Anonymous. (2002). Impact of September 11 attacks on workers in the vicinity of the World Trade Center – New York City. *MMWR Morbidity and Mortality Weekly Report*, **51 Spec No**, 8–10.

Anthony, J. C. & Helzer, J. E. (1991). Syndromes of drug abuse and dependence. In *Psychiatric Disorders in America: The Epidemiologic Catchment Area Study*, eds. L. N. Robins & D. A. Regier, pp. 116–154. New York: The Free Press.

Arata, C. M., Picou, J. S., Johnson, G. D. & McNally, T. S. (2000). Coping with technological disaster: an application of the conservation of resources model to the Exxon Valdez oil spill. *Journal of Traumatic Stress*, **13**, 23–39.

Associated Press (2001). Poll: Americans depressed, sleepless. Available at http://www.chron.com/cs/CDA/story.hts/special/terror/impact/1055126. Accessed April 3, 2007.

Baker, D. R. (2002). A public health approach to the needs of children affected by terrorism. *Journal of the American Medical Women's Association*, **57**, 117–118, 123.

Bartholomew, R. E. & Wessely, S. (2002). Protean nature of mass sociogenic illness: from possessed nuns to chemical and biological terrorism fears. *British Journal of Psychiatry*, **180**, 300–306.

Baum, A., Fleming, R. & Davidson, L. M. (1983). Natural disaster and technological catastrophe. *Environment and Behavior*, **15**, 333–354.

Beigel, A. & Berren, M. (1985). Human-induced disasters. *Psychiatric Annals*, **15**, 143–150.

Blanchard, E. B., Rowell, D., Kuhn, E., Rogers, R. & Wittrock, D. (2005). Posttraumatic stress and depressive symptoms in a college population one year after the September 11 attacks: the effect of proximity. *Behavior Research and Therapy*, **43**, 143–150.

Bland, R. C. (1998). Psychiatry and the burden of mental illness. *Canadian Journal of Psychiatry*, **43**, 801–810.

Bland, S. H., O'Leary, E. S., Farinaro, E. *et al.* (1997). Social network disturbances and psychological distress following earthquake evacuation. *Journal of Nervous and Mental Disease*, **185**, 188–195.

Blazer, D. G., Hughes, D., George, L. K., Swartz, M. & Boyer, R. (1991). Generalized anxiety disorder. In *Psychiatric Disorders in America: The Epidemiologic Catchment Area Study*, eds. L. N. Robins & D. A. Regier, pp. 180–203. New York: The Free Press.

Bowler, R. M., Mergler, D., Huel, G. & Cone, J. E. (1994a). Aftermath of a chemical spill: psychological and physiological sequelae. *Neurotoxicology*, **15**, 723–729.

Bowler, R. M., Mergler, D., Huel, G. & Cone, J. E. (1994b). Psychological, psychosocial, and psychophysiological sequelae in a community affected by a railroad chemical disaster. *Journal of Traumatic Stress*, **7**, 601–624.

Boxer, P. A. & Wild, D. (1993). Psychological distress and alcohol use among fire fighters. *Scandinavian Journal of Work and Environmental Health*, **19**, 121–125.

Brady, K. T. & Randall, C. L. (1999). Gender differences in substance use disorders. *Psychiatric Clinics of North America*, **22**, 241–252.

Bravo, M., Rubio-Stipec, M., Canino, G. J., Woodbury, M. A. & Ribera, J. C. (1990). The psychological sequelae of disaster stress prospectively and retrospectively evaluated. *American Journal of Community Psychology*, **18**, 661–680.

Breslau, N. (1998). Epidemiology of trauma and posttraumatic stress disorder. In *Psychological Trauma*, ed. R. Yehuda, pp. 1–29. Washington, D.C.: American Psychiatric Press.

Breslau, N. (2001). The epidemiology of posttraumatic stress disorder: what is the extent of the problem? *Journal of Clinical Psychiatry*, **62**, 16–22.

Breslau, N. (2002). Gender differences in trauma and posttraumatic stress disorder. *Journal of Gender Specific Medicine*, **5**, 34–40.

Breslau, N. & Davis, G. C. (1992). Posttraumatic stress disorder in an urban population of young adults: risk factors for chronicity. *American Journal of Psychiatry*, **149**, 671–675.

Breslau, N., Davis, G. C., Andreski, P. & Peterson, E. (1991). Traumatic events and posttraumatic stress disorder in an urban population of young adults. *Archives of General Psychiatry*, **48**, 216–222.

Breslau, N., Kessler, R. C., Chilcoat, H. D. *et al.* (1998). Trauma and posttraumatic stress disorder in the community: the 1996 Detroit area survey of trauma. *Archives of General Psychiatry*, **55**, 626–632.

Breslau, N., Peterson, E. L., Kessler, R. C. & Schultz, L. R. (1999). Short screening scale for DSM-IV posttraumatic stress disorder. *American Journal of Psychiatry*, **156**, 908–911.

Brewin, C. R., Andrews, B. & Valentine, J. D. (2000). Meta-analysis of risk factors for posttraumatic stress disorder in trauma-exposed adults. *Journal of Consulting and Clinical Psychology*, **68**, 748–766.

Bromet, E. J., Parkinson, D. K. & Schulberg, H. C. (1982). Mental health of residents near the Three Mile Island reactor: a comparative study of selected groups. *Journal of Preventive Psychiatry*, **1**, 225–276.

Bucholz, K. (1999). Nosology and epidemiology of addictive disorders and their comorbidity. *Psychiatric Clinics of North America*, **22**, 221–240.

Canino, G., Bravo, M., Rubio-Stipec, M. & Woodbury, M. (1990). The impact of disaster on mental health: prospective and retrospective analyses. *International Journal of Mental Health*, **19**, 51–69.

Cardeña, E. (1994). The domain of dissociation. In *Dissociation: Clinical and Theoretical Perspectives*, eds. S. Lynn & J. Rhue, pp. 15–31. New York: Guilford.

Chen, C. C., Yeh, T. L., Yang, Y. K. *et al.* (2001). Psychiatric morbidity and post-traumatic symptoms among survivors in the early stage following the 1999 earthquake in Taiwan. *Psychiatric Research*, **105**, 13–22.

Covello, C. T., Peters, R. G., Wojteki, J. G. & Hyde, R. C. (2001). Risk communication, the West Nile virus, and bioterrorism: responding to the challenges posed by the intentional or unintentional release of a pathogen in an urban setting. *Journal of Urban Health*, **87**, 382–391.

David, D., Mellman, T. A., Mendoza, L. M. *et al.* (1996). Psychiatric morbidity following Hurricane Andrew. *Journal of Traumatic Stress*, **9**, 607–612.

Doyle, C. R., Akhtar, J., Mrvos, R. & Krenzelok, E. P. (2004). Mass sociogenic illness – real and imaginary. *Veterinary and Human Toxicology*, **46**, 93–95.

Eaton, W. W., Dryman, A. & Weissman, M. M. (1991). Panic and phobia. In *Psychiatric Disorders in America: The Epidemiologic Catchment Area Study*, eds. L. N. Robins & D. A. Regier, pp. 155–179. New York: The Free Press.

Epstein, R., Fullerton, C. & Ursano, R. (1998). Posttraumatic stress disorder following an air disaster: a prospective study. *American Journal of Psychiatry*, **155**, 934–938.

Feinstein, A. & Dolan, R. (1991). Predictors of post-traumatic stress disorder following physical trauma: an examination of the stressor criterion. *Psychological Medicine*, **21**, 85–91.

Ford, C. A., Udry, J. R., Gleiter, K. & Chantala, K. (2003). Reactions of young adults to September 11, 2001. *Archives of Pediatrics and Adolescent Medicine*, **157**, 572–578.

Frazier, P. A., Byrne, C. & Klein, C. (1995). Resilience among sexual assault survivors. New York City: Presented at the 103rd Annual Convention of the American Psychological Association, 11–15 August, New York.

Frederick, C. J. (1980). Effects of natural vs. human-induced violence upon victims. *Evaluation and Change*, Special Issue, 71–75.

Fullerton, C. S., Ursano, R. J., Epstein, R. S. *et al.* (2001). Gender differences in posttraumatic stress disorder after motor vehicle accidents. *American Journal of Psychiatry*, **158**, 1486–1491.

Galea, S., Ahern, J., Resnick, H. *et al.* (2002). Psychological sequelae of the September 11 terrorist attacks in New York City. *New England Journal of Medicine*, **346**, 982–987.

Galea, S., Vlahov, D., Resnick, H. *et al.* (2003). Trends of probable post-traumatic stress disorder in New York City after the September 11 terrorist attacks. *American Journal of Epidemiology*, **158**, 514–524.

Gibbs, M. S. (1989). Factors in the victim that mediate between disaster and psychopathology: a review. *Journal of Traumatic Stress*, **2**, 489–514.

Gleser, G. C., Green, B. L. & Winget, C. N. (1981). *Prolonged Psychosocial Effects of Disaster: A Study of Buffalo Creek*. New York: Academic Press.

Green, B. L. (1993). Identifying survivors at risk: trauma and stressors across events. In *International Handbook of Traumatic Stress Syndromes*, eds. J. P. Wilson & B. Raphael, pp. 135–144. New York: Plenum Press.

Green, B. L. & Linday, J. D. (1994). Post-traumatic stress disorder in victims of disasters. *Psychiatric Clinics of North America*, **17**, 301–309.

Green, B. L., Lindy, J. D., Grace, M. C. *et al.* (1990). Buffalo Creek survivors in the second decade: stability of stress symptoms. *American Journal of Orthopsychiatry*, **60**, 43–54.

Green, B. L., Lindy, J. D., Grace, J. C. & Leonard, A. C. (1992). Chronic posttraumatic stress disorder and diagnostic comorbidity in a disaster sample. *Journal of Nervous and Mental Disease*, **180**, 760–766.

Hassling, P. (2000). Disaster management and the Goteborg Fire of 1998: when first responders are blamed. *International Journal of Emergency Mental Health*, **2**, 267–273.

Helzer, J. E., Robins, L. N. & McEvoy, L. (1987). Post-traumatic stress disorder in the general population. Findings of the epidemiologic catchment area survey. *New England Journal of Medicine*, **317**, 1630–1634.

Helzer, J. E., Burnam, A. & McEvoy, L. T. (1991). Alcohol abuse and dependence. In *Psychiatric Disorders in America: The Epidemiologic Catchment Area Study*, eds. L. N. Robins & D. A. Regier, pp. 81–115. New York: The Free Press.

Hocking, F. (1970). Psychiatric aspects of extreme environmental stress. *Diseases of the Nervous System*, **31**, 542–545.

Jacobsen, L. K., Southwick, S. M. & Kosten, T. R. (2001). Substance use disorders in patients with posttraumatic stress disorder: a review of the literature. *American Journal of Psychiatry*, **158**, 1184–1190.

Johnes, M. (2000). Aberfan and the management of trauma. *Disasters*, **24**, 1–17.

Jones, T. F. (2000). Mass psychogenic illness: role of the individual physician. *American Family Physician*, **62**, 2649–**2653**, 2655–2656.

Joseph, S., Yule, W., Williams, R. & Hodgkinson, P. (1993). Increased substance use in survivors of the Herald of Free Enterprise disaster. *British Journal of Medical Psychology*, **66**, 185–191.

Kasl, S. V., Chisholm, R. E. & Eskenazi, B. (1981). The impact of the accident at Three Mile Island on the behavior and well-being of nuclear workers. *American Journal of Public Health*, **71**, 472–495.

Kessler, R. C., Sonnega, A., Bromet, E., Hughes, M. & Nelson, C. B. (1995). Posttraumatic stress disorder in the National Comorbidity Survey. *Archives of General Psychiatry*, **52**, 1048–1060.

Koppel, S. & McGuffin, P. (1999). Socio-economic factors that predict psychiatric admissions at a local level. *Psychological Medicine*, **29**, 1235–1241.

Lamberg, L. (2005). Terrorism assails nation's psyche. *Journal of the American Medical Association*, **294**, 544–546.

Lenze, E. L., Miller, A., Munir, Z., Pornoppadol, C. & North, C. S. (1999). Psychiatric symptoms endorsed by somatization disorder patients in a psychiatric clinic. *Annals of Clinical Psychiatry*, **11**, 73–79.

Liao, W. C., Lee, M. B., Lee, Y. J. *et al.* (2002). Association of psychological distress with psychological factors in rescue workers within two months after a major earthquake. *Journal of the Formosan Medical Association*, **101**, 169–176.

Lindy, J. D., Grace, M. C. & Green, B. L. (1981). Survivors: outreach to a reluctant population. *American Journal of Orthopsychiatry*, **51**, 468–478.

Linley, P. A., Joseph, S., Cooper, R., Harris, S. & Meyer, C. (2003). Positive and negative changes following vicarious exposure to the September 11 terrorist attacks. *Journal of Traumatic Stress*, **16**, 481–485.

Lopez-Ibor, J. J., Jr., Canas, S. F. & Rodriguez-Gamazo, M. (1985). Psychological aspects of the toxic oil syndrome catastrophe. *British Journal of Psychiatry*, **147**, 352–365.

Maes, M., Mylle, J., Delmeire, L. & Janca, A. (2001). Pre- and post-disaster negative life events in relation to the incidence and severity of post-traumatic stress disorder. *Psychiatry Research*, **105**, 1–12.

Marcus, A. (2001). Attacks spark rise in substance abuse treatment; group says stress-related drug, alcohol problems will worsen. HealthScout News. www.healthscout.com, accessed December 5, 2001.

Marks, T. A. (1993). Birth defects, cancer, chemical, and public hysteria. *Regulatory Toxicology and Pharmacology*, **2** (Pt 1), 44.

McFarlane, A. C. (1989). The aetiology of post-traumatic morbidity: predisposing, precipitating and perpetuating factors. *British Journal of Psychiatry*, **154**, 221–228.

McFarlane, A. C. (1998). Epidemiological evidence about the relationship between PTSD and alcohol abuse: the nature of the association. *Addictive Behaviors*, **23**, 813–825.

McFarlane, A. C. & Papay, P. (1992). Multiple diagnoses in posttraumatic stress disorder in the victims of a natural disaster. *Journal of Nervous and Mental Disease*, **180**, 498–504.

McMillen, J. C. (1999). Better for it: how people benefit from adversity. *Social Work*, **44**, 455–468.

McMillen, J. C., Smith, E. M. & Fisher, R. H. (1997). Perceived benefit and mental health after three types of disaster. *Journal of Consulting and Clinical Psychiatry*, **6**, 733–739.

McMillen, J. C., North, C. S. & Smith, E. M. (2000). What parts of PTSD are normal: intrusion, avoidance, or arousal? Data from the Northridge, California earthquake. *Journal of Traumatic Stress*, **13**, 57–75.

McNally, R. J., Clancy, S. A., Schacter, D. L. & Pitman, R. K. (2000). Cognitive processing of trauma cues in adults reporting repressed, recovered, or continuous memories of childhood sexual abuse. *Journal of Abnormal Psychology*, **109**, 355–359.

Merskey, H. (1995). *The Analysis of Hysteria: Understanding Conversion and Dissociation*, 2nd edn. London: Gaskell.

Moore, H. E. & Friedsam, H. J. (1959). Reported emotional stress following a disaster. *Social Forces*, **38**, 135–138.

Moscrop, A. (2001). Mass hysteria is seen as main threat from bioweapons. *British Medical Journal*, **323**, 1023.

National Academy of Sciences Institute of Medicine (2003). *Preparing for the Psychological Consequences of Terrorism: A Public Health Strategy*. Washington, D.C.: National Academy Press.

National Research Council (1999). *Chemical and Biological Terrorism: Research and Development to Improve Civilian Medical Response*. Washington, D.C.: National Academy Press.

Newman, J. P. & Foreman, C. (1987). The Sun Valley Mall disaster study. Presented at the Annual Meeting of International Society for Traumatic Stress Studies. Baltimore, MD.

Norris, F. H., Friedman, M. J. & Watson, P. J. (2002a). 60,000 disaster victims speak: Part II. Summary and implications of the disaster mental health research. *Psychiatry*, **65**, 240–260.

Norris, F. H., Friedman, M. J., Watson, P. J. *et al.* (2002b). 60,000 disaster victims speak: Part I. An empirical review of the empirical literature, 1981–2001. *Psychiatry*, **65**, 207–239.

North, C. S. (1995). Human response to violent trauma. *Ballieres Clinical Psychiatry*, **1**, 225–245.

North, C. S. (2001). Psychosocial consequences of disasters: a longitudinal study. Final report to NIMH for Grant R01

MH 040025. St. Louis, Mo: Washington University School of Medicine, Department of Psychiatry.

North, C. S. & Hong, B. A. (2000). Project C.R.E.S.T.: a new model for mental health intervention after a community disaster. *American Journal of Public Health*, **90**, 1–2.

North, C. S. & Pfefferbaum, B. (2002). Research on the mental health effects of terrorism. *Journal of the American Medical Association*, **288**, 633–636.

North, C. S., Smith, E. M., McCool, R. E. & Lightcap, P. E. (1989). Acute post-disaster coping and adjustment. *Journal of Traumatic Stress*, **2**, 353–360.

North, C. S., Smith, E. M. & Spitznagel, E. L. (1994). Post-traumatic stress disorder in survivors of a mass shooting. *American Journal of Psychiatry*, **151**, 82–88.

North, C. S., Smith, E. M. & Spitznagel, E. L. (1997). One-year follow-up of survivors of a mass shooting. *American Journal of Psychiatry*, **154**, 1696–1702.

North, C. S., Nixon, S. J., Shariat, S. *et al.* (1999). Psychiatric disorders among survivors of the Oklahoma City bombing. *Journal of the American Medical Association*, **282**, 755–762.

North, C. S., Spitznagel, E. L. & Smith, E. M. (2001). A prospective study of coping after exposure to a mass murder episode. *Annals of Clinical Psychiatry*, **13**, 81–87.

North, C. S., McMillen, J. C., Pfefferbaum, B. *et al.* (2002a). Coping, functioning, and adjustment of rescue workers after the Oklahoma City bombing. *Journal of Traumatic Stress*, **15**, 171–175.

North, C. S., Tivis, L., McMillen, J. C. *et al.* (2002b). Psychiatric disorders in rescue workers after the Oklahoma City bombing. *American Journal of Psychiatry*, **159**, 857–859.

North, C. S., Pfefferbaum, B., Tivis, L. *et al.* (2004). The course of posttraumatic stress disorder in a follow-up study of survivors of the Oklahoma City bombing. *Annals of Clinical Psychiatry*, **16**, 209–215.

Norwood, A. E., Holloway, H. C. & Ursano, R. J. (2001). Psychological effects of biological warfare. *Military Medicine*, **166**, 27–28.

Pastel, R. H. (2001). Collective behaviors: mass panic and outbreaks of multiple unexplained symptoms. *Military Medicine*, **166**, 44–46.

Pfefferbaum, B. & Doughty, D. E. (2001). Increased alcohol use in a treatment sample of Oklahoma City bombing victims. *Psychiatry*, **64**, 296–303.

Pfefferbaum, B., Nixon, S. J., Krug, R. S. *et al.* (1999). Clinical needs assessment of middle and high school students following the 1995 Oklahoma City bombing. *American Journal of Psychiatry*, **156**, 1069–1074.

Pfefferbaum, B., Seale, T. W., McDonald, N. B. *et al.* (2000). Posttraumatic stress two years after the Oklahoma City bombing in youths geographically distant from the explosion. *Psychiatry*, **63**, 358–370.

Pfefferbaum, B., Pfefferbaum, R. L., North, C. S. & Neas, B. R. (2002). Does television viewing satisfy criteria for exposure in posttraumatic stress disorder? *Psychiatry*, **65**, 306–309.

Pfefferbaum, B., Seale, T. W., Brandt, E. N. *et al.* (2003). Media exposure in children one hundred miles from a terrorist bombing. *Annals of Clinical Psychiatry*, **15**, 1–8.

Pfefferbaum, B., North, C. S. & Pfefferbaum, R. L. (2005). Psychosocial issues in bioterrorism. In *Biodefense: Principles and Pathogens*, eds. M. S. Bronze & R. A. Greenfield. Norfolk, England: Horizon Bioscience.

Pincinelli, M. & Wilkinson, G. (2000). Gender differences in depression. Critical review. *British Journal of Psychiatry*, **177**, 486–492.

Prigerson, H. G., Maciejewski, P. K. & Rosenheck, R. A. (2001). Combat trauma: trauma with highest risk of delayed onset and unresolved posttraumatic stress disorder symptoms, unemployment, and abuse among men. *Journal of Nervous and Mental Disease*, **189**, 99–108.

Ramsay, R. (1990). Post-traumatic stress disorder: a new clinical entity? *Journal of Psychosomatic Research*, **34**, 355–365.

Ramsay, R., Gorst-Unsworth, C. & Turner, S. (1993). Psychiatric morbidity in survivors of organised state violence including torture. *British Journal of Psychiatry*, **162**, 55–59.

Regehr, C., Hemsworth, D. & Hill, J. (2001). Individual predictors of posttraumatic distress: a structural equation model. *Canadian Journal of Psychiatry*, **46**, 156–161.

Robins, L. N., Fishbach, R. L., Smith, E. M. *et al.* (1986). Impact of disaster on previously assessed mental health. In *Disaster Stress Studies: New Methods and Findings*, ed. J. H. Shore, pp. 22–48. Washington, D.C.: American Psychiatric Association.

Roy, W. (1982). Risk factors for suicide in psychiatric patients. *Archives of General Psychiatry*, **39**, 1089–1095.

Rubonis, A. V. & Bickman, L. (1991). Psychological impairment in the wake of disaster: the disaster–psychopathology relationship. *Psychological Bulletin*, **109**, 384–399.

Rutter, M. (2003). Poverty and child mental health: natural experiments and social causation. *Journal of the American Medical Association*, **290**, 2063–2064.

Saxon, A. J., Davis, T. M., Sloan, K. L. *et al.* (2001). Trauma, symptoms of posttraumatic stress disorder, and associated problems among incarcerated veterans. *Psychiatric Services*, **52**, 959–964.

Schlenger, W. E., Caddell, J. M., Ebert, L. *et al.* (2002). Psychological reactions to terrorist attacks: findings from the National Study of Americans' Reactions to September 11. *Journal of the American Medical Association*, **288**, 581–588.

Schuster, M. A., Stein, B. D., Jaycox, L. *et al.* (2001). A national survey of stress reactions after the September 11, 2001, terrorist attacks. *New England Journal of Medicine*, **345**, 1507–1512.

Shalev, A. Y., Tuval-Mashiach, R. & Hadar, H. (2004). Posttraumatic stress disorder as a result of mass trauma. *Journal of Clinical Psychiatry*, **65** (Suppl 1), 4–10.

Shimizu, S., Aso, K., Noda, T. *et al.* (2000). Natural disasters and alcohol consumption in a cultural context: the Great Hanshin Earthquake in Japan. *Addiction*, **95**, 529–536.

Shore, J. H., Tatum, E. L. & Vollmer, W. M. (1986a). Psychiatric reactions to disaster: the Mount St Helens experience. *American Journal of Psychiatry*, **143**, 590–595.

Shore, J. H., Tatum, E. L. & Vollmer, W. M. (1986b). The Mount St. Helens stress response syndrome. In *Disaster Stress Studies: New Methods and Findings*, ed. J. H. Shore, pp. 77–97. Washington, D.C.: American Psychiatric Press.

Shore, J. H., Vollmer, W. M. & Tatum, E. L. (1989). Community patterns of posttraumatic stress disorders. *Journal of Nervous and Mental Disease*, **177**, 681–685.

Silver, R. C., Holman, E. A., McIntosh, D. N., Poulin, M. & Gil-Rivas, V. (2002). Nationwide longitudinal study of psychological responses to September 11. *Journal of the American Medical Association*, **288**, 1235–1244.

Sims, A. & Sims, D. (1998). The phenomenology of posttraumatic stress disorder. A symptomatic study of 70 victims of psychological trauma. *Psychopathology*, **31**, 96–112.

Sloan, P. (1988). Posttraumatic stress in survivors of an airplane crash-landing: a clinical and exploratory research intervention. *Journal of Traumatic Stress*, **1**, 211–229.

Smith, D. W., Christiansen, E. H., Vincent, R. & Hann, N. E. (1999). Population effects of the bombing of Oklahoma City. *Journal of the Oklahoma State Medical Association*, **92**, 193–198.

Smith, E. M., Robins, L. N., Przybeck, T. R., Goldring, E. & Solomon, S. D. (1986). Psychosocial consequences of a disaster. In *Disaster Stress Studies: New Methods and Findings*, ed. J. H. Shore, pp. 49–76. Washington, D.C.: American Psychiatric Association.

Smith, E. M., North, C. S., McCool, R. E. & Shea, J. M. (1990). Acute postdisaster psychiatric disorders: identification of persons at risk. *American Journal of Psychiatry*, **147**, 202–206.

Smith, E. M., North, C. S. & Spitznagel, E. L. (1993). Posttraumatic stress in survivors of three disasters. *Journal of Social Behavior and Personality*, **8**, 353–368.

Solomon, S. D., Smith, E. M., Robins, L. N. & Fischbach, R. L. (1987). Social involvement as a mediator of disaster-induced stress. *Journal of Applied Social Psychology*, **17**, 1092–1112.

Southwick, S. M., Yehuda, R. & Giller, E. L. (1993). Personality disorders in treatment-seeking combat veterans with posttraumatic stress disorder. *American Journal of Psychiatry*, **150**, 1020–1023.

Sprang, G. (2001). Vicarious stress: patterns of disturbance and use of mental health services by those indirectly affected by the Oklahoma City bombing. *Psychological Reports*, **89**, 331–338.

Steinglass, P. & Gerrity, E. (1990). Natural disasters and posttraumatic stress disorder: short-term vs. long-term recovery in two disaster-affected communities. *Journal of Applied Social Psychology*, **20**, 1746–1765.

Steinglass, P., Weisstub, E. & De-Nour, A. K. (1988). Perceived personal networks as mediators of stress reactions. *American Journal of Psychiatry*, **145**, 1259–1264.

Sungur, M. & Kaya, B. (2001). The onset and longitudinal course of a man-made post-traumatic morbidity: survivors of the Sivas disaster. *International Journal of Psychiatry in Clinical Practice*, **5**, 195–202.

Tennant, C., Goulston, K. & Dent, O. (1986). Australian prisoners of war of the Japanese: post-war psychiatric hospitalization and psychological morbidity. *Australia and New Zealand Journal of Psychiatry*, **20**, 334–340.

Viel, J. F., Curbakova, E., Eglite, M., Zvagule, T. & Vincent, C. (1997). Risk factors for long-term mental and psychosomatic distress in Latvian Chernobyl liquidators. *Environmental Health Perspectives*, **105**, 1539–1544.

Vlahov, D., Galea, S., Resnick, H. *et al.* (2002). Increased use of cigarettes, alcohol, and marijuana among Manhattan, New York, residents after the September 11th terrorist attacks. *American Journal of Epidemiology*, **155**, 988–996.

Weisaeth, L. (1985). Post-traumatic stress disorder after an industrial disaster. In *Psychiatry-The State of the Art*, eds. P. Pichot, P. Berner, R. Wolf & K. Thau, pp. 299–307. New York: Plenum Press.

Weisaeth, L. (2001). Acute posttraumatic stress: non-acceptance of early intervention. *Journal of Clinical Psychiatry*, **62**, 35–40.

Weissman, M. M., Bruce, M. L., Leaf, P. J., Florio, L. P. & Holzer, I. C. (1991). Affective disorders. In *Psychiatric Disorders in America: The Epidemiologic Catchment Area Study*, eds. L. N. Robins & D. A. Regier, pp. 53–80. New York: The Free Press.

Wetzel, R. D., Clayton, P. J., Cloninger, C. R. *et al* (2000). Diagnosis of posttraumatic stress disorder with the MMPI: PK scale scores in somatization disorder. *Psychological Reports*, **87**, 535–541.

World Health Organization (1991). *Psychosocial Guidelines for Preparedness and Intervention in Disaster*. Geneva: World Health Organization.

Zatzick, D. F., Roy-Byrne, P., Russo, J. E. *et al.* (2001). Collaborative interventions for physically injured trauma survivors: a pilot randomized effectiveness trial. *General Hospital Psychiatry*, **23**, 114–123.

3

Children and disasters: public mental health approaches

Robert S. Pynoos, Alan M. Steinberg, & Melissa J. Brymer

Introduction

It has been estimated that, each year between 1990 and 1999, an average of 188 million people world-wide were affected by disaster, six times more than the average of 31 million people affected annually by conflict (International Strategy for Disaster Reduction, 2005). These figures for disasters do not include estimates for smaller disasters that typically are under-reported. Of particular concern around the world is that weather-related disasters have increased over the past decade, as evidenced by the devastating hurricanes across the Gulf Coast in the United States. Along with natural disasters, the possibility of Weapons of Mass Destruction (WMD) terrorism places significant numbers of children and families at enormous risk for psychosocial morbidity, and places extreme demands on shelters, schools, primary care settings, health and mental health care facilities, as well as federal, state and local agencies and organizations that play a role in coordinating or participating in disaster response. Children have unique risks from WMDs due to various physiological and psychological factors, including susceptibility to radiation, propensity to become hypothermic from mass decontamination, inadequate availability of pediatric emergency care and equipment, contraindications for pediatric use of standard treatments, and possible greater risk from the biological agents themselves (Pynoos *et al.*, 2005a). Pandemic flu represents another type of catastrophic scenario, with special mental health aspects for children and families, including issues of potential quarantine for long periods.

To date, there are no reliable large-scale epidemiological data on the morbidity or mortality of children exposed to terrorism and disaster. However, individual studies of children and adolescents affected by acts of terrorism and specific disasters have begun to document a range of adverse mental health consequences. After massive trauma, a large segment of the child and adolescent population may experience post-traumatic stress reactions and traumatic grief. As evidenced by exceedingly high rates of chronic psychiatric morbidity among children after the devastating 1988 earthquake in Armenia (Goenjian *et al.*, 1995; Pynoos *et al.*, 1993), the existence of thousands of traumatized children in different stages of recovery may place special burdens on society. These may include widespread disturbances in moral development and conscience functioning (Goenjian *et al.*, 1999), impairment in school, peer, family and community functioning, and diminished resilience to future stress. Changes in outlook on the future may not only affect the individual child, but on a massive scale permeate and transform cultural expectations, altering the social ecology of the next generation.

Disaster is one of the few life stresses for which early access to affected children and their families in the United States is authorized as a public health measure. Section 413 of the US Disaster Relief Act mandates such immediate assistance to states and local agencies within the disaster area "to help preclude possible damaging physical or psychological effects" (US Government, 1976). Subsequent to the Public Health Security and Bioterrorism Preparedness and Response Act of 2002, federal guidance directs all states to address the unique needs of children and families in recognition that children are more susceptible to the untoward consequences of disasters because of a host of special circumstances, including biological and psychological vulnerability. As a result, there has been a significant modernization of public child and family mental health approaches to terrorism and disaster preparedness, response and recovery. This chapter will review some of these advances, placing particular emphasis on the importance of maintaining a child and adolescent developmental perspective.

Key concepts

Recent theoretical and empirical work has contributed to a clarification of several key concepts that are central to discussion of the impact of disasters on children, and issues related to public mental health approaches to preparedness, response and recovery (see Table 3.1). The following deserve special consideration.

Danger apparatus refers to the systems of the brain and associated cognitions, emotions and behaviors that underlie evolving appraisal of and response to danger situations. Trauma is a subcategory in which efforts to prevent or protectively intervene to preclude the consequences of danger have failed. These systems undergo substantial maturation during the course of child and adolescent development, influenced by genetics, neurobiology, and experience (Pynoos *et al.*, 1997). Understanding the appraisal of and intervention considerations for children at different points of development, and under different environmental and cultural ecologies informs all aspects of disaster child mental health.

Table 3.1 Key concepts

Danger apparatus – system of biological and experiential maturation that underlies evolving appraisal and response to danger situations

Degree of exposure – level of severity of objective and subjective features of the disaster and loss experience

Vulnerability/risk – susceptibility to increased distress and impairment

Resistance – capacity to buffer the impact on distress and impairment

Resilience – capacity for early, effective adjustment, restoration and progression

Adjustment – appropriate efforts to cope with effects over time

Exertion – effort needed for adjustment

Maladjustment – inadequate or ineffective efforts to cope with effects over time

Developmental compromise – adverse developmental ramifications

Degree of exposure refers to the nature and severity of disaster-related experiences and losses, including life-threat to self and others, injury to self, injury and death of others, witnessing of mutilation or grotesque injury and death, and loss of family members, friends, property, and community. A major objective feature of disaster exposure for children is separation from parents, siblings and other caretakers during the disaster and its immediate aftermath.

Exposure factors may also include subjective features associated with the appraisal of danger, including the experience of extreme fear, horror, and helplessness. In addition to these categories, hearing unanswered cries of distress from victims trapped in rubble can create unalleviated empathic arousal in children (Goenjian, 1993). Young children can experience an intolerable sense of passivity in the face of disaster; older children may endure a painful sense of ineffectiveness, even cowardliness; and adolescents can experience disturbing existential dilemmas over protection for themselves versus others, as well as struggles over engagement in efforts at rescue. Another key subjective experience for young children is often the disruption of an expectation of a protective shield, where children's belief in parental protection is shattered. Numerous studies among children after disasters have indicated that both objective and subjective features of exposure make independent contributions to the severity and persistence of postdisaster distress and impairment (Goenjian *et al.*, 2001). That is to say, the higher the level of exposure, the more severe and persistent the subsequent distress and impairment.

Vulnerability/risk refers to an increased susceptibility to distress and adverse psychological, behavioral, functional, biological, and developmental outcomes attendant to a given level of exposure. It is worth noting that these factors may include both positive and negative mental health attributes, as, for example, capacity for empathy may serve as a vulnerability factor for increased distress, whereas disturbances in attachment may do the opposite. Vulnerability factors can include both child intrinsic characteristics (e.g., gender, age, neurobiological maturation, for example of the startle reflex, anxiety sensitivity, prior attachment disturbances, prior history of trauma and loss, and coping repertoire, including prior disaster experiences), and child extrinsic circumstances, (e.g., postdisaster stresses and adversities, prior and current family disruption, disturbed parent/child communication, parental substance abuse, caregiver psychological distress, physiological arousal and compromised functioning, caregiver physical disability or illness, and pervasiveness of trauma and loss reminders in the postdisaster ecology) (Pynoos *et al.*, 1995, 1999).

Resistance refers to the capacity of children and their families to buffer detrimental effects typically associated with exposure to disaster, thereby maintaining relative equilibrium and preserved psychological, behavioral, functional, biological, and developmental progression. Factors contributing to resistance can include child intrinsic factors as well as features of the child's family, school, and community.

Resilience refers to the capacity to adapt to and recover from disaster-related distress and developmental disruption in a timely and effective manner (Pynoos & Steinberg, 2006; Steinberg & Ritzmann, 1990). Children and adolescents vary in their ability to tolerate postdisaster symptoms and distress without interference in daily functioning and disturbance in the acquisition of developmental competencies. Many of the same features noted above that contribute to vulnerability and resistance may also play a role in resilience. Children who are excessively anxious or have preexisting anxiety disorder provide an example of the interplay of vulnerability and potential reduced resilience. These children may subjectively experience more catastrophic thoughts during the disaster disproportionate to their level of exposure, thereby increasing the severity of their post-traumatic stress symptoms. In the aftermath, they may also respond to reminders with more catastrophic thinking, be less responsive to reassurance or to seeking appropriate clarifying information or, through excessive clinging, reduce appropriate social support over time, all of which may negatively affect their ability to recover. In addition to the concept of "bouncing back," resilience can also include notions of "moving forward" developmentally, including postdisaster increased empathic capacity, accelerated moral development, and engagement in pro-social activity (Goenjian *et al.*, 1999).

Adjustment refers to appropriate and effective ongoing efforts to contend with disaster-related experiences and postdisaster stresses and adversities. There is a growing body of literature on the use and effectiveness of various coping and problem-solving strategies among children exposed to disaster (Almqvist & Hwang, 1999; Compas *et al.*, 2001; Halcon *et al.*, 2004; Kline & Mone, 2003; Vernberg *et al.*, 1996).

Exertion refers to the energy expended (costs to the child and family) in what are often extensive efforts at ongoing postdisaster adjustment. These efforts can seriously interfere with the resolution of postdisaster distress, and impact many areas of child and family functioning and development (Goenjian *et al.*, 1995). The co-occurrence of post-traumatic stress and grief reactions can significantly tax the emotional resources of both child and family. The course of exertion is often difficult to predict in the aftermath of a disaster because of the potential for ongoing danger, the challenge of unexpected reminders, and the changing ecology of postdisaster hardships and adversities.

Maladjustment refers to inadequate or ineffective adjustment over time, thereby initiating a cascade of changes that may result in a complex constellation of adverse psychological, behavioral, functional, biological, and developmental outcomes.

Developmental compromise refers to adverse developmental ramifications for children and families after exposure to disaster. Developmental progression can be compromised through different, yet often interdependent pathways. There can be direct loss of recently acquired development achievements, interference with the acquisition of developmental competencies, decreased developmental opportunities associated with failure to acquire age-related skills, and decreased initiative to take on developmental challenges. These key concepts can be summarized as follows:

The concept of "degree of exposure" is central to any discussion of resistance, vulnerability, resilience, and adjustment. Researchers and clinicians have typically drawn mistaken conclusions from data across exposure groups that show that a majority of children or adolescents are "resilient" or only temporarily distressed, experiencing an unproblematic course of recovery. In an early study of children exposed to a sniper attack at an elementary school, strong dose-of-exposure effects were found over time (Pynoos et al., 1987). Children who were in the direct line of fire in the playground were significantly more likely to have severe and persistent post-traumatic reactions over the next year, whereas children who were trapped in classrooms, one step removed from the direct assault, showed nearly the same levels of distress initially, but recovered at a much faster rate. Although there was some variability in recovery among the most-exposed group, their reactions did not subside commensurately with those of children with lower levels of exposure (Nader et al., 1990; Pynoos et al.,

1987). Thus, care must be taken not to overuse the concept of "resilience" without adequately controlling for dose of exposure.

For example, it has been reported that 25% of children after disaster will typically remain distressed over time (Vogel & Vernberg, 1993). However, the rate can be nearly 90%–95% among children buried by a mudslide following a hurricane (Goenjian et al., 2001). Whereas the rate of postdisaster distress at 3 months for children within the epicenter of the 1994 Northridge earthquake was under 40%, among the few hundred children who had been trapped the rate was 85% (UCLA Report to Los Angeles Unified School District, unpublished data, 1995). A structural equation model using data from a large cohort of adolescents exposed to war in Bosnia and Herzegovina showed that among those who experienced direct threats to their lives, injuries and/or traumatic war-related deaths of immediate family members, there was an unmoderated pathway to levels of current distress and impairment (Layne et al., 2001).

Impact of disasters on children and adolescents

Studies of the biological, psychological, and behavioral impact of natural disasters on children and adolescents have been growing steadily since the early 1990s, with earthquakes and hurricanes being the most widely investigated disasters. More recently, there has been a growing body of scientific literature concerning the adverse effects of political violence and terrorism. Such research is imperative if we are to better understand the full range of consequences of catastrophic events on this vulnerable population, and put in place effective preparedness and response programs to foster resilience and promote recovery.

More recent studies have included the September 11 terrorist attacks (Fairbrother et al., 2004; Hoven et al., 2005; Stuber et al., 2005), the Oklahoma City bombing (Pfefferbaum et al., 1999), Cambodian refugees exposed to war traumas (Kinzie et al., 1998; Mollica et al., 1997; Sack et al., 1995; Savin et al., 1996),

Hurricane Andrew (Shaw *et al.*, 1995; Vernberg *et al.*, 1996), the Three Mile Island nuclear disaster (Hanford *et al.*, 1986), the earthquake in Armenia (Goenjian *et al.*, 1995, 1997; Pynoos *et al.*, 1993), the earthquake in Greece (Roussos *et al.*, 2005) the Northridge Earthquake (Asarnow *et al.*, 1999), Hurricane Mitch in Nicaragua (Goenjian *et al.*, 2001), and Iraqi SCUD missile attacks on Israeli civilians (Laor *et al.*, 1997, 2001). Although reported rates have varied widely, traumatized children across studies have been found to have high prevalence rates of mental health problems. Table 3.2 indicates the adverse psychological reactions that have been reported.

From a developmental perspective, it is important to recognize that differing profiles of response are age-related. Young children may exhibit extreme fear of being alone, and reactions of helplessness or passivity. They may be confused about what happened and the danger being over, as they overhear things from adults or older children, see things on television, or just imagine that it is happening again. They are most susceptible to experiencing a failure in a "protective shield," which may require a substantial period of psychological recovery, during which they may act insecure in their attachments, separation behaviors and beginning sense of self-efficacy. They may regress to earlier stages of development that represent greater security, including reverting to thumb-sucking. Physiological regressions may also occur and contribute to symptoms such as bedwetting. School-age children are susceptible to major interruptions in their emerging self-efficacious behavior in regard to safety and danger. They can assume excessive responsibility or a sense of cowardliness, and experience deep shame and guilt. Their traumatic play many incorporate many efforts at successful protection and intervention, even through assuming extraordinary human powers. This age group often reports the most somatic complaints, with traumatic reminders rekindling similar somatic experiences that occurred during the disaster experience. Adolescents are more fully aware of their capacity to address danger directly, and can experience both heroic and anti-

Table 3.2 Adverse psychological reactions

- Acute stress disorder (ASD)
- Post-traumatic stress disorder (PTSD)
- Depression
- Anxiety
- Separation anxiety disorder
- Incident-specific new fears
- Agoraphobia
- Phobic disorder
- Traumatic bereavement
- Somatization
- Hostility/irritability
- Dissociative reactions
- Sleep disturbances
- Diminished perceived self-efficacy and self-esteem
- Reduced self-care
- Learning problems, diminished school interest
- Distressing reactivity to trauma and loss reminders
- Disturbances in moral development and conscience functioning
- Traumatic expectations/maladaptive cognitions (including those concerning interpersonal relationships, future orientation, career ambitions, plans for family life, trust in government and the social contract)

heroic feelings. They often feel self-conscious about their post-traumatic stress reactions, considering them to feel childlike, and respond to traumatic reminders with engagement in high-risk behaviors and substance abuse. Radical changes in attitudes about danger and the future can instigate substantial changes in an adolescent's and young adult's future plans, and traumatic loss experiences can initiate abrupt changes in interpersonal relationships with peers and family members. A change in perception of danger after disasters can shift the prevalence of separation anxiety into school-age and adolescent-age groups, where it is less expected (Goenjian *et al.*, 1995; Hoven *et al.*, 2005).

It is important to be careful about over-diagnosing phobia among school-age children, where the development of incident-specific new fears is common (Yule *et al.*, 1990). Of importance, sleep disturbance across all age groups has major consequences, as it can be associated with interference with concentration, attention, learning, and school failure. It is important to differentiate traumatic grief from post-traumatic stress disorder (PTSD) (Brown & Goodman, 2005; Cohen & Mannarino, 2004; Pynoos, 1992). Traumatic grief includes continued preoccupation with the circumstances of the death. This preoccupation can interfere with, or delay, the course of grief reactions, the ability to positively reminisce, and adaptation to the loss.

Research is also beginning to examine factors within the post-disaster ecology that mediate or moderate children's recovery (see Table 3.3).

Frequency of exposure to trauma reminders can significantly influence recovery postdisaster reactions are evoked by trauma reminders that are often pervasive in the postdisaster ecology. After disaster, children continue to encounter places, people, sights, sounds, and smells, and experience feelings that remind them of what happened. Reminders bring on distressing mental images, thoughts, and emotional/physical reactions. Common examples include: direct references to the type of disaster (e.g., high winds or rain after a hurricane), signs of physical damage (including destroyed buildings or debris), signs of injury (seeing people with disabilities), signs of people in distress (e.g., sirens of ambulances), specific locations, time or day associated with the disaster experience, and ongoing, often unexpected, encounters with television or radio news about the disaster and its consequences or stories about future dangers. Three months after the Northridge earthquake, having increasing difficulty calming down following aftershocks among children, parents and teachers was significantly associated with high levels of post-traumatic stress reactions, independent of degree of exposure (UCLA Report to Los Angeles Unified School District, 1995). Studies in Bosnia and Herzegovina suggest that post-war family conflicts may themselves be significantly mediated by the frequency of occurrence of trauma reminders (Layne *et al.*, 2006).

Of special importance is the difficulty in contending with family members who may themselves serve as reminders of disaster-related experiences

Table 3.3 Factors that mediate or moderate children's recovery

- Frequency of exposure to trauma reminders
- Frequency of exposure to loss reminders
- Type and severity of secondary stresses and adversities
- Impairment in caregiver functioning
- Quality of family functioning
- Overcrowded or adverse living conditions
- School and community milieu
- Quality of peer relationships
- Physical injury, disability, and rehabilitation
- Inter-current trauma and loss

and losses. This dynamic can perpetuate a sense of estrangement and of being misunderstood, and impede family communication. Loss reminders need to be differentiated from trauma reminders, and refer to times a child or adolescent may be reminded of the absence of a family member or friend. These reminders may induce unspoken grief reactions, including acting out, or more silent depressive responses.

Major studies have indicated that, as adversities accrue, there is a measurable increase in a range of child psychopathology, partly dependent on family or genetic history. Disasters can produce substantial adversities within a short period of time that persist over weeks, months or years. In addition, specific adversities, for example unemployment, reduced family income, overcrowded living situations, and parental disagreement over how to respond to adversities, is associated with increased risk of marital conflict, domestic violence, and child abuse. Often overlooked is the importance of the school community as a recovery environment for children and adolescents. Course of recovery may vary significantly due to variations in school administration support for additional school-related learning activities and sustained school-based disaster-specific mental health interventions. Physical injury and rehabilitation not only present their own challenges, but also serve as ongoing trauma reminders. Studies have indicated that inter-current trauma and loss, especially in the first year or two of recovery, are important factors that can adversely influence outcome (Nader *et al.*, 1990).

This body of research on children and disasters has some distinct limitations (Steinberg *et al.*, 2006). Most studies to date have assessed reactions more than three months after the disaster, leaving a gap in our understanding of acute reactions and their course. Most studies have been "one-shot" or cross-sectional in design, lacking information about predisaster status and course of recovery. Of studies that were longitudinal, most began after the disaster, again making the findings of rates of distress and impairment difficult to interpret. Most studies have also had too few participants, with sampling strategies that were less than optimal, and without long-term follow-up. In addition, there have been too few studies in which young children have been included, and in which youth and adults have been sampled and compared in the same study. Finally, there are too few studies evaluating postdisaster interventions among children and adolescents (Cohen *et al.*, 2006).

The next decade of research should expand a narrow focus on symptoms to better characterize a broad range of impact and outcome, and assess factors that moderate or mediate these. Outcome domains need to be broadened to include: biological alterations and physical health; developmental disruptions; disturbances in peer and social relationships; family conflict; impairments in academic functioning; and effects on pro-social behavior, citizenship and motivation for learning and career. Among many others, moderating or mediating factors that need to be studied include: physical injury and disability; severity of postdisaster adversities; frequency of exposure to trauma and loss reminders; prior traumatic experiences and losses; history of psychopathology; coping repertoire and style; and level of peer, family, and social support.

A good deal of research is also needed to evaluate the effectiveness of mitigation, preparedness, response, and recovery strategies in schools, communities and nationally, as well as the effectiveness of acute, intermediate, and long-term interventions in promoting the recovery of children and adolescents. In this regard, one study has shown positive results (Chemtob *et al.*, 2002a, 2002b), and a more recent longitudinal study has shown the beneficial effects at $5\frac{1}{2}$ years postdisaster of a trauma/grief-focused intervention delivered 1 year postdisaster (Goenjian *et al.*, 2005).

An important area for research is the impact of media, especially television viewing, on the recovery of children and adolescents (Fairbrother *et al.*, 2003; Pfefferbaum *et al.*, 2001). Research on the effectiveness of risk communication and emergency public information is especially needed in regard to scenarios involving WMDs. There is also a need for more research among special populations, including orphans, unaccompanied minors, homeless children, children with special needs, refugees and displaced children, and children who have been exposed to multiple disasters and losses.

Stages and strategies of postdisaster intervention

A modern public mental health approach to the postdisaster recovery of children, adolescents, adults, and families recognizes the importance of conceptualizing stages of disaster response (Pynoos *et al.*, 1995, 1998, 2005b). Although the timing, setting and service providers for delivery of acute, intermediate, and longer-term postdisaster interventions will vary by type of disaster and post-disaster ecology, it is generally accepted that different levels of intervention are needed for each of these stages. For children and families, schools represent a major setting for many modalities of intervention (individual, classroom, group, family).

Acute interventions are typically brief, and provided in the days and weeks post-event, while intermediate-stage interventions are offered over the first 18 months following a disaster. Children, adolescents, and adults who continue to experience difficulties months to years after a disaster can benefit from longer-term, more comprehensive trauma/grief-focused treatment that also addresses concomitant comorbid conditions and rehabilitation of developmental disruptions.

Table 3.4 Stages of postdisaster intervention

Psychological First Aid
Skills for psychological recovery
Enhanced services
Treatment

These different stages of interventions represent more in-depth and extended efforts that encompass similar objectives, so that the main foci of intervention remain constant. For example, although postdisaster stresses and adversities may evolve over time, a focus on these remains an integral component across all stages of recovery. The same may be said for a focus on reactivity to trauma and loss reminders, despite the fact that the nature and frequency of exposure to reminders may vary over the course of recovery. The following sections provide an overview of the basic principles and goals of each of these staged interventions (see Table 3.4).

Psychological First Aid

Negative findings and controversy over the effectiveness of critical incident stress debriefing techniques have left a gap in the disaster field regarding effective acute interventions (McNally *et al.*, 2003). In response, the National Child Traumatic Stress Network and the National Center for PTSD has developed a Psychological First Aid (PFA) Field Operations Guide, second edition for the provision of early psychological assistance to children, adolescents, adults, and families after disaster and terrorism (Brymer *et al.*, 2006, National Child Traumatic Stress Network and National Center for PTSD, 2005). In the aftermath of Hurricane Katrina, with the enormous number of children and families directly affected and evacuated, PFA was released for use in the disaster-affected regions, including areas across the United States with large numbers of displaced children and families. The PFA Field Operations Guide was initially designed for use by mental health professionals. However, it has been widely used by individuals from a variety of backgrounds. There are currently adaptations of PFA being developed for use by school crisis teams, clergy, first responders, emergency room personnel, pediatricians, and by the Medical Reserve Corps. The PFA Guide and various adaptations will be available on the website of the National Child Traumatic Stress Network, www.nctsn.org.

In developing the protocol, our group took advantage of numerous materials available from many agencies and organizations that coordinate or participate in disaster response, and from the current research literature and national and international experience in regard to principles that were found to be most effective in providing acute assistance after disasters. A distinct advantage of the PFA protocol is that, in contradistinction to most materials available, it includes interventions designed for both children and adults, and provides in-depth description of recommended strategies to accomplish the intervention goals, along with specific examples of what to say and do.

Psychological First Aid is deliverable in diverse settings. Such settings may include shelters, schools, hospitals, homes, faith-based locations, staging areas, feeding locations, family assistance centers, and other community settings. Following WMD events, PFA may be delivered in mass casualty collection points, hospitals, and in field decontamination and mass prophylaxis locations. The PFA Guide includes basic information-gathering techniques to help providers make rapid assessments of survivors' immediate needs and concerns, and to tailor interventions in a flexible manner. Of importance, concepts such as "clinical evaluation," "diagnosis," "symptoms," "disorder," and "psychopathology" are not components of the provision of immediate assistance provided through PFA.

The PFA Guide was developed to be as strongly evidence-informed as possible, and constructed from within a sound developmental and cultural framework (Pynoos *et al.*, 1995, 1998). Important features of PFA are the use of information-gathering strategies to tailor the intervention to the specific needs and concerns of affected children and families, and informational handouts that are provided to those affected by disaster. The basic PFA objectives include:

1. Making contact
2. Ensuring immediate safety and comfort
3. Helping with stabilization
4. Gathering information
5. Providing practical assistance
6. Promoting use and provision of social support
7. Providing information on coping
8. Linking with collaborative services.

Handouts are included in PFA that provide information about common reactions after disasters, seeking and giving support, positive and negative coping strategies, tips for parents on assisting children at the preschool, school-age, and adolescent levels, basic relaxation techniques, alcohol use and abuse after disasters, and self-care strategies for providers implementing the PFA protocol. These materials allow survivors to continue to get assistance over the weeks and months of recovery by providing important information that they can use over time. The overarching approach is to empower children, adolescents, and families to actively utilize their natural recovery and support systems, and engage in proactive problem-solving to facilitate their own recovery. An important component of PFA is to help children and families understand expectable reactions, and how to connect with behavioral health and social services if these are needed in the future. Importantly, in light of findings regarding debriefing, the guide provides specific cautions about engaging children and adults in discussing details of their disaster-related trauma and loss experiences.

In clarifying disaster-related traumatic experiences, the Psychological First Aid provider should avoid asking for in-depth description of traumatic experiences as this may provoke unnecessary additional distress. It is especially important to follow the lead of the survivor in discussing what happened during the event. Individuals should not be pressed to disclose details of any trauma or loss. On the other hand, if individuals are anxious to talk about their experiences, let them know politely and respectfully that what would be most helpful now is to get some *basic*

information to be able to help with what is currently needed and plan for future care. Let them know that the opportunity to discuss their experiences in a proper professional setting can be arranged for the future.

The guide also recommends that, in providing assistance to disadvantaged and culturally diverse populations, providers consult local community leaders to better understand local customs in regard to specific religious and mourning rituals, social connectedness, and coping strategies.

The nature and course of grief is strongly influenced by family, cultural and religious beliefs and rituals related to mourning. You should inform yourself about cultural norms with the assistance of community cultural leaders who best understand local customs. Remember that it is important for families to decide from their own tradition of practices and rituals how to honor the death.

A special feature to be added to the PFA Guide is an evaluation component integrated within the intervention that also serves a therapeutic function. For example, in gathering information about concerns, worries, distress, and immediate needs of children, adults and families, survivors will be asked to rate their level of current distress, "put a number to it." At the conclusion of the intervention, providers will again obtain a rating in these areas to ascertain the intervention's immediate impact. There is a critical need for this type of evaluation, as well as longer-term follow-up studies, to begin to establish an evidence base for acute interventions.

Skills for Psychological Recovery

This intervention, "Skills for psychological recovery" (SPR), which is currently under development, is more extended and in-depth than PFA, and is designed to meet criteria for mental health interventions that are provided through the Crisis Counseling Program funded by the FEMA/Center for Mental Health Services (CMHS). SPA is designed for the weeks and months following a disaster. It includes more in-depth and systematic gathering of information to identify specific risks for post-disaster distress and problems, and to tailor the intervention to the specific needs of children, adolescents, adults, and families. It also includes a wider range of strategies to accomplish the intervention objectives. As with PFA, SPR is organized around major goals, specific objectives within each goal, and provides operationalized strategies that can be employed to accomplish each of the objectives. As this is an intermediate postdisaster intervention, important additional objectives include:

- Assistance with problem-solving and coping with ongoing postdisaster stresses and adversities (e.g., coping with prolonged displacement, unemployment, physical rehabilitation)
- Strengthening capacity to manage on-going trauma and loss reminders, including in anticipation, during and after
- Focused assistance with singularly troubling aspects of disaster experience (e.g., preoccupation with action or inaction, or postdisaster viewing of a dead relative)
- Helping to restore family functioning and normal routines, including helping primary caregivers in enhancing effective parenting roles and responsibilities even during their own recovery course
- Assisting children and families in managing ongoing grief reactions and emerging depressive responses
- Promoting linkage with mental health, health, and social services
- Promoting youth and family developmental progression (e.g., integration into a new or reconstituted school system and peer group, and resumption of family activities)
- Enhancing information acquisition and management skills in regard to ongoing safety information (e.g., air quality, hazardous areas, quarantine and other public health measures, rebuilding efforts)
- Promoting constructive activities that improve peer, social, and community ecology.

Enhanced Services

A child and adolescent Enhanced Services model is a brief mental health intervention program for children and adolescents who continue to experience moderate to severe reactions months to years after large-scale disasters. These interventions represent an intermediate step between crisis counseling services and longer-term mental health treatment. The goals are to accelerate recovery from ongoing or phasic distress toward a predisaster level, to mitigate long-term mental health difficulties or disorders, and to promote adaptive functioning. Enhanced Services interventions for children and adolescents have included 10–12 sessions that can be delivered individually or in a group setting. Enhancing parental understanding, family communication and disaster recovery parenting skills are an important component. In Florida for the 2004 hurricanes, Enhanced Services were developed for Project Recovery using a ten-session manualized protocol for children 8 years old and above (Allen *et al.*, 2006). Because of prior empirical evidence regarding the increased risk of anxiety-prone children to persistent and more severe post-hurricane distress, this intervention included addressing anticipatory anxiety and fear of recurrence, and provided hurricane-specific psychoeducation and anxiety management in regard to reactivity to hurricane-related reminders. A unique feature of this intervention involved the child and parents describing a timeline of their disaster-related experiences to promote a shared understanding of both overlap and differences in their objective and subjective experience and responses. Unlike PFA and SPR, Enhanced Services includes the use of instruments to evaluate baseline and postintervention levels of post-traumatic stress, anxiety, depression, and coping. An Enhanced Services intervention is currently being developed for preschool children and their caretakers.

Treatment

Over the past decade, there have been considerable advancements in the treatment of children and adolescents exposed to disaster. Approaches have included individual, family, group, and classroom modalities. Randomized studies among school-age children have primarily examined trauma- and loss-focused cognitive-behavioral and interpersonal approaches. For example, using a staggered start comparison group, March and colleagues (1998) reported a robust beneficial effect of an 18-week cognitive-behavioral therapy (CBT) intervention after an industrial fire. There was a significant improvement in PTSD symptoms, depression, anxiety, and a reduction in anger. Two studies reported on the effectiveness of a brief six-session school-based trauma-focused intervention after a large-scale earthquake (Goenjian *et al.*, 1997, 2005). At both 3 years and 5 years post-earthquake, the treated group showed significant improvement in PTSD and stable depressive symptoms, whereas untreated adolescents suffered a worsening of PTSD and exacerbation of depression. The significance of these longitudinal studies from Armenia is that treatment gains persisted over a 4-year period post-treatment. After the sinking of the *Jupiter*, Yule (1992) reported that a CBT treatment for girls was associated with lower PTSD, depressive, and fear symptoms at 9 months postdisaster, compared with a no-treatment group. Another study, conducted after Hurricane Iniki using a psychosocial intervention in a randomized control design, found a significant reduction in trauma-related symptoms that was maintained at 10–12 months follow-up (Chemtob *et al.*, 2002a, 2002b). Layne *et al.* (2001) reported a significant reduction in PTSD, depression, and traumatic grief reactions among war-traumatized students from Bosnia-Herzegovina 2 years after a 20-session adolescent group, school-based intervention. Although open studies have identified medications with promise for use among traumatized children and adolescents, there have been no studies evaluating the effectiveness of medications in the recovery of children and youths after disasters (Cohen, 2005).

Postdisaster interventions for children and adolescents have included the following components: psychoeducation, anxiety management, problem-solving and coping skills, extended trauma narrative reprocessing, enhancing emotional regulation,

Table 3.5 Primary therapeutic foci

Traumatic experiences
Trauma and loss reminders
Trauma-related bereavement
Postdisaster adversities
Developmental progression

progressive review of disturbing appraisals, cognitions and expectations, relapse prevention, and techniques for enhancing social support. Specific parent–child/youth sessions are incorporated into many of the treatment protocols. Five primary therapeutic foci have emerged as important components of postdisaster intervention for youth (see Table 3.5). These foci are briefly described below.

First, a comprehensive intervention for children and adolescents exposed to disaster must systematically address disaster-related *traumatic experiences*, both their objective and subjective features. This focus includes psycho-education about age-appropriate reactions to trauma and loss. This is essential in order to help children identify trauma/loss-related distress reactions and difficulties, and to reduce perception that reactions are related to personal shortcomings. Treatment must also include repeated opportunities to revisit the traumatic experience through trauma narrative exercises that promote remembering with immediacy. Children are guided to produce a coherent, temporally ordered narrative of their subjective experience. These sessions enhance understanding of the child's moment to moment appraisals, intervention considerations, somatic experience and emotional challenges. Progressive verbal and visual representations serve to enhance emotional regulation, especially in regard to "worst moments." Particular attention is also paid to attributions of excessive responsibility, moments of estrangement from others, failures of protective intervention and maladaptive beliefs. Two additional goals are to better identify sources of potential trauma reminders embedded in the experience, and points of disruption in a sense of a "protective shield" that will require psychological repair over time.

Second, *trauma and loss reminders* are features of the child's environment that trigger intrusive distressing thoughts, feelings, and memories. Reminders are often associated with strong emotional and physiological reactivity, traumatic avoidance, and reenactment behaviors that, at times, can be dangerous. Treatment must assist children in identifying current and future trauma/loss reminders, and in understanding the links between their disaster-related traumatic experience(s), reactions, and current maladaptive behavior. Efforts to increase coping and adaptive responses can include facilitating contextual discrimination between the present and past, increasing tolerance for expectable reactivity, reducing unnecessary exposures to unnecessary reminders, and the development of appropriate support-seeking and anxiety-management skills for the periods before, during, and after exposure to distressing reminders.

Third, when traumatic circumstances accompany the death of a family member or close friend, there is often interplay between trauma and bereavement. Normal grieving requires the ability to positively reminisce about the deceased. Often, loss of loved ones due to terrorism and disaster involves extreme traumatic elements. As a consequence, the grieving child may avoid thinking about the deceased because such efforts result in upsetting and painful memories. The result is a form of traumatic grief, with prolonged symptoms and maladaptive coping responses. The sequencing of therapeutic efforts is first to promote the receding of traumatic aspects that maintain preoccupation with details of the death; then, second, to facilitate the appropriate child's or adolescent's grief within the context of their individual, family, and cultural background. Specific therapeutic tasks undertaken toward this goal include psycho-education about grief reactions and the course of bereavement, framing grief reactions and bereavement as beneficial processes that facilitate accommodation to the ongoing absence of the loved one, and, in cases in which traumatic intrusions interfere with positive reminiscing, construction of a non-traumatic mental representation of the deceased.

Other goals include increasing tolerance for current and future loss reminders, making healthy changes to further accommodate to the loss, and addressing conflicts over past interactions that evoke regret, guilt, or shame. This therapeutic work serves to promote acceptance of traumatic losses, and mobilize adaptive coping responses. Disasters and terrorism can further complicate adaptation to loss when there is no recovery of the deceased body or delay or disturbing aspects of body identification. Confirming the physical reality of the death has been reported to be important in the grieving process of even young children (Furman, 1973).

Fourth, effective treatment for children after disaster must focus on *postdisaster adversities*. Typically, a series of adverse life changes follow in the wake of disaster, including financial hardship, medical treatment and physical rehabilitation, relocation, and loss of friends, school, and community. Intervention for children is focused on enhancing coping skills, identifying current difficulties, developing pragmatic coping and problem-solving strategies to contend with adversities, and enhancing the social skills needed to communicate appropriately about trauma and loss to others (and handle uninvited social inquiries), and to seek appropriate forms of support. A group format has proven especially advantageous to improving constructive problem solving, especially among adolescents.

Fifth, it is critical that a comprehensive trauma-grief treatment program address ways in which trauma or grief-related reactions may have contributed to disturbance in *developmental progression*, including withdrawing from developmentally important activities and relationships, difficulties in academic and interpersonal life at school, and risk behaviors, often with newly formed maladaptive peer groups. Guided by an understanding of normative developmental competencies, tasks, transitions and expectations, a treatment program must identify missed developmental opportunities, support resumption of compromised developmental activities, address traumatic expectations governing current and future behavior, and facilitate prosocial activities and constructive future planning.

Three tiers of postdisaster intervention

A three-tier model for providing postdisaster mental health interventions for children and families (Saltzman *et al.*, 2003; Pynoos & Steinberg, 2006; Pynoos *et al.*, 2005b) includes general psychosocial support to a broad population, specialized interventions for those with severe, persistent distress and impairment, and specialized treatment for high-risk cases that need more intensive psychiatric care. The following is a brief outline of some of the major characteristics of each tier.

Tier 1: broad-scale intervention

- The primary objective is to promote adaptive adjustment and normal developmental progression among children and adolescents, and prevent the onset of psychological, behavioral, functional, and developmental problems.
- The target population includes children, adolescents, and their indigenous support networks, including parents, family members, teachers, and school administrators.
- Implementation sites include schools, community mental health agencies, religious institutions, after-school programs.
- Implementing personnel can include trained teachers, school counselors, community mental health professionals, clergy.
- Program content can include presentations and/or printed materials designed to provide general, broad-spectrum information on common postdisaster distress reactions, coping skills, support-seeking and support-providing skills, and descriptions of signs suggesting the need for professional evaluation.
- Intervention modalities can include individual sessions, classroom-based interventions, school-wide presentations, parent meetings, school staff meetings, and discussions with peer support groups and mentorship programs, web-based informational material, and official risk communications.

Tier 2: specialized intervention

- The primary objective is to reduce psychological distress, promote normal developmental progression, and adaptive postdisaster adjustment among moderately to severely affected children and adolescents, and to provide early tertiary prevention of severe and persisting psychological, behavioral, functional, and developmental difficulties.
- The target population includes children and adolescents with severe levels of disaster-related trauma exposure and loss deemed at risk for chronic, severe distress reactions (especially PTSD, depression, and grief) and behavioral, functional, and developmental disturbance.
- Implementing personnel can include trained school counselors or community mental health professionals.
- Program content can include semi-structured risk screening interviews, and trauma/grief-focused group intervention protocols.
- Intervention modalities can include individual counseling, trauma/grief-focused individual or group interventions and family-based interventions.

Tier 3: highly specialized intervention

- The primary objective is to reduce severe psychological distress, suicidal risk, and other high-risk behaviors as tertiary prevention of severe psychological, behavioral, or developmental difficulties.
- The target population includes children and adolescents with severe psychiatric disorders whose specialized needs exceed the resources available at local schools. Markers of risk include signs or symptoms of severe depression, high suicide risk, antisocial behavior, extreme risk-taking, severe substance abuse, and psychosis.
- Implementation sites for youths who may be identified through risk screening methods at schools typically include community-based mental health agencies, although certain types of Tier-3 services may be provided at schools (e.g., a

psychiatrist may see students at a school-based health clinic), or combined with Tier 2 services (e.g., a psychiatrist may prescribe and monitor antidepressant medication for a student participating in school-based group intervention).

- Implementing personnel can include community mental health specialists (e.g., psychiatrists, psychologists).
- Program content includes traditional psychiatric/psychological treatments. These may be supplemented by concurrent or subsequent Tier 2 interventions.

Stages of postdisaster data collection

Public concern regarding the impact of disasters on children, adolescents and their families has led to efforts to develop measures that can accurately identify youths whose exposure to traumatic situations, subjective responses, loss of loved ones and property, and post-event adversities increases their risk for severe, persisting distress, functional impairment and biological/behavioral/developmental disturbance. The focus on assessment is related to the importance of making an early estimate of the nature, extent, and severity of the postdisaster adverse impact, in order to plan for public mental health interventions to promote the recovery of different trauma/loss/adversity-exposed groups. Data collection can also inform ongoing efforts to monitor the course of recovery, the added impact of post-event circumstances, and the effectiveness of services and interventions. Stages of data collection can be categorized as follows:

1. Pre-event surveillance
2. Acute post-impact/triage
3. Needs assessment
4. Ongoing surveillance
5. Screening
6. Clinical evaluation
7. Outcome evaluation.

Pre-event surveillance can be systematically carried out through periodic national representative surveys of children and adolescents to track demographically related rates of various types of exposure to trauma and loss, symptomatic response, functional impact, and help-seeking behavior. Such data can be invaluable in providing population-based baseline information for statistical comparison in interpreting findings from data collection efforts post-event. Collection of acute post-impact triage data from members of an affected population as they appear in a variety of acute emergency response settings can be effectively used to obtain early information about the impact of the event and its population distribution, and to link survivors early on with available services.

Needs assessment involves systematic data collection from a representative sample of an affected population to make a rigorous determination of the scope and impact of the disaster. Such data can be used for planning needed response strategies and resources. Ongoing surveillance is conducted to monitor the course of recovery among an affected population and the impact of new events and ongoing adversities. Screening more systematically targets members of an affected population for linkage with available recovery resources.

Clinical evaluation and intervention outcome data involve the rigorous clinical evaluation of affected individuals, and are used to examine the contribution of interventions to the course of recovery. These stages of data collection can be conceptualized as increasingly including more detailed metrics about objective and subjective features of trauma exposure, loss and traumatic bereavement, post-event stresses and adversities, ongoing distress, and behavioral, social and functional/developmental impairment.

There are a number of factors that strongly affect these data collection methods and respective metrics. These factors include: type of event, setting in which data are collected, individuals collecting the data, available resources and services, ethical issues, and available funding for data collection efforts.

The initial screening items typically capture basic exposure information about where children were during the event, and what happened to them and those around them. This is followed by specific questions about high-risk experiences; for example, direct life-threat, being trapped or injured, witnessing grotesque injury, hearing screams of distress, being separated from family members or caretakers, or injury or death of family members. Additional exposure questions address the child's subjective appraisal of the event and associated emotional responses. These exposure questions are complemented by a brief evaluation of prior trauma and loss, prior mental health problems and substance abuse, family disturbances, and post-traumatic

For some of the continuous scales, psychometric studies have been conducted to determine their sensitivity and specificity in detecting PTSD. Abbreviated versions of instruments can be used to make an initial assessment of a child's level of distress. For example, Project Liberty in New York City used an abbreviated version of the UCLA PTSD Reaction Index for DSM IV (Steinberg *et al.*, 2004). Where sensitivity and specificity are high, abbreviated scales provide an efficient means for needs assessment and screening. For example, rating frequency of occurrence over the past month, eight items from the UCLA PTSD Index do

	None	Some	Little	Much	Most
I get very upset, afraid or sad when something makes me think about what happened.	☐0	☐1	☐2	☐3	☐4
I have upsetting thoughts or pictures of what happened come into my mind when I do not want them to.	☐0	☐1	☐2	☐3	☐4
I feel grouchy, or I am easily angered.	☐0	☐1	☐2	☐3	☐4
I try not to talk about, think about, or have feelings about what happened.	☐0	☐1	☐2	☐3	☐4
I have trouble going to sleep, or wake up often during the night.	☐0	☐1	☐2	☐3	☐4
I have trouble concentrating or paying attention.	☐0	☐1	☐2	☐3	☐4
I try to stay away from people, places, or things that make me remember what happened.	☐0	☐1	☐2	☐3	☐4
I felt as if it hadn't happened or was unreal.	☐0	☐1	☐2	☐3	☐4

stress, depressive, anxiety, and grief reactions.

Both structured diagnostic instruments and continuous-scale child and adolescent PTSD measures have been employed after disasters. Structured instruments provide estimates of rates of disorder, while continuous scales invariably show greater sensitivity to exposure parameters.

almost as well as the full scale in predicting PTSD. These items include:

Ideally, collaborating community, state and federal systems should carry out data collection in the context of a broader public mental health response and recovery program, a "disaster system of care" (Pynoos & Steinberg, 2006). These systems can include emergency medical services, disaster relief organizations (such as the American Red Cross), first responders, state and county public and mental health, and schools.

A body of data has emerged which suggests several important factors that should be taken into account whenever conducting postdisaster mental health assessments of children and adolescents. These factors include: the necessity of assessing multiple disorders; independent assessment of children's behaviors; assessment of family members, especially mothers; functional status; pre-existing risk factors; and cross-cultural differences (Balaban et al., 2005).

There are a variety of instruments that have been specifically designed to assess levels of exposure to various types of disasters including wars, hurricanes, earthquakes, and fires. These questionnaires provide an important way to identify children and adolescents who may be at higher risk for developing postdisaster reactions. Event-specific exposure items vary with the type of event, i.e., earthquake, hurricane, catastrophic school violence or forms of terrorism. Before designing specific exposure items, interviews with key informants must be conducted to ascertain salient event-specific features of exposure. During the acute post-impact phase, exposure variables can be of use in identifying subgroups of an affected population that are at increased risk for severe and persistent distress reactions and behavioral and functional impairment. The inclusion of post-event adversity variables may add incremental validity to the assessment battery. Another important part of the exposure section of any postdisaster battery are questions related to loss of loved ones, along with questions about normal grief and complicated grief reactions (Layne et al., 2001).

Postdisaster assessment should not be limited to the prevalence of any single psychological disorder. There is evidence that the prevalence of PTSD in children and adolescents may be related to the severity of the original trauma, while rates of depression may be related to ongoing secondary adversities. This suggests that different assessments and interventions may be needed in the aftermath of disasters (Goenjian et al., 1995; Sack et al., 1994, 1995).

Assessing child mental health often requires input from several informants. Adults, in contrast, are generally reliable observers of children's behaviors, but have a tendency to underestimate children's internal distress. Whenever possible, assessments of children should include an adult's assessment of the child's behavior. Parent- and/or teacher-completed behavior rating scales can provide reliable, inexpensive, and easy to administer measures of children's disruptive behaviors.

If possible, the mental health status of primary caretakers should be assessed at the same time as children, as parental adjustment is an important predictor of children's mental health outcomes, particularly maternal reactions. Whenever possible, instruments that include questions about social and behavioral functioning should be used when assessing children and adolescents in disaster contexts. Empirical data on the relationship between psychopathology and functional status for children are still very limited, but it has been estimated that only between one-half and one-third of children with a DSM diagnosis show some significant impairment at home, in school or with peers (Sack et al., 1995). A number of studies have reported the prevalence of psychiatric diagnoses, but not the proportion of those with impaired functioning. Further, appropriate and adaptive behaviors may be very different in the aftermath of disasters. Consequently, the presence of symptoms does not always indicate functional disability, nor does the absence of reported symptoms indicate lack of distress (e.g., Ahmad et al., 2000; Jones & Kafetsios, 2002; Terr, 1983).

In addition to traditional categories related to psychological sequelae, recent postdisaster data collection efforts among children and adolescents have assessed a broader range of potential behavioral and functional outcomes (depending on developmental stage). These have included:

- Alcohol and drug use
- Delinquency and antisocial behavior
- Teenage sexual activity
- School underachievement and failure
- Empathic and pro-social behavior/citizenship
- Quality of peer relationships
- Quality of family relationships
- Quality of romantic relationships
- Quality of work performance
- Physical health.

Although the contribution of age to children's post-traumatic reactions, behavior, and psychopathology still needs to be clarified, it is critically important that any assessment instruments be appropriate to age and stage of development.

As the strength of association between trauma exposure and distress may be influenced by psychological and socio-environmental factors, a number of vulnerability and resilience factors have been investigated. Data collection in the aftermath of disasters can usefully include items that relate to potential mediating or moderating variables to increase the predictive accuracy and inform public mental health and clinical strategies. As noted above, vulnerability and resilience factors have been suggested to include child intrinsic factors, family factors, and extra-familial/community factors. For terrorism, additional specific factors that may mediate or moderate outcome include emergency public information, levels of federal, state and community emergency response capability for multi-hazards (adequate evacuation plans, decontamination, mass prophylaxis) school emergency response plans and capacity, surge capacity of the emergency medical system specific to children, and availability of timely effective mental health services for children and families. A number of postdisaster studies among children and adolescents have strongly suggested that severe postdisaster adversities can exacerbate post-traumatic stress reactions, interfere with recovery from post-traumatic stress

reactions, and contribute independently to the presence and severity of other comorbid conditions, including depression, grief, anxiety, somatization, hostility, etc. (Goenjian *et al.*, 1995; Layne *et al.*, 2001).

Factors embedded within the postdisaster ecology that may be etiologic, or mediate/moderate the impact of disaster on intermediate and long-term recovery include:

- Frequency of exposure to trauma reminders
- Frequency of exposure to loss reminders
- Type and severity of secondary adversities, including:
  - Impairment in caregiver mental health
  - Quality of family functioning
  - Overcrowded or adverse living conditions
  - School and community milieu
  - Quality of peer relationships
  - Physical injury, disability, rehabilitation.

The methodological problems of psychological assessment are complex in the context of ethnic and cultural groups who may have differing levels of exposure to previous traumas, differing vulnerabilities and strengths, differing levels of coping resources, and differing cultural mores of the expression of mourning and grief. Scales must be used with caution when the population being assessed differs from that in which the validation of the instrument was established. Many assessment instruments may not be appropriately sensitive to culture and ethnicity. Of course, simply translating an instrument into another language does not guarantee that the same symptoms or the same disorders are being assessed. Since nearly all tests have been validated in Western, clinical populations, this is a serious problem for cross-cultural research. Other methodological issues that can arise in these settings include issues of translation, relevance of cultural categories of mental health and illness, biases against confiding personal feelings to people from other cultures, and difficulty in finding control groups of nontraumatized populations (Jones *et al.*, 2006).

REFERENCES

Ahmad, A., Sofi, M. A., Sundelin-Wahlsten, V. & von Knorring, A. L. (2000). Posttraumatic stress disorder in children after the military operation "Anfal" in Iraqi Kurdistan. *European Child and Adolescent Psychiatry*, **9**, 235–243.

Allen, A., Saltzman, W. R., Brymer, M. J., Oshri, A. & Silverman, W. K. (2006). An empirically informed intervention for children following exposure to severe hurricanes. *Behavior Therapist*, **29**, 118–124.

Almqvist, K. & Hwang, P. (1999). Iranian refugees in Sweden. Coping processes in children and their families. *Childhood*, **6**, 167–188.

Asarnow, J., Glynn, S., Pynoos, R. S. *et al.* (1999). When the earth stops shaking: earthquake sequelae among children diagnosed for pre-earthquake psychopathology. *Journal of the American Academy of Child and Adolescent Psychiatry*, **38**, 1016–1023.

Balaban, V. F., Steinberg, A. M., Brymer, M. J. *et al.* (2005). Screening and assessment for children's psychosocial needs following war and terrorism. In *Promoting the Psychosocial Well-Being of Children Following War and Terrorism*, eds. M. J. Friedman & A. Mikus-Kos, pp. 121–161. Amsterdam: IOS Press.

Brown, E. J. & Goodman, R. F. (2005). Childhood traumatic grief: an exploration of the construct in children bereaved on September 11. *Journal of Clinical Child and Adolescent Psychology*, **34**, 248–259.

Chemtob, C. M., Nakashima, J. & Carlson, J. G. (2002a). Brief treatment for elementary school children with disaster-related posttraumatic stress disorder: a field study. *Journal of Clinical Psychology*, **58**, 99–112.

Chemtob, C. M., Nakashima, J. P., Roger, S. & Hamada, S. (2002b). Psychosocial intervention for post-disaster trauma symptoms in elementary school children. *Archives of Pediatric and Adolescent Medicine*, **56**, 211–216.

Cohen, J. A. (2005). Treating traumatized children: current status and future directions. *Journal of Trauma and Dissociation*, **6**, 109–121.

Cohen, J. A. & Mannarino, A. P. (2004). Treatment of childhood traumatic grief. *Journal of Clinical Child and Adolescent Psychology*, **33**, 819–831.

Cohen, J. A., Mannarino, A. P., Gibson, L. E. *et al.* (2006). Interventions for children and adolescents following disasters. In *Interventions Following Mass Violence and Disaster: Strategies for Mental Health Practice*, eds. E. C. Ritchie, P. J. Watson & M. J. Friedman, pp. 227–256. New York: Guilford.

Compas, B. E., Connor-Smith, J. K., Saltzman, H., Thomsen, A. H. & Wadsworth, M. E. (2001). Coping with stress during childhood and adolescence: problems, progress, and potential in theory and research. *Psychological Bulletin*, **127**, 87–127.

Fairbrother, G., Stuber, J., Galea, S., Fleischman, A. R. & Pfefferbaum, B. (2003). Posttraumatic stress reactions in New York City children after the September 11, 2001, terrorist attacks. *Ambulatory Pediatrics*, **3**, 304–311.

Fairbrother, G., Stuber, J., Galea, S., Pfefferbaum, B. & Fleischman, A. R. (2004). Unmet need for counseling services by children in New York city after the September 11 attacks on the World Trade Center: implications for pediatricians. *Pediatrics*, **113**, 1367–1374.

Furman, R. (1973). A child's capacity for mourning. In *The Child in his Family: The Impact of Disease and Death*, eds. E. J. Anthony & C. Koupernik, pp. 225–231. New York: John Wiley & Sons.

Goenjian, A. K. (1993). A mental health relief programme in Armenia after the 1988 earthquake: implementation and clinical observations. *British Journal of Psychiatry*, **163**, 230–239.

Goenjian, A. K., Pynoos, R. S., Steinberg, A. M. *et al.* (1995). Psychiatric comorbidity in children after the 1988 earthquake in Armenia. *Journal of the American Academy of Child and Adolescent Psychiatry*, **34**, 1174–1184.

Goenjian, A. K., Pynoos, R. S., Karayan, I. *et al.* (1997). Outcome of psychotherapy among pre-adolescents after the 1988 earthquake in Armenia. *American Journal of Psychiatry*, **154**, 536–542.

Goenjian, A. K., Stilwell, B. M., Steinberg, A. M. *et al.* (1999). Moral development and psychopathological interference with conscience functioning among adolescents after trauma. *Journal of the American Academy of Child and Adolescent Psychiatry*, **38**, 376–384.

Goenjian, A. K., Molina, L., Steinberg, A. M. *et al.* (2001). Posttraumatic stress and depressive reactions among Nicaraguan adolescents after hurricane Mitch. *American Journal of Psychiatry*, **158**, 788–794.

Goenjian, A. K., Walling, D., Steinberg, A. M. *et al.* (2005). Five years post-disaster: a prospective study of posttraumatic stress and depressive reactions among treated and untreated adolescents. *American Journal of Psychiatry*, **12**, 2302–2308.

Green, B. L., Korol, M., Grace, M. C. *et al.* (1991). Children and disaster: age, gender, and parental effects of PTSD symptoms. *Journal of the American Academy of Child and Adolescent Psychiatry*, **30**, 945–951.

Guarnaccia, S., Canino, G., Rubio-Stipec, M. & Braro, M. (1993). The prevalence of ataques de nerrios in the Puerto Ricodisaster study. The role of culture in psychiatric epidemiology. *Journal of Nervous and Mental Diseases*, **181**, 157–165.

Halcon, L. L., Robertson, C. L., Savik, K. *et al.* (2004). Trauma and coping in Somali and Oromo refugee youth. *Journal of Adolescent Health*, **35**, 17–25.

Hanford, H. A., Mayes, S. D., Mattison, R. E. *et al.* (1986). Child and parent reactions to the Three Mile Island nuclear accident. *Journal of the American Academy of Child and Adolescent Psychiatry*, **25**, 346–356.

Hoven, C. W., Duarte, C. S., Lucas, C. P. *et al.* (2005). Psychopathology among New York city public school children 6 months after September 11. *Archives of General Psychiatry*, **62**, 545–552.

International Strategy for Disaster Reduction. (2005). Available at www.unisdr.org.

Jones, L. & Kafetsios, K. (2002). Assessing adolescents' mental health in war-affected societies: the significance of symptoms. *Child Abuse and Neglect*, **26**, 1059–1080.

Jones, R. T., Hadder, J. M., Carvajal, F. *et al.* (2006). Conducting research in diverse, minority, and marginalized communities. In *Methods for Disaster Mental Health Research*, eds. F. Norris, S. Galea, M. Friedman & P. Watson. New York: Guilford Press.

Kinzie, J. D., Boehnlein, J. & Sack, W. H. (1998). The effects of massive trauma on Cambodian parents and children. In *International Handbook of Multigenerational Legacies of Trauma. The Plenum Series on Stress and Coping*, ed. Y. Danieli, pp. 211–222. New York: Plenum Press.

Kline, P. M. & Mone, E. (2003). Coping with war: three strategies employed by adolescent citizens of Sierra Leone. *Child and Adolescent Social Work Journal*, **20**, 321–333.

Laor, N., Wolmer, L., Mayes, L. C. *et al.* (1997). Israeli preschool children under Scuds: a 30-month follow-up. *Journal of the American Academy of Child and Adolescent Psychiatry*, **36**, 349–356.

Laor, N., Wolmer, L. & Cohen, D. J. (2001). Mothers' functioning and children's symptoms 5 years after a SCUD missile attack. *American Journal of Psychiatry*, **158**, 1020–1026.

Layne, C. M., Pynoos, R. S., Saltzman, W. R. *et al.* (2001). Trauma/grief-focused group psychotherapy: school-based postwar intervention with traumatized Bosnian adolescents. *Group Dynamics Theory, Research and Practice*, **5**, 277–290.

Layne, C. M., Warren, J. S., Saltzman, W. S. *et al.* (2006). Contextual influences on posttraumatic adjustment: retraumatization and the roles of revictimization, posttraumatic adversities and distressing reminders. In *Psychological Effects of Catastrophic Disasters: Group Approaches to Treatment*, eds. L. A. Schein, H. I. Spitz, G. M. Burlingame & P. R. Muskin, pp. 235–286. New York: Haworth Press.

March, J. S., Amaya-Jackson, L., Murry, M. C. & Schulte, A. (1998). Cognitive-behavioral psychotherapy for children and adolescents with posttraumatic stress disorder after an industrial fire. *Journal of the American Academy of Child and Adolescent Psychiatry*, **37**, 585–593.

McNally, R. J., Bryant, R. A. & Ehlers, A. (2003). Does early psychological intervention promote recovery from posttraumatic stress? *Psychological Science in the Public Interest*, **4**, 45–79.

Mollica, R. F., Cui, X., McInnes, K. & Massagli, M. P. (2002). Science-based policy for psychosocial interventions in refugee camps: a cambodian example. *Journal of Nervous and Mental Diseases*, **190**, 158–166.

Nader, K., Pynoos, R., Fairbanks, L. & Frederick, C. (1990). Children's PTSD reactions one year after a sniper attack at their school. *American Journal of Psychiatry*, **147**, 1526–1530.

Pfefferbaum, B., Nixon, S. J., Krug, R. S. *et al.* (1999). Clinical needs assessment of middle and high school students following the 1995 Oklahoma City bombing. *American Journal of Psychiatry*, **156**, 1069–1074.

Pfefferbaum, B., Nixon, S. J., Tivis, R. D. *et al.* (2001). Television exposure in children after a terrorist incident. *Psychiatry*, **64**, 202–211.

Pynoos, R. S. (1992). Grief and trauma in children and adolescents. *Bereavement Care*, **11**, 2–10.

Pynoos, R. S. & Steinberg, A. M. (2006). Recovery of children and adolescents after exposure to violence: a developmental ecological framework. In *Interventions for children Exposed to Violence*, eds. A. F. Lieberman & R. DeMartino, pp. 17–44. New Jersey: Johnson & Johnson Pediatric Institute.

Pynoos, R. S., Frederick, C., Nader, K. *et al.* (1987). Life threat and posttraumatic stress in school-age children. *Archives of General Psychiatry*, **44**, 1057–1063.

Pynoos, R. S., Goenjian, A., Tashjian, M. *et al.* (1993). Posttraumatic stress reactions in children after the 1988 Armenian earthquake. *British Journal of Psychiatry*, **163**, 239–247.

Pynoos, R. S., Steinberg, A. M. & Wraith, R. (1995). A developmental model of childhood traumatic stress. In *Manual of Developmental Psychopathology: Risk, Disorder and Adaptation*, eds. D. Cicchetti & D. J. Cohen, pp. 72–93. New York: John Wiley & Sons.

Pynoos, R. S., Steinberg, A. M., Ornitz, E. M. & Goenjian, A. K. (1997). Issues in the developmental neurobiology of traumatic stress. *Annals of the New York Academy of Sciences*, **821**, 176–193.

Pynoos, R. S., Goenjian, A. K. & Steinberg, A. M. (1998). A public mental health approach to the postdisaster treatment of children and adolescents. *Child and Adolescent Psychiatric Clinics of North America*, **7**, 195–210.

Pynoos, R. S., Steinberg, A. M. & Piacentini, J. C. (1999). A developmental psychopathology model of childhood traumatic stress and intersection with anxiety disorders. *Biological Psychiatry*, **46**, 1542–1554.

Pynoos, R., Schreiber, M. D., Steinberg, A. M. & Pfefferbaum, B. J. (2005a). Impact of terrorism on children. In *Comprehensive Textbook of Psychiatry*, 8th edn., eds. B. J. Sadock & V. A. Sadock, pp. 3551–3564. Philadelphia: Lippincott Williams & Wilkins.

Pynoos, R. S., Steinberg, A. M., Schreiber, M. D. & Brymer, M. (2005b). Children and families: a new framework for preparedness and response to danger, terrorism and trauma. In *Psychological Effects of Catastrophic Disasters: Group Approaches to Treatment*, eds. L. A. Schein, H. I. Spitz, G. M. Burlingame & P. R. Mushkin, pp. 83–112. New York: Haworth Press.

Roussos, A., Goenjian, A. K., Steinberg, A. M. *et al.* (2005). Posttraumatic stress and depressive reactions among children and adolescents after the 1999 Ano Liosia earthquake in Greece. *American Journal of Psychiatry*, **162**, 530–537.

Sack, W. H., Clarke, G. N., Kinney, R. *et al.* (1995). The Khmer Adolescent Project. II: Functional capacities in two generations of Cambodian refugees. *Journal of Nervous and Mental Disease*, **183**, 177–181.

Saltzman, W. R., Layne, C. M., Steinberg, A. M., Arslanagic, B. & Pynoos, R. S. (2003). Developing a culturally and ecologically sound intervention program for youth exposed to war and terrorism. *Child and Adolescent Psychiatric Clinics of North America*, **12**, 319–342.

Savin, D., Sack, W. H., Clarke, G. N., Meas, N. & Richart, I. (1996). The Khmer Adolescent Project: III. A study of trauma from Thailand's Site II refugee camp. *Journal of the American Academy of Child and Adolescent Psychiatry*, **35**, 384–391.

Shaw, J. A., Applegate, B., Tanner, S. *et al.* (1995). Psychological effects of Hurricane Andrew on an elementary school population. *Journal of American Academy of Child and Adolescent Psychiatry*, **34**, 1185–1192.

Steinberg, A. M. & Ritzmann, R. F. (1990). A living systems approach to understanding the concept of stress. *Behavioral Science*, **35**, 138–146.

Steinberg, A. M., Brymer, M. J., Decker, K. & Pynoos, R. S. (2004). The UCLA PTSD Reaction Index. *Current Psychiatry Reports*, **6**, 96–100.

Steinberg, A. M., Brymer, M. J., Steinberg, J. R. & Pfefferbaum, B. (2006). Conducting research with children and adolescents after disaster. In *Methods for Disaster Mental Health Research*, eds. F. Norris, S. Galea, M. Friedman & P. Watson. New York: Guildford.

Stuber, J., Galea, S., Pfefferbaum, B. *et al.* (2005). Behavior problems in New York City's children after the September 11, 2001, terrorist attack. *American Journal of Orthopsychiatry*, **75**, 190–200.

Terr, L. (1983). Chowchilla revisited: the effects of psychic trauma four years after a schoolbus kidnapping. *American Journal of Psychiatry*, **140**, 1543–1550.

US Government (1976). Rules and regulations for the Disaster Relief Act. PL 93–288, Section 413. Federal Register, November 6, 1976.

Vernberg, E. M., Silverman, W. K., La Greca, A. M. & Prinstein, M. J. (1996). Prediction of posttraumatic stress symptoms in children after Hurricane Andrew. *Journal of Abnormal Psychology*, **105**, 237–248.

Vogel, M. & Vernberg, E. M. (1993). Psychological responses of children to natural and human-made disasters: I. Children's psychological reactions to disasters. *Journal of Clinical Child Psychology*, **22**, 464–484.

Yule, W. (1992). Post-traumatic stress disorder in child survivors of shipping disasters; the sinking of the "Jupiter." *Psychotherapy and Psychosomatics*, **57**, 200–205.

Yule, W., Udwin, O. & Murdoch, K. (1990). The "Jupiter" sinking: effects on children's fears, depression and anxiety. *Journal of Child Psychology and Psychiatry and Allied Disciplines*, **31**, 1051–1061.

4

Disaster ecology: implications for disaster psychiatry

James M. Shultz, Zelde Espinel, Sandro Galea, & Dori B. Reissman

The nature of disaster from an ecological perspective

When disaster strikes, individuals, families, and entire communities are subjected to powerful forces of harm. Yet, exposure to disaster impact is only the opening salvo. As the disaster unfolds, and far into the aftermath, affected populations grapple with loss and change, consequences that persevere long after the risk for physical harm has dissipated. This trilogy of forces – exposure to hazard, massive personal and societal loss, and profound and enduring life change – characterizes the nature of disaster. Thus we define a disaster as an encounter between a hazard (forces of harm) and a human population in harm's way, influenced by the ecological context, creating demands that exceed the coping capacity of the affected community (Landesman, 2001; Noji, 1997a; Quarantelli, 1985, 1995, 1998; Shultz et al., 2007; Somasundaram et al., 2003; World Health Organization, 1999).

Disasters are population-based phenomena. According to Raphael (2000), "Disasters can have widespread and devastating impact on individuals, families, communities and nations." Disasters are collective, community-wide events, necessitating simultaneous consideration of issues residing within a person, or between persons, or between persons and their community and society. We propose an ecological frame of reference to concurrently consider the interplay of these factors as they pertain to

disaster's forces of harm: exposure, loss, and change. Our disaster ecological approach aligns with the tidal shift now occurring within the field of public health that recognizes that human health status is determined not only at the individual level, but just as powerfully by a broad, multi-layered spectrum of factors comprising the social and environmental "context" (Blakely & Woodward, 2000; Kaplan, 1999, 2004; Karpati et al., 2002; Krieger, 1994, 2001; Mackenbach, 1993; McMichael, 1999; Pearce, 1996; Poundstone et al., 2004; Susser, 1994, 1998; Sussser & Susser, 1996; Woodward, 1996). Disaster ecology examines the interrelationships and interdependence of the social, psychological, anthropological, cultural, geographic, economic, and human context surrounding disasters and extreme public health events such as severe storms, earthquakes, acts of terrorism, industrial accidents, and disease epidemics (Kaplan, 1999).

Psychosocial reactions to trauma are recognized to be among the most long-term and debilitating outcomes of disasters (Norris, 2005; Ursano et al., 1994). The extent and extremity of psychosocial responses, ranging from transient fear and distress to chronic psychopathology, relate directly to the nature of disaster itself and to the complex interplay of factors including the exposure of vulnerable human communities to massive forces of harm or widespread perception of imminent threat. Exposure, loss, and change – the forces of harm – represent disaster consequences and powerful stressors (Table 4.1).

Table 4.1 Forces of harm: exposure to hazard, loss, and change

Disaster stressors associated with the forces of harm		
Exposure to hazard	Loss	Change
• Perceived threat of harm	• Bereavement	• Disruption of services
• Disaster warning	• Separation from loved ones	• Physical displacement
• (or) Lack of warning	• Physical harm: pain, debility	• Separation from essential health care,
• Shopping/stockpiling	• Loss of function	medications
• Evacuation/sheltering	• Loss of home, worksite	• Lack of utilities
• Perception of personal threat to life	• Property damage	• Lack of transportation
• Exposure to physical force of disaster	• Lack of basic necessities	• Unemployment, job change
• Personal physical harm	• Loss of personal possessions	• School closure
• injury	• Loss of social support	• Displacement
• disease	• Resource loss/financial loss	• Financial hardship
• Witnessing	• Loss of employment, income	• Disruption of community
• widespread destruction	• Loss of independence	• Personal, community bereavement
• mass casualties	• Loss of control	• Shortages, rationing
• death/injury of others		• Occupying forces/military rule
• Exposure to		• Refugee conditions
• grotesque scenes		• Social violence
• noxious agents		• Community poverty
• Human causality		• Postdisaster disease outbreaks

This chapter describes the evolution of a disaster ecological framework for portraying the impact of disasters on human populations. We begin with a detailed look at exposure to hazards – categorized by type, intensity, time, and place factors – providing the most extensive presentation on this topic within this volume. Issues of loss and change are discussed in detail throughout many chapters and are treated briefly here. We discuss the multiple levels of factors that may influence disaster-related public health outcomes on a proximal to distal continuum, including individual/family, community, and societal/structural levels. Examples of individual/family factors are demographics, family structure, socioeconomic position, disaster-specific behaviors, and response roles. Community context includes community infrastructure and disaster preparedness, social support networks, social environment, civic society, and community socioeconomic status. Societal/structural context includes the physical and built environment, political structure and governance, cultural context, and national or multinational disaster preparedness and response.

Evolution of a disaster ecology framework

Along the historical path toward a disaster ecology model, two conceptual formulations have provided critical building blocks, the "epidemiological triad" (Fox, 2003; Last, 2001) and the Haddon matrix (Haddon, 1972, 1980). We discuss both prior to outlining our disaster ecology model (Figure 4.1).

Epidemiological triad: causal or exposure pathway models

Epidemiology is defined as "the study of the distribution of a disease or a physiological condition

Epidemiological Triad

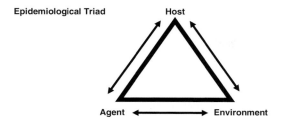

Haddon Matrix

	Host	Vector	Environment
Pre-event			
Event			
Post-event			

Figure 4.1 Epidemiological triad and Haddon matrix

in human populations and of the factors that influence this distribution" (Lilienfeld & Stolley, 1994). Epidemiology originated as the study of infectious disease epidemics. The classic "epidemiological triad," consisting of agent, host, and environment, was introduced to explain the spread of disease throughout a community, to identify points of intervention to halt transmission, and to guide field epidemiologic investigations. For example, the influenza virus (*infectious disease agent*) is readily spread to susceptible humans (*host*) through respiratory exposure in communal settings or public gatherings (*environment*). As we comprehended more about the causal or exposure pathway of disease transmission, a fourth element was added to depict intermediaries (i.e., vehicles or vectors) essential for transmission of certain infectious agents through the environment. Some biological agents infect susceptible hosts via such "vehicles" as contaminated water (cholera), food (salmonella), or blood (hepatitis B). Other infectious agents rely upon a living arthropod "vector" (mosquito or tick) to harbor, transport, and mechanically inject the agent when feeding upon an unsuspecting human host. The infectious agents that cause malaria (*Plasmodium* species), West Nile disease (West Nile virus), and Lyme disease (*Borrelia burgdorferi*) are transmitted in this manner

(Butler *et al.*, 2003; Reissman *et al.*, 2005; Rundell & Christopher, 2004).

Applying the agent–host–environment triad to the realm of disasters requires bridging the chasm from infectious disease agents to physical forces of harm. Such an analysis was performed to investigate earthquake-related traumatic injuries (Logue *et al.*, 1981; Peek-Asa *et al.*, 2003; Ramirez & Peek-Asa, 2005). Depicting the *agent* as the energy transferred from the earthquake, the *environment* as the buildings and structures in which humans are located at the time of ground shaking, and *host factors* as the demographics, behavioral response, and physiological robustness of individuals, these investigators examined interactions among the three components to elucidate the "causal pathway to injury" (Ramirez & Peek-Asa, 2005).

The Haddon matrix: analyzing the triad factors by event phase

Haddon (1972, 1980) extended the epidemiologic triad to the field of injury prevention and control. In an automobile crash, the motor "vehicle" itself serves as the object for an injurious transfer of kinetic energy (*agent*) to the driver (*host*) with the likelihood and severity of harm strongly influenced by such elements as road conditions, vehicle speed, and use of seatbelt (*environment*). Haddon's primary contribution was to examine the anatomy of a motor vehicle crash, and associated human injury, in time sequence: pre-event, event, and post-event. He considered the interrelation of agent, host, and environment within each phase in order to identify strategies for injury prevention and intervention. His analysis was structured as a two-dimensional table with columns labeled "host," "vehicle," and "environment" and rows representing pre-event, event, and post-event time phases, an elegant formulation that bears his name, the Haddon matrix (Figure 4.1). Runyan (1998) proposed a third dimension to the model, giving a cubic appearance to the matrix.

In 2003, the authors of the Institute of Medicine (IOM) report *Preparing for the Psychological Consequences of Terrorism* (Butler *et al.*, 2003), a landmark publication in the field of disaster psychiatry, extended the Haddon matrix analysis to acts of terrorism – and specifically to psychosocial outcomes. Within their framework, terrorists (*vector*) perpetrate a threat or violent act (*agent*), targeting individuals or populations (*host*), within a "physical and social environment." A more sophisticated analysis might view psychological "terror" as the agent, with terrorists using the threat or overt infliction of harm as the vehicle to incite terror.

The IOM expert panel populated a Haddon matrix to map the psychosocial impact of a terrorist attack. Their 3-by-3 matrix included disaster phase (pre-event, event, post-event) as one dimension and the triad of affected populations, "terrorist and injurious agent," and "physical and social environment" as the others. The same array was also used to map intervention strategies that might be implemented to mitigate the psychosocial impact of a future event.

Others have used the Haddon matrix for public health readiness and response planning, including pandemic influenza preparedness, and have expanded the columns to treat physical and social environments separately (Barnett *et al.*, 2005a, 2005b). The Centers for Disease Control and Prevention (CDC) used modified Haddon matrices to promote strategic planning for public health response and recovery functions and to help map out a comprehensive research agenda. Innovations applied to the model included the concept of "collective efficacy" and community resilience as part of the environmental context to describe proactive, community-based health protection strategies (Pfefferbaum *et al.*, 2006; Reissman *et al.*, 2005; Ritchie *et al.*, 2005).

Disaster ecology model

To model disaster ecology, we will apply a causal and exposure pathways approach incorporating the elements portrayed in the epidemiologic triad and Haddon matrix. To account for the diverse types of disasters and emergency events, we will use disaster-specific terminology that is applicable across all hazards.

We recast agent in terms of "hazard" or "forces of harm." Host expands to "affected communities and populations," the term used in the IOM report. The physical and social environment acquires multiple dimensions and layers of "ecological context" to account for a variety of socio-cultural relationships and the interdependence within and between communities (Figure 4.2).

Second, we recommend strengthening the emphasis on what historically has been the short stump of the triad's three-legged stool of the epidemiologic triad, the "environment." We propose to expand environment to ecological context and to greatly strengthen the focus on this component. Consider for example, at a time of intensive focus on terrorism, that the socio-cultural context is the dominant determinant of what sets terrorists on their course, while the interaction between the mechanism of harm (an explosive, for example) and persons in harm's way is quite secondary when considering intervention strategies.

Fortunately, the emphasis on ecological context is gaining momentum as increasing numbers of investigations and sophisticated analyses are conducted from the perspectives variously described as eco-social (Krieger, 1994), eco-epidemiological (Susser & Susser, 1996), and social-epidemiological (McMichael, 1999).

To the progressive evolution of the triad and matrix formulations, the disaster ecology perspective offers the prospect of disaster-specific focus and terminology coupled with full appreciation for the co-equal, and sometimes predominant, importance of the ecological context dimension. Also, the simple clarity offered by the Haddon matrix, with its appeal for planning and preparedness, can be supplemented by more in-depth, multi-level analyses being developed by social epidemiologists that will better define points for intervention to diminish disaster likelihood, in the case of human-generated events, and the devastating impact of disasters of all types.

The disaster ecology model, depicted in Figures 4.2 and 4.3, serves as the basis for the remaining discussion that will focus sequentially on hazard factors,

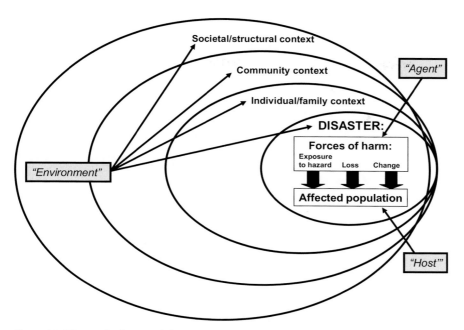

Figure 4.2 Disaster Ecology Model

followed by three levels of ecological context factors: individual/family, community, and societal/structural.

Disaster ecology model: exposure to hazards (the forces of harm)

Exposure to the forces of harm represents the defining disaster event and a strong predictor of adverse medical and psychological effects (Galea & Resnick, 2005). This is represented as the inner circle on the disaster ecology diagram (Figure 4.2). The spectrum of hazards can be described across multiple dimensions of type, magnitude, frequency, and locale; each of these descriptors provides a measure of exposure for human populations encountering these harmful forces. Directly relevant to the field of disaster psychiatry, the degree of psychosocial impact varies by disaster type and generally increases with increasing magnitude and frequency of disaster occurrence (Norris *et al.*, 2002a, 2002b).

Moreover, loss and change associated with disaster are powerful forces of harm that create overt hardship and exacerbate stress, continuing the psychosocial impact of disasters far beyond the period of time when the disaster hazards are exerting their effects (Table 4.1). The protraction of loss and the relative permanence of change partially explain why psychosocial effects are prolonged relative to the time of direct exposure and physical harm. Through loss, many more persons are affected psychologically than physically, extending the reach of the disaster numerically, temporally, and geographically. These forces are integrated into the discussion of the multiple levels of context and are a principal focus of other chapters.

Forces of harm: disaster type

An expansive range of events qualify as disasters, capable of exerting destructive force and causing damage, injury, disease, death, and loss of infrastructure (Noji, 1997a). The universe of extreme events is frequently divided into two broad

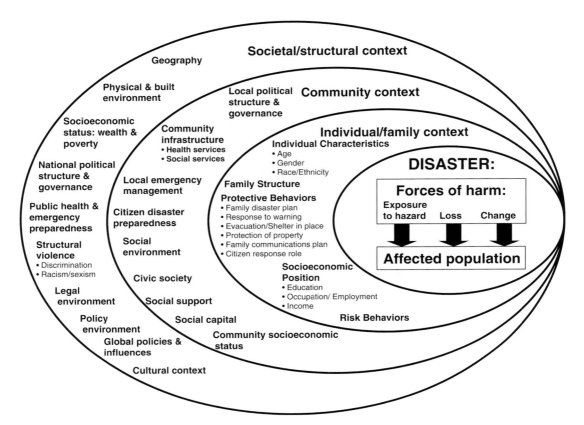

Figure 4.3 Detailed disaster ecology model

categories, natural disasters and human-generated disasters (Rutherford & de Boer, 1983) (Table 4.2). Norris and colleagues determined that disaster type matters (Norris & Kaniasty, 2004; Norris *et al.*, 2002a, 2002b). These reviewers conclude that large-scale, mass-violence events, in which harm is intentionally perpetrated, are associated with more severe psychosocial impairment than are natural disasters and that, within developed nations, technological disasters are more harmful psychologically than are natural disasters.

Natural disasters

Natural disasters, in which harm to human populations is primarily caused by the forces of nature, can be further categorized into hydro-meteorological

disasters (typically weather-related) such as floods and windstorms; geophysical disasters such as earthquakes and tsunamis, and volcanic eruptions; droughts and related phenomena; and pandemic waves of disease (Centre for Research on the Epidemiology of Disasters, 2005; Guha-Sapir *et al.*, 2004).

The United Nations Development Program provides a strong statement regarding the impact of natural disasters: "In the last two decades, more than 1.5 million people have been killed by natural disasters. Worldwide, for every person killed, about 3 000 people are exposed to natural hazards. Some 75 percent of the world's population lives in areas affected at least once by earthquake, tropical cyclone, flood or drought between 1980 and 2000. At the global level, and with respect to large- and medium-scale disasters, these four hazard types (earthquakes,

Table 4.2 Disaster classification

Natural disasters
  Hydrometeorological disasters (Weather-related)
    Floods and related disasters
      Floods
      Landslides/mudslides
      Avalanches
    Windstorms
      Tropical cyclones (hurricanes, cyclones, typhoons, tropical storms)
      Tornadoes
      Storms: thunderstorms, winter storms
  Geophysical disasters
    Earthquakes
    Volcanic eruptions
    Tsunamis/tidal waves
  Droughts and related disasters
    Extreme temperatures
    Wildfires
    Droughts
    Famine
    Insect infestation
  Pandemic diseases
Human-generated disasters
  Nonintentional/technological
    Industrial accidents
    Transportation accidents
    Ecological/environmental destruction
    Miscellaneous accidents
  Intentional
    Declared war
    Civil strife
    Ethnic conflict
    Mass gatherings
    Terrorism
  Complex emergencies

tropical cyclones, floods and droughts) account for approximately 94 percent of total mortality." (United Nations Development Program, 2004).

Human-generated disasters

Disasters caused or exacerbated by human action are subdivided into intentional versus nonintentional events based upon the presence or absence of purposeful human causation. Industrial disasters, transportation disasters, and progressive or precipitous destruction of ecosystems reflect failures or side-effects of human-devised technologies (frequently referenced as "technological disasters"), failures of human judgment, or even flagrant human neglect. However, harm and destruction are not intentionally perpetrated. Several particularly memorable technological disasters are the accidental toxic gas release in Bhopal, India and the nuclear meltdown in Chernobyl, Russia.

In contrast, intentional harm is a defining feature during acts of mass violence including declared war, civil strife, ethnic or religious conflict, and acts of terrorism. Terrorist actions threaten harm, or overtly inflict harm, with the intent of provoking widespread fear that extends beyond those who are directly targeted (Butler *et al.*, 2003; Ursano, 2002). Civilians, rather than soldiers or police, are increasingly targeted, and represent a growing proportion of casualties from all types of mass violence, especially acts of terrorism.

Disasters have been described as "extreme event(s) at the interface of natural and human systems," (Sarewitz & Pielke, 2001). Some extreme events generate compounding consequences and pervasive human suffering on a scale that warrants use of the term "complex emergency." According to the World Health Organization and United Nations, a complex emergency has been defined as:

a humanitarian crisis in a country, region or society where there is considerable breakdown of authority resulting from internal or external conflict which requires an international response that goes beyond the mandate or capacity of any single agency ... complex emergencies are typically characterized by: excessive violence and loss of life; massive displacements of people; widespread damage to societies and economies; the need for large-scale, multifaceted humanitarian assistance; the hindrance or prevention of humanitarian assistance by political and military constraints; and considerable security risks for humanitarian relief workers in some areas. (United Nations Development Program, 2004; World Health Organization, 2005).

Disaster consequences frequently derive from interaction between both natural and human factors. Tropical cyclones are particularly disastrous when they strike densely populated, low-lying coastal areas where many live in structurally vulnerable, ramshackle housing (Shultz *et al.*, 2005). In the case of Hurricane Katrina in 2005, New Orleans sustained damage but withstood the pummeling storm surge and battering hurricane winds. However, post-storm failure of the human-engineered levee system produced massive flooding which was to become the major hazard, claiming more than 1 000 lives and devastating infrastructure. New Orleans essentially survived the natural disaster, but succumbed to a technological catastrophe.

The reverse pattern was observed following twin explosions at the Chernobyl nuclear reactor on April 26, 1986 (Hatch *et al.*, 2005). Radioactive cesium^{137} was released from the incinerating site for 10 days, a classic human-generated event. However, geographical dispersion of airborne radioactive material extended over much of the former Soviet Union, Scandinavia, and Europe, a function of strong and highly variable winds.

In a similar vein, The United Nations Development Program described the term "hazard" as "a natural or human-made event that threatens to adversely affect human life, property, or activity to the extent of causing a disaster," (World Health Organization, 1999) and offered the following five-fold typology:

Natural-physical	hydrometeorological and geophysical disasters
Natural biotic, biological	pest infestations, epidemics, pandemics
Socio or pseudo natural	human transformation of the natural environment
Man-made technological	contamination, explosions, conflagrations
Social	conflict including war, civil strife, violence.

Forces of harm: magnitude

Globally, the cumulative impact of disasters can be estimated using multiple measures. The public health consequences of disasters can be assessed in terms of mortality, morbidity (injury, disease, psychosocial impact), and disruption of health care infrastructure. During the 1995–2004 decade, cumulative disaster-associated mortality associated with 5 989 registered disasters totaled 901 177 deaths, an average of 150 deaths per disaster (Centre for Research on the Epidemiology of Disasters, 2005) worldwide (Table 4.1). These disasters generated 2.5 billion person-events in which an individual was affected by disaster (physical harm, displacement, property loss), with some individuals affected by multiple disaster events. Injury predominates as the major form of disaster-associated morbidity but disasters may also involve infectious disease outbreaks as the defining event. The precise pattern of morbidity is dependent upon the type and intensity of the event interacting with the vulnerabilities of the affected populations. Disasters are also expensive; Centre for Research on the Epidemiology of Disasters (CRED) has estimated total economic costs associated with the 5 989 disasters occurring during 1995–2004 at $739 billion.

Absolute magnitude

Increased physical magnitude of a hazard is associated with increased physical harm and destruction, and concomitant psychosocial impact. Specifically, severe, lasting, and pervasive psychological effects are likely when a disaster causes extreme and widespread damage to property, serious and ongoing problems for the community, and there is a high prevalence of trauma in the form of injuries, threat to life, and loss of life (Norris *et al.*, 2002a, 2002b).

However, examined from the opposite perspective, Norris and colleagues (2002a, 2002b) offer the following insightful caveat: events (1) that involve few deaths or injuries, (2) that create limited destruction and property loss, (3) during which social support systems remain intact and function well, and (4) that involve no indication of human neglect or malicious intent are likely to have minimal psychosocial impact on the affected population. A high proportion of disaster events fulfill these criteria. Disaster events of such magnitude that they cause great harm, necessitate large-scale response, and generate extensive media attention are relatively few in number; yet these exceptional incidents tend to become the focus for published research studies regarding physical and psychosocial consequences.

Relative magnitude

Events of identical type and equal physical magnitude may pose very different challenges for populations of different sizes, and for communities with ample versus limited response capacity (United Nations Development Program, 2004). Norris and colleagues (2002a, 2002b) noted that the scale of the disaster relative to the size of the community is relevant. Describing this phenomenon as the "impact ratio" the point made is that a disaster that causes harm to 100 persons has a very different level of impact for a community of 500 versus a community of 500 000.

This point finds its way to the very core of disaster terminology. Quarantelli (1985) defined disaster as a "crisis occasion where demands exceed capabilities," and he offered the following continuum of labels for disasters of varying magnitude relative to community resources (Quarantelli, 2006):

Crisis	Capacity exceeds demands – with capacity to spare
Emergency	Capacity meets or somewhat exceeds demands
Disaster	Demands exceed capacity
Catastrophe	Demands overwhelm and may destroy capacity.

Immediately following the extreme damage wrought by Hurricane Katrina along the Gulf Coast, Quarantelli (2005) described six distinctions that place catastrophe in a qualitatively different realm from disaster: (1) much of the built structure of the community is damaged or destroyed including operational headquarters for emergency response

organizations; (2) local officials are unable to perform their usual job functions; (3) destruction is frequently so widespread that nearby communities are impacted and unable to offer aid; (4) community functions and vital services are markedly disrupted and shortages may become acute; (5) mass media "socially construct" the event, selectively broadcasting negative consequences, antisocial behaviors, and damaging rumors to a national audience while local coverage is limited or absent; and (6) the expansive magnitude of the event demands attention from national leaders, infusing the catastrophe with political implications of blame and responsibility. While disaster preparedness has become a major theme of homeland security initiatives in developed nations, catastrophe preparedness remains beyond reach by the very nature of the capacity-obliterating destruction that defines such an event (Lakoff, 2005).

Measures of magnitude

The greater the magnitude of the hazard, the greater is the potential for causing harm, but the hazard must impact vulnerable human populations to precipitate disaster. Consider that while more than 500 000 earthquakes are detected by ultra-sensitive instrumentation each year, the majority are of minimal intensity or occur far from human habitation. Less than 1% (3 000) is even perceptible to human populations, among which 7–11 will cause significant loss of life (Alexander, 1996; International Federation of Red Cross and Red Crescent Societies, 1996; Ramirez & Peek-Asa, 2005).

It is apparent that forces of harm come in gradations. Scales have been devised to measure magnitude and intensity. For hurricanes, the Saffir–Simpson Scale classifies tropical cyclones into tropical depressions, tropical storms, and five categories of hurricanes based on specific cut-points of wind speed and central pressure (Shultz *et al.*, 2005). Accompanying the scale are estimates of the height of coastal storm surge and a narrative description of the degree of damage likely to be sustained by physical structures subjected to the full brunt of the storm. Similarly, the Fujita scale provides an intensity assessment for tornadoes, describing the width of the tornado's destructive swath and the distance traveled along the ground, accompanied by wind speed and damage estimates.

Magnitude and intensity are measures of an earthquake's strength. *Magnitude*, measured on the Richter scale, is the total energy from seismic or elastic waves radiating from the epicenter (Alexander, 1993; Ramirez & Peek-Asa, 2005). However, as a single, summary exposure measure for the entire earthquake event, this metric is not useful for predicting harm to individuals who are distributed over a broad geography. Measures of *intensity* such as peak ground acceleration and Modified Mercalli Intensity (MMI) assess the earthquake effect at specific locations (Noji, 1997b) and, where sensors are available, these measures may accurately predict earthquake injury and death (Mahue-Giangreco *et al.*, 2001; Peek-Asa *et al.*, 2000, 2003; Shoaf *et al.*, 1998).

For human-generated events, quantity measures are often used to denote magnitude or dose of exposure. For example, the destructive force of bombs and blast devices is measured as a multiple of the explosive power of a ton of dynamite (trinitrotoluene). The greater the quantity of explosive, chemical, nuclear, or biological agent released, the greater will be the destructive potential.

Forces of harm: the time dimension

Generally, harm, destruction, and psychosocial impact will increase with increasing frequency and duration of disaster events, and subsequent destruction of infrastructure and services leading to prolonged disruption. Multiple simultaneous or serial events will have a more profound, and possibly synergistic, impact than single events. Concatenation and compounding of multiple forces of harm will extend the impact period, expand the magnitude of destruction, and exacerbate the complexity of the recovery process. Multiplicity may come into play with or without hazard impact; the perception of ongoing threat and possible distortion of one's sense of safety may be prompted, for example, by the approach of a series of menacing hurricanes

during a highly active tropical storm season, or by sporadic ominous statements released by a terrorist organization.

Lack of warning precludes defensive or protective actions that could mitigate the approaching forces of harm or move citizens from harm's way. In contrast, knowledge that certain types of hazards are rare or that the hazards are cyclical, restricted to specific seasons, or are preceded by ample warning periods, increases predictability and perceived control – and diminishes stress.

Frequency and trends

Disasters are common phenomena. Once every 19 h, a natural disaster is recorded in the international disaster registry located at CRED in Brussels, Belgium (CRED, 2005). Once every 25 h, a human-generated "technological" disaster is registered.

CRED maintains the EM-DAT Emergency Disasters Data Base (CRED, 2005), as the mechanism for compiling and sharing information on disasters worldwide. To be included as a disaster recorded in the EM-DAT data base, at least one of the following four criteria must be met: (1) 10 or more people reported killed, (2) 100 or more people reported affected, (3) declaration of a state of emergency, or (4) request for international assistance. Greater attention to disasters and an increasing sophistication in our ability to detect them produce the appearance of an explosive, exponential increase in disasters (Figure 4.4).

Technological advances and expansion of international communications coupled with enhanced global cooperation have increased the completeness of disaster reporting (Guha-Sapir *et al.*, 2004). Furthermore, a significant trend toward increased reporting of small- and medium-impact disasters has swelled the numbers of disaster records. The largely artifactual upsurge in numbers of disaster events, particularly from the 1960s forward, also coincides with the emergence of the field of disaster management (Kirschenbaum, 2004). Proliferation of governmental, nongovernmental, and university-based disaster management and

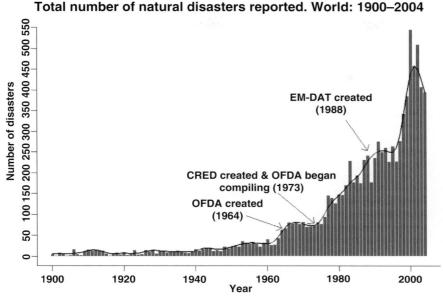

Figure 4.4 Frequency of reported and registered disasters

response services has generated intensive demand for disaster reporting, since the very announcement of a disaster launches these programs into action.

EM-DAT organizes and counts disaster events by country. Thus disasters affecting many nations generate multiple registrations. Hurricane Mitch, a single tropical cyclone that ravaged Central America in 1998, appears in the EM-DAT data base as a collection of seven country-specific disaster records. The tsunami of December 26, 2004, the highest fatality event of its type in recorded history, generated 12 country-specific disaster entries. Approximately one-in-six disasters in the data base is a multi-country event (Guha-Sapir *et al.*, 2004).

It is the aim of EM-DAT to systematically define and routinely report disasters in a timely manner with high fidelity and consistency worldwide. It is anticipated that the number of natural disasters annually will reach something resembling a steady state, or perhaps a gradual upward trend, as

increasing numbers of persons continue to migrate and settle in disaster-prone regions. During the 5 years 2000–2004, 3 199 natural disasters and 2 790 technological disasters were registered with CRED. On average, for each of these 5 years, 9 cyclones, 12 hurricanes, 17 typhoons, 11 tornadoes, 32 earthquakes, 154 floods, 20 landslides, 57 industrial accidents, and 225 transportation disasters were recorded. While EM-DAT does not track terrorist events, the recently established U.S. Department of Homeland Security's Counter-Terrorism Center compiles such incidents and reported an average of eight terrorist events per day in 2004.

Seasonality and cyclicity

Many types of natural disasters, particularly the large class of hydrometeorological events, tend to be seasonal. Tropical cyclone seasons are determined by annual fluctuations in ocean temperature (Figure 4.5). Winter storms are seasonal by

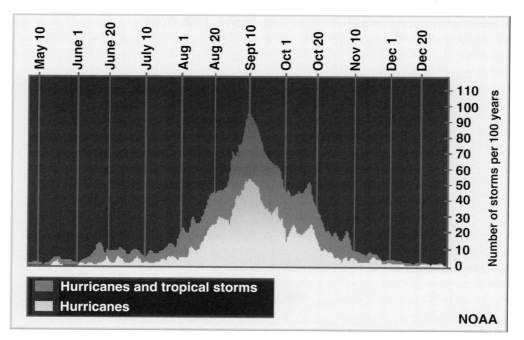

Figure 4.5 Seasonality: Atlantic Hurricane Basin tropical storms and hurricanes

definition and flooding occurs with spring thaws, rainy seasons, or monsoons. Some infectious diseases such as influenza circulate globally, rising and falling on a seasonal basis within a particular geographic area.

Severity of certain forces of harm may also vary over multi-year periods. One notable example is the 20- to 40-year cycle of hurricane frequency and intensity. Increases in numbers of named tropical storms, hurricanes, and major (Category 3 or higher) hurricanes occurred in the Atlantic Hurricane Basin during the 1940s, 1970s, and again during the early 2000s. As another example, influenza causes illness and death on a seasonal basis annually. Influenza viruses periodically emerge from animal reservoirs and mutate in such a fashion to cause infection in humans. When antigenic shift or adaptive mutations result in a highly virulent strain, an influenza pandemic erupts (as no humans have immunity). This has led to deadly flu pandemics three times in the past century; thus highlighting current concerns

about the evolving avian flu designated H5N1 from Southeast Asia.

Duration of impact/duration of disruption

Time factors of great import are duration of impact and duration of disruption. Impact varies from seconds (earthquakes and landslides, conventional bomb blasts) to minutes (tornadoes, flash floods, tsunamis) to hours and days (hurricanes) to weeks and months (riverine flooding, volcanic eruption, pandemics and bioterrorist disease outbreaks) to years (famine, drought) to decades and centuries (radioactive contamination). Moreover, the period of disruption of vital services may be protracted if power is disrupted, and schools and businesses are closed due to damage. Population displacement is one of the hallmarks of humanitarian crises and complex emergencies. In some cases persons can never return home due to physical destruction so catastrophic that the area is deemed unsalvageable. Events such as extreme contamination, profound depletion of vital resources, or change in ownership following warfare or ongoing militant threat may displace and dispossess persons in a manner that may be life-long.

Multiplicity

While isolated, discrete disaster events may produce widespread consequences, multiple events exert a greater effect than do single events. This has been explicated in relation to terrorism (Butler et al., 2003; Ursano, 2002). We distinguish three patterns of multiplicity: simultaneous, sequential (consecutive), and cascading (Shultz et al., 2007). Multiple events may occur simultaneously. A signature tactic of the terrorist organization Al Qaeda involves same-time strikes on multiple targets: (1) bombing two American embassies in Kenya and Tanzania in 1998; (2) hijacking four civilian aircraft on September 11, 2001; (3) attacking three hotels in Amman, Jordan in 2005. Another variation on the theme of multiplicity involves repetitive assaults over time, especially when it is difficult to assess the individual risk of being targeted. This was demonstrated with the serial sniper shootings in the metropolitan areas of Washington D.C., Maryland, and Virginia in 2002 (Grieger et al., 2003), and the anthrax bioterrorism in 2001 involving spore-laden envelopes mailed through the US Postal Service (Jernigan et al., 2002) – both events were protracted over several months. In the realm of natural disasters, repeated strikes by the same type of disaster are not uncommon. From August through November of 2004, the State of Florida was struck by a succession of four destructive hurricanes (Centers for Disease Control and Prevention, 2004). Similarly, Guam endured a series of five consecutive typhoons in 1992 (Staab et al., 1996).

Multiplicity may appear as a cascade or concatenation of disaster events. The succession of the forces of harm related to Hurricane Katrina striking the Gulf Coast in 2005 included extraordinary storm surge, inundating rains, powerful hurricane force winds, levee failure, massive flooding, and onshore flow of hazardous materials from damaged oil platforms. These hazards amplified and compounded into overwhelming health concerns and significant doubts about economic and socio-cultural recovery.

Predictability

The time factor is also relevant in terms of warning periods. Most types of natural disasters provide minimal warning periods (tornadoes, tsunamis, flash floods, volcanoes) or none at all (earthquakes, slides, tsunamis in areas without warnings systems). Notable exceptions are tropical cyclones, riverine floods, and winter storms, events that provide sufficient warning to prepare and protect lives and property. Acts of terrorism and many acts of warfare are conducted without warning to maximize both the devastation and the terror provoked.

Forces of harm: the place dimension

There are definable geographical boundaries that prescribe where disasters may – and may not – occur and, by extension, which populations may sustain impact. Similarly, terrain and topographic features mark areas of risk for certain types of disasters.

Geography and topography

One of the most distinguishing features of disaster occurrence is geographic distribution. For example, tropical cyclones form seasonally in seven hurricane basins distributed as twin belts just north and south of the equator. Tropical cyclones require multiple simultaneous climatic conditions for cyclogenesis, most fundamental of which is warm ocean water. Human populations susceptible to powerful hurricane strikes are those living in coastal regions at the perimeter of the hurricane basins. Populations living in vast inland areas and along coastal areas that border perennially cool waters are spared from the worst ravages of hurricanes, typhoons, and cyclones (Shultz et al., 2005).

While tropical systems can maintain momentum over considerable distances inland, the destructive

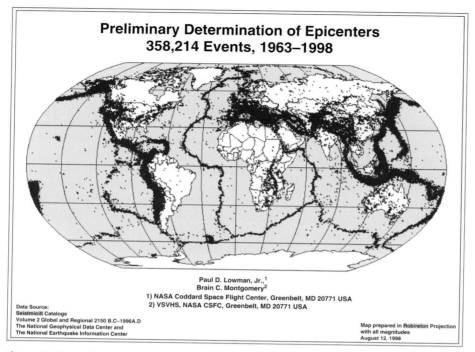

Figure 4.6 Place characteristics: worldwide seismic activity

force of tsunamis is restricted to several miles inland from the coast, yet the affected coastline may extend for thousands of miles along the perimeter of multiple continents. Likewise, earthquakes are concentrated in regions where the tectonic plates that compose the Earth's surface abut and interact (Adams, 1990; Kious & Tilling, 1996; Noji, 1997b; Simkin *et al.*, 2004) (Figure 4.6). Ramirez and Peek-Asa (2005) describe the geospatial dimensions of earthquake risk, "Populations located above plate activity are at greatest risk of earthquake-related morbidity and mortality, such as communities along the Pacific Rim ..., along island chains ..., and boundaries between certain continents."

Tornadoes form at the intersection of unstable air masses and the most active tornado belt on Earth is in the United States Midwest. Landslides and mudslides require steep, mountainous terrain while winter storms and avalanches occur in low temperatures and high elevations. Flash floods and riverine floods,

the most deadly of natural disasters, require a combination of meteorological and geographical features for their propagation.

The World Bank's *Natural Disaster Hotspots: A Global Risk Analysis* displays a series of composite maps and corresponding analyses of the worldwide distribution of risk for single and multiple hazards, disaster mortality, and economic loss (World Bank, 2005). Graphical depiction demonstrates that portions of the world's population are at heightened risk and high vulnerability for the onslaught of a variety of disasters while other populations live in zones of nominal risk.

The Asia–Pacific region experiences the greatest absolute and proportional mortality due to earthquakes, tropical cyclones, and floods. The only comparable loss of life is sustained in Africa associated with drought and exacerbated by the dynamics of complex emergency including armed conflict, extremes of poverty and epidemic disease

(United Nations Development Program, 2004). Africa also sustains loss of life from flooding. Latin America and the Caribbean are principally affected by tropical cyclones, flooding, and associated landslides and mudslides.

Currently, wars and civil conflict are raging in multiple venues. Refugee and internally displaced populations frequently reside in makeshift housing at elevated risk for harm, vulnerable to the ravages of natural hazards. Acts of terrorism likewise have geographic foci; much of the world's surface is spared from such atrocities while certain pockets remain hotbeds for frequent acts of terror. Within nations threatened by terrorism, risk for attack varies remarkably by locale; a function of terrorist tactics, target selection, and population concentration.

Extending the previous discussion, topography further defines the boundaries for disaster occurrence. Low-lying areas are susceptible to flooding, while coastal areas are prey to wave action and storm surge. Steep terrain and mountainous areas are prone to landslides and mudslides in response to heavy rains or seismic activity. In northern latitudes and high altitudes, avalanches may occur. Dust storms and sand storms sweep arid plains and deserts. Regarding acts of terrorism, terrain, geology, and topography are all relevant factors in determining availability and choice of targets, availability and choice of weapons materials, and availability of remote and inaccessible hiding places where terrorists may lurk between attacks.

Area and path

The area of impact may be geographically focalized, or may expand to cover a vast area, or may extend over extraordinary linear distances. The September 11 attack on the United States was geographically constrained to several dozen blocks in lower Manhattan, Pentagon City, and a small acreage in Shanksville, Pennsylvania. Hurricane Katrina, in contrast, affected 600 miles of Gulf of Mexico coastline and pierced deep into the southern states

before losing force and momentum. The track of destruction of hurricanes and tornadoes can extend for hundreds of miles over land. The tsunami of December 2004 devastated coastlines on multiple continents and the entire circumference of the island nation of Sri Lanka. Drought, such as that in the Darfur area of Sudan, may stretch over large territorial expanses.

Forces of harm: summary

Forces of harm are powerful primary stressors in their own right, and the consequences of disaster impact typically result in disruption of function that creates a cascade of secondary stressors. Hurricane Katrina, striking the US Gulf Coast in 2005, provides a "forceful" example of the hazard or forces of harm dimension (Table 4.3).

Forces of harm associated with a disaster can be considered from many perspectives. The degree and extent of harm are directly related to the type of disaster, the magnitude and intensity of the event, the frequency and duration of exposure to the forces of harm, and the geographic scope and scale – and so too are the psychosocial impacts (Norris *et al.*, 2002a, 2002b; *Science*, 2005).

Disaster ecology model: the ecological context of disaster risk and protective factors

Disaster risk is the product of hazard and vulnerability. We now describe multiple levels of factors that influence disaster risk with the disaster ecology model, providing illustrations of factors that populate each of the layers. Individual and family factors are viewed as relatively proximal. Community context and societal/structural context factors are described in later sections. It is important to understand that many factors come into play at multiple levels. For this discussion, we present a flexible layering of factors; risk and protective factors are richly and dynamically interconnected. For simplicity, we have

Table 4.3 Hazards: forces of harm: Hurricane Katrina, Gulf Coast, USA, 2005

Type	Definition	Catastrophe/complex emergency
	Classification	Hurricane (tropical cyclone)
Magnitude	**Intensity**	Florida landfall: Category 1
	Saffir–Simpson Scale	Peak intensity: Gulf of Mexico: Category 5
		Louisiana landfall: Category 3–4
		Mississippi landfall: Category 3
	Size	Large storm: 500-mile diameter
Time dimension	**Frequency**	No previous strike of this magnitude in recorded history. However, hurricanes repeatedly strike the area
	Multiplicity	Multiple tropical storms and hurricanes have struck Florida and the Gulf Coast each year recently. During 2005, the Gulf Coast was impacted by T. S. Arlene, T. S. Cindy, Hurricane Dennis prior to Hurricane Katrina and by Hurricane Rita later in the season Sequence of impacts: storm surge, rain, wind, eyewall impact, wind, rain, flood from levee break
	Seasonality	Atlantic Basin hurricane season: June 1–November 30
	Cyclicity	Strike occurred during the peak of a 30- to 40-year cycle of increased hurricane frequency
	Predictability	Predictable with days of advanced warning. Unpredicted change of course – striking the Florida coast and moving sharply southwest over Miami-Dade County (forecast track was due west). Track in Gulf of Mexico toward New Orleans held very steady on the middle of the predicted storm path
	Duration of impact	*Florida* Surge: 1 day; wind: several hours *Gulf Coast* Surge: 2 days; wind: 1 day; flood: weeks
	Duration of disruption	*Florida* 1 week *Gulf Coast* undetermined – months to lifetime
Place dimension	**Geography**	Atlantic Basin Hurricane Increasing intensity in Gulf of Mexico due to passing over Northern Loop Current of warm water New Orleans surrounded on all sides by bodies of water
	Topography	Concave shoreline of Gulf of Mexico produces very high storm surge Below water level construction Inadequate construction of levees to contain flooding
	Scale/scope	500-mile diameter storm Impact along 600 miles of Gulf Coast shoreline Total 1000 mile trajectory: Caribbean; Atlantic; Florida peninsula; Gulf of Mexico; landfall in Louisiana; Mississippi and Alabama; continuation of strong storm into northern United States

categorized factors into just three levels – individual/family, community, and societal/structural; other socio-ecological models have created a more detailed set of tiers (Figures 4.2, 4.3).

Ecological context: individual/family factors

Forces of harm – exposure to hazard, loss, and change – are brought closest to home within the realm of individual and family factors. Frequently families weather the storm or battle the pandemic on the home front. Losses are most acute when harm or death comes to a spouse, child, or other close family member. Losses for one family member ripple through the household, the extended family unit, and the neighborhood. Change is also experienced with particular intensity by partners, families, and close gatherings of friends.

Disaster impact on citizens and whole populations varies by individual and family characteristics such as age, gender, race/ethnicity, education, occupation, employment status, and income. Gender and race/ethnicity will be discussed as examples. Also highly relevant are the disaster mitigation, preparedness, response, and recovery activities and behaviors in which individuals and families engage. This includes such protective actions as developing a family disaster plan, stockpiling survival supplies, responding to disaster warnings, evacuating when instructed, sheltering in place, protecting property from harm, and developing a family contact and communications plan. Also included at this level, we consider the opposing risk behaviors that place individuals in harm's way (e.g., failure to heed warnings or evacuate, risk-taking during impact and postimpact periods). A proportion of the community is composed of full-time disaster response professionals. Many other community members will assume emergency response functions within their occupational roles at the time of a disaster. Others will train to develop disaster volunteer skills. Despite ample options for citizen engagement in personal, family, and community preparedness, the stark reality is that few

nations have a broadly trained public that can mobilize rapidly in time of disaster.

Gender

Gender inequalities are notable throughout many cultures and contribute to disparities in disaster impacts (Kumar-Range, 2001; World Health Organization, 2002). Women bear a disproportionate burden of disaster vulnerability due to biological and gender role differences. World Health Organization (2002) notes that gender differences are pervasive throughout all aspects of the disaster cycle: "The differential impact of disasters on men and women may be due to socially determined differences in women's and men's roles and status, due to biological differences between the sexes, or due to an interaction of social and biological factors."

Women's heightened vulnerability is related to their lower socioeconomic status, limiting abilities to provide adequately for their families, and access to critical resources. Moreover, a higher proportion of women live in poverty, greatly diminishing their ability to protect themselves against disaster hazards. Within the family, women's control over life decisions for themselves and their children may be severely restricted. Within the community, women lack political influence, a byproduct of disempowerment. Women are more vulnerable in the wake of disaster when care-giving demands increase, and access to resources decrease (Kumar-Range, 2001). Conversely, the care-giving roles (that ironically increase women's susceptibility), and women's ability to establish formal and informal networks are instrumental for household and community recovery following disasters (Morrow, 1997).

While most studies highlight the relative disadvantage for women in disasters, men's "protector" roles may demand considerable risk-taking during rescue and recovery phases placing men at elevated risk at such times (World Health Organization, 2002).

Race/ethnicity

Review of the literature paints a picture of increased vulnerability to and risk of disasters for racial and ethnic communities in the United States. Fothergill *et al.* (1999) contend that, "In terms of racial and ethnic communities, we believe that there are links between racism, vulnerability and economic power in the disaster context." Based on earlier work (Fothergill, 1996), these authors expand "the cyclical framework of the human ecology perspective which uses the following categories: preparedness, response, recovery, and mitigation," to a typology of eight categories based on the stages of a disaster. They reviewed the scientific literature and found mixed results generally trending toward disadvantage for race/ethnic minority populations for each of the disaster stages: (1) heightened perception of personal disaster risk; (2) lack of preparedness; (3) less access and response to warning systems; (4) increased physical impacts due to substandard housing; (5) poorer psychological outcomes; (6) cultural insensitivity on the part of emergency responders; (7) marginalization, lower socioeconomic status, and less familiarity with support resources leading to protracted recovery; and (8) diminished standard of living, job loss, and exacerbated poverty during reconstruction (Fothergill *et al.*, 1999).

Ecological context: community-level factors

When thinking about disasters, the local "environment," or perhaps better put, the local "context" may determine the likelihood of a disaster itself and the rates of disaster consequences. These features of the local context interact with, and shape, one another and may be considered as features of a socioecological model that explains the consequences of disasters. We discuss key features of the local environment that are critical to our thinking about the epidemiology of disasters and its consequences.

Elements subsumed under community context include the local political structure and governance, and related community infrastructure including health and social services and local emergency management. Gaining increasing emphasis in recent years is the concept of citizen training and empowerment to assume disaster response roles through

such mechanisms as Community Emergency Response Teams (CERT) and Medical Reserve Corps (MRC). Key elements of community context that will receive expanded discussion are social support, community socioeconomic status, social environment, and civic society.

Social support

Substantial research has demonstrated a central role for social support as a resource influencing risk of psychopathology postdisaster (Kaniasty & Norris, 1993; Norris & Kaniasty, 1996). In a longitudinal study in China, social support was associated with lower prevalence of post-traumatic stress disorder (PTSD) throughout a 1-year follow-up of earthquake victims (Zhao *et al.*, 2000) and social support moderated stress processes after the Three Mile Island disaster (Chisholm *et al.*, 1986). One study showed that although social support was protective for psychiatric disorders after the Three Mile Island disaster, it was not protective for the development of affective disorders (Solomon, 1985). Social support that individuals receive from postdisaster mobilization efforts is thought to counter the diminishing expectations of support often experienced by victims of major life events (Fullerton *et al.*, 1992). One study has suggested that a disaster fortifies social cohesion with a tendency towards perseverance and strengthening of core values (Norris & Kaniasty, 1996). The relation between these factors and others, discussed here, that may predispose groups toward vulnerability or resilience is likely complex.

Community socioeconomic status

Postdisaster evidence has demonstrated an association between individual poverty and lower perception of risk, poorer preparedness, limited warning communication, greater physical and psychological impacts, and more limited access to emergency response and recovery resources after disasters (Fothergill & Peek, 2004). While the disaster literature has focused almost exclusively on *individual* poverty, rather than community deprivation, an abundance of public health research demonstrates that aggregate community socio-economic status is associated with health, independent of individual socioeconomic position. Community socioeconomic status encompasses multiple domains including high rates of poverty and unemployment (Berkman & Kawachi, 2000), and lower education and income levels (Berkman & Kawachi, 2000; Krieger, 1994).

Empirically, low community socioecological status, frequently also referred to as community deprivation, is a determinant of health outcomes including health-related behaviors, mental health, infant mortality rate, adult physical health, coronary heart disease and mortality; even after accounting for individual level factors (Diez-Roux, 2001; Diez-Roux et al., 1997; Pickett & Pearl, 2001).

Community deprivation may be associated with differential access to quality medical care (Mandelblatt et al., 1999), limited availability of other salutary resources, such as healthy food (Cheadle et al., 1991; Sooman et al., 1993), and psychosocial stress accompanying chronic shortage of essential resources (Williams et al., 1994). These mechanisms influence health in the disaster context. Postdisaster, when both formal and informal resources are limited, societies with a priori fewer resources are less likely to have access to health and social services or food reserves. Similarly, postdisaster circumstances are more likely to heighten pre-existing stressors and potentially lead to poor coping and health-compromising behaviors (e.g., substance abuse). An example of these mechanisms at work is provided by the differential response capacities and recovery trajectories of two towns impacted by the 1992 earthquakes in Humboldt County, California; with the less affluent community unable to mount a sufficient response, resulting in a more constrained and prolonged recovery phase (Rovai, 1994).

Social environment

The social environment has been broadly defined to include, " . . . occupational structure, labor markets, social and economic processes, wealth, social, human, and health services, power relations, government, race relations, social inequality, cultural practices, the arts, religious institutions and practices, and beliefs about place and community" (Barnett & Casper, 2001, p. 465). This definition, by its very complexity, suggests that there are multiple ways in which the social environment may affect health. Limited social cohesion may predispose persons to less adaptive coping and adverse health consequences (Kawachi & Berkman, 2001; McLeod & Kessler, 1990).

Social capital effects are thought to offer general economic and social support on an ongoing basis and also to make specific resources available at times of stress. Social capital has been shown to be associated with lower all-cause mortality (Kawachi et al., 1997; Skrabski et al., 2004), reduced violent crime (Kennedy et al., 1998), and self-reported health status (Subramanian et al., 2002). Persons who live in segregated communities may have disproportionate exposure, susceptibility, and response to economic and social deprivation, toxic substances, and hazardous conditions (Williams & Collins, 2002).

Predisaster community cohesion is a basis upon which postdisaster recovery can be built (Oliver-Smith, 1996; Pfefferbaum et al., 2006; Reissman et al., 2005; Torry, 1986). In addition, pre-existing social stressors, influenced by racial/ethnic and socioecological strains, may influence postcrisis interactions during the recovery phase. Pre-existing social stressors may also influence social interactions between disaster-affected communities and those attempting to provide postdisaster aid. This was evident in the aftermath of Hurricane Katrina in New Orleans in September 2005, as national television captured relief workers repeatedly exacerbating tensions in a racially segregated city. Also, in the context of limited postdisaster resources, some of the social stressors could be mitigated by enforcing or rewarding equitable distribution of resources.

Civic society

Although related to features of the social and cultural environment, civic society frequently plays a distinct role in shaping a context that is salutary for population health. Civic society defines the space not controlled by government or the market where residents interact to achieve common goals. Several participants in civil society influence the health of populations. Community-based organizations (CBOs) or nongovernmental organizations (NGOs) have a long history of working to improve living conditions both in their own home countries and internationally (Halpern, 1995). CBOs such as neighborhood associations and tenant groups who provide services, mobilize populations, and advocate for resources could be re-purposed during a crisis to work in concert with each other to protect the health and safety of the community (Reissman *et al.*, 2005).

Places of worship and faith-based organizations offer social support, a safe space, and political leadership (Lincoln & Mamiya, 1990; Thomas *et al.*, 1994). In many instances, civic society may well be the only formal societal structure standing in the aftermath of a disaster that has the population's respect and trust. Particularly in human-made disasters when public suspicion of formal governmental authority may be high, civic society can serve as an honest broker and cultural ambassador, delivering aid and helping to rebuild the social and physical environments. For example, during the extended conflict between Israel and Lebanon in the 1980s and 1990s, local civic institutions, many predating the conflict, played a central role in providing health and social services to local populations in contested territory.

Ecological context: societal/structural factors

Beyond the community level, broader societal and structural factors influence disaster severity and consequences. Here we revisit geography, discussed previously during the explication of the hazard component of the ecological model, and now viewed as part of the environmental context. The physical, engineered and built environment is an important factor in relation to human settlement patterns. Cultural context, political structure and governance, and health and social services infrastructure resonate across all levels but are discussed here as societal/structural factors. Related factors include the legal and policy environment at national and international levels, socioeconomic status and development, and issues such as structural violence within and across populations.

Geography

Although disasters are a global phenomenon, the impact of disasters remains grounded in local context. As noted earlier in this chapter, geographic factors render specific areas to a particularly high risk of disasters. Areas that are below sea level or close to bodies of water that change levels frequently (e.g., the Gulf Coast region in the US, river Deltas in Bangladesh) are particularly prone to flooding. Similarly, human settlements in arid areas (e.g., Southern Australia) are vulnerable to fires (Gillen, 2005). The threat of disasters in such areas is endemic, and floods, bushfires, and earthquakes are cyclical events, with varying degrees of intensity in different seasons. In some areas, the exigencies of geography dictate the unavoidable risk for recurrent disasters; complete resettlement of human populations into lower risk areas is the sole option for elimination of disaster risk.

Geography also plays an important role in structuring the postdisaster response. News of a disaster event in isolated communities may take far longer to reach aid agencies or the media, as in the case of the Darfur famine of 2004–2005, than in more accessible locations. The ability of agencies to provide aid may be limited in geographically distant or difficult locales. For example, it took more than a week for aid efforts to reach some victims of the devastating 2005 earthquakes in the Kashmir region of Pakistan that killed an estimated 54 000 people (Agence France Presse, 2005).

Physical environment

There are multiple features of the physical environment that are associated with human health, with a vast empiric literature demonstrating links between the physical (human-engineered and natural) environment and well-being, within the physical, psychological, and spiritual realms.

The physical environment is a central feature of context for postdisaster recovery. As an immediate consequence of a disaster, structures such as buildings, bridges, and skyscrapers may be vulnerable to natural or human-made disasters, as recent earthquakes in Japan and Iran and the September 11, 2001 terrorist attacks on New York City demonstrated respectively. Features of the physical environment directly influence disaster outcomes (Daley *et al.*, 2005). The cities of Kobe, Japan and Bam, Iran sustained earthquakes of comparable magnitude in 1995 and 2003, respectively. While the buildings in Kobe were structurally engineered to withstand earthquake tremors, those in Bam collapsed wholesale. Absolute numbers of deaths and mortality rates were substantially higher in Bam. Infrastructure can be damaged after an earthquake or hurricane, straining already taxed systems and contributing to adverse health consequences. Lengthy time periods for reconstruction of the local physical environment may contribute to prolonged community suffering after a disaster, limited job opportunities, and a torrent of other factors slowing, and possibly compromising, the recovery of population physical and mental health.

Cultural context

The impact of culture on health-related beliefs and practices is difficult to describe and quantify, especially in the postdisaster period. "Culture" as a notion lends itself to diverse definitions and interpretations. For the purposes of this chapter we consider culture to be "shared, learned behaviors and meanings that are transmitted socially" (Marsella & Christopher, 2004, p. 529). Social relationships associated with formal civic and religious institutions are elements of the cultural context that may shape health. Similarly, religiously sanctioned or endorsed behaviors and practices have the potential to influence health in the predisaster context. For example, religious prohibition of alcohol use is associated with much lower rates of alcohol dependence among Muslims compared to non-Muslims (Cochrane & Bal, 1990). Evidence suggests that other manifestations of a dominant culture, such as patterns of social congregation in public places, are associated with social transmission of health behavior and norms (Henrich & McElreath, 2003). Complex social security networks, which serve to minimize the risk of resource shortfalls, have also been identified as important informal sources of assistance that are called upon during disasters (Shipton, 1990). Importantly, this "moral economy" of sharing is also linked to community socioeconomic status, which, in turn, influences the efficacy of informal support networks. Less affluent communities may be less able than more affluent communities to mobilize material resources (i.e., instrumental social support) to assist others (Hadley *et al.*, under review, 2006). Strong cultural norms about societal organization, altruism, and diversity may influence social cohesion postdisaster and contribute to communal efforts to restore symbolic structures, social hierarchies, and services to their predisaster state. Conversely, destruction of culturally significant places may be associated with communal grief (Bode, 1989), that has been in turn associated with elevated rates of depression in the aftermath of disasters (Goenjian *et al.*, 2001).

Political structure and governance

Political structures and systems of governance establish the parameters (e.g., taxation, federal–state relations) that shape many of the other contextual factors that have an impact on health. Democratic governance is associated with greater governmental openness and responsiveness to domestic criticism and there is some evidence that such regimes are less prone to state failures. For example, analyses of state failures in Liberia and

Somalia that predisposed their citizens to disasters show that these events are more likely to occur in partial as compared to fully democratic regimes (Esty & Ivanova, 2002). There is also evidence that disasters occurring in alternate political systems are substantially mitigated by effective governance.

A feature of political structures that relates directly to the mitigation of disaster is the *effectiveness* of political structures and governance. At the extreme, there are a few societies worldwide without an effective government of any sort. For example, Somalia has not had a central government since 1993. In its stead, informal organizations established along clan lines provide a loose form of governance and respond to mass disasters such as famines by providing relief for persons in affected communities and brokering international aid. Within well-established national political structures, there have been several recent examples of both effective and ineffective governmental response to disasters. In the US as an example, some environmental and consumer regulations have been loosened, and many previously public services (e.g., sanitation, water, health care) have been privatized (Gans, 1995; Katz, 1989). Limited regulation of municipal water supplies has been considered, at least in part, responsible for water-borne disease outbreaks in different North American cities (Corso *et al.*, 2003; Garrett, 2000; Krewski *et al.*, 2002). Problems with the domestic response to Hurricane Katrina in August/September 2005 have been widely attributed to significant changes within central governmental authority and to poor coordination among federal, state, and municipal levels of government (Nates & Moyer, 2005).

Health and social services infrastructure

Predisaster availability of health and social resources is inextricably linked to postdisaster recovery. Affluent countries and communities are characterized by a broader array of health and social services compared with poorer counterparts (Casey *et al.*, 2001; Felt-Lisk *et al.*, 2002). In the US, even the poorest communities have dozens of social agencies, each with a distinct mission and service package. Many of the public health successes in wealthy countries over the past few decades, including reductions in human immunodeficiency virus (HIV) transmission and tuberculosis control, have depended in part on the efforts of these groups (Freudenberg *et al.*, 2000). In poor communities, or less wealthy countries, social and health services are frequently susceptible to changing national and donor fiscal realities and service reductions frequently coincide with times of greater need in the population (Felt-Lisk *et al.*, 2002; Friedman, 1989).

The scope and magnitude of disasters are associated with the extent of disruption of health and social services. When health and social services continue to function postdisaster, the contribution of these resources to preserving or restoring health in a population is self-evident. However, these pre-existing resources are also relevant in devastating disasters where most formal resources are destroyed because local health and social service practitioners have indigenous knowledge, acceptance by local community members, and are much more likely to be able to provide continuity of care than are services provided by outside aid agencies (Fissel & Haddix, 2004).

Ecological context: summary

The rich complexity of environmental features at community and societal levels interactiong across all phases of disaster mitigation, preparedness, response, and recovery. Consideration of the context is instrumental for disaster psychiatrists and providers of disaster behavioral health support. Context largely determines the extent of disaster impact, and, in turn, the extent of natural supports and community resources that can be tapped in times of disaster.

Concluding comments

Systematic consideration of the defining components of disaster, presented from a socioecological perspective, can guide efforts aimed at mitigating the consequences of these events, diminishing the pervasive psychosocial impacts, and improving the health of populations worldwide. We have advocated for promoting an ecological approach to better understand the avenues of prevention, mitigation, and recovery. Doing so will facilitate the ongoing movement to integrate public health and behavioral health strategies for disaster preparedness and will allow us to identify and leverage other sectors of government and civic life, whose interdependence and interrelatedness are essential in times of disaster such that we can protect and improve community or population-level health and well-being. Understanding the dynamic nature of disasters as the collision between forces of harm – exposure to hazard, loss, and change – and vulnerable human populations in harm's way, richly influenced by the ecological context, is a fundamental underpinning for the effective practice of disaster psychiatry.

REFERENCES

Adams, R. D. (1990). Earthquake occurrence and effects. *Injury*, **21**, 17–20.

Agence France Presse (2005). Musharraf defends handling of devastating pakistan quake. Available at: http://web.lexis-nexis.com/universe/document?_m=6509211fbe72cf882063e380faffa66e&_docnum=1&wchp=dGLbVlz-zSkVb&_md5=715c332a1eb5c90f4eeb04ec85375da7. Accessed October 27, 2005.

Alexander, D. (1993). *Natural Disasters*. New York: Chapman & Hall.

Alexander, D. (1996). The health effects of earthquakes in the mid-1990s. *Disasters*, **20**, 231–247.

Barnett, D. J., Balicer, R. D., Blodgett, D. *et al.* (2005a). The application of the Haddon Matrix to public health readiness and response planning. *Environmental Health Perspectives*, **113**, 561–566.

Barnett, D. J., Balicer, R. D., Lucey, D. R. *et al.* (2005b). A systematic analytic approach to pandemic influenza preparedness planning. *PLoS Medicine*, **2**, 1235–1241.

Barnett, E. & Casper, M. (2001). A definition of "social environment." *American Journal of Public Health*, **91**, 465.

Berkman, L. & Kawachi, I. (eds.) (2000). *Social Epidemiology*. New York: Oxford University Press.

Blakely, T. A. & Woodward, A. J. (2000). Ecological effects in multi-level studies. *Journal of Epidemiology and Community Health*, **54**, 367–374.

Bode, B. (1989). *No Bells to Toll Destruction and Creation in the Andes*. New York: Scribners.

Butler, A. S., Panzer, A. M. & Goldfrank, L. R. (2003). Institute of Medicine Committee on Responding to the Psychological Consequences of Terrorism Board of on Neuroscience and Behavioral Health. *Preparing for the Psychological Consequences of Terrorism: A Public Health Approach*. Washington, D.C.: National Academies Press.

Casey, M. M., Thiede Call, K. & Klingner, J. M. (2001). Are rural residents less likely to obtain recommended preventive healthcare services? *American Journal of Preventive Medicine*, **21**, 182–188.

Centers for Disease Control and Prevention (2004). Epidemiologic assessment of the impact of four hurricanes – Florida, 2004. *MMWR Morbidity and Mortality Weekly Report*, **54**, 693–697.

Center for Research on the Epidemiology of Disasters (CRED) (2005). *EM-DAT Data Base*. Brussels: Universite Catholique de Louvain.

Cheadle, A., Psaty, B. M., Curry, S. *et al.* (1991). Community-level comparisons between the grocery store environment and individual dietary practices. *Preventive Medicine*, **20**, 250–261.

Chisholm, R. F., Kasl, S. V. & Mueller, L. (1986). The effects of social support on nuclear worker responses to the Three Mile Island accident. *Journal of Occupational Behaviour*, **7**, 179–193.

Cochrane, R. & Bal, S. (1990). The drinking habits of Sikh, Hindu, Muslim and white men in the west midlands: a community survey. *British Journal of Addictions*, **85**, 759–769.

Corso, P. S., Kramer, M. H., Blair, K. A. *et al.* (2003). Cost of illness in the 1993 waterborne cryptosporidium outbreak, Milwaukee, Wisconsin. *Emerging Infectious Diseases*, **9**, 426–431.

Daley, R. W., Brown, S., Archer, P. *et al.* (2005). Risk of tornado-related death and injury in Oklahoma, May 3, 1999. *American Journal of Epidemiology*, **161**, 1144–1150.

Diez-Roux, A. V. (2001). Investigating neighborhood and area effects on health. *American Journal of Public Health*, **91**, 11783–11789.

Diez-Roux, A. V., Nieto, F. J., Muntaner, C. *et al.* (1997). Neighborhood environments and coronary heart disease: a multilevel analysis. *American Journal of Epidemiology*, **146**, 48–63.

Esty, D. C. & Ivanova, I. (eds.) (2002). *Global Environmental Governance: Options and Opportunities*. New Haven, CT: Yale School of Forestry and Environmental Studies.

Felt-Lisk, S., McHugh, M. & Howell, E. (2002). Monitoring local safety-net providers: do they have adequate capacity? *Health Affairs*, **21**, 277–283.

Fissel, A. & Haddix, K. (2004). Traditional healer organizations in Uganda should contribute to AIDS debate. *Anthropology News*, **45**, 10–11.

Fothergill, A. (1996). Gender, risk and disaster. *International Journal of Mass Emergencies and Disasters*, **3**, 49–56.

Fothergill, A. & Peek, L. A. (2004). Poverty and disasters in the United States: a review of recent sociological findings. *Natural Hazards*, **32**, 89–110.

Fothergill, A., Maestas, E. G. M. & DeRoune, J. A. (1999). Race, ethnicity and disasters in the United States: a review of the literature. *Disasters*, **23**, 156–173.

Fox, A. (2003). Glossary of epidemiological terms. *International Journal of Pediatrics and Neonatalogy*, **3**(1).

Freudenberg, N., Silver, D., Carmona, J. M. *et al.* (2000). Health promotion in the city: a structured review of the literature on interventions to prevent heart disease, substance abuse, violence and HIV infection in U. S. metropolitan areas, 1980–1995. *Journal of Urban Health*, **77**, 443–457.

Friedman, F. (1989). Donor policies and third world health. *International Health Development*, **1**, 16–17.

Fullerton, C. S., McCarroll, J. E., Ursano, R. J. & Wright, K. M. (1992). Psychological responses of rescue workers: fire fighters and trauma. *American Journal of Orthopsychiatry*, **62**, 371–378.

Galea, S. & Resnick, H. (2005). Post-traumatic stress disorder in the general population after mass terrorist incidents: considerations about the nature of exposure. *CNS Spectrums*, **10**, 107–115.

Gans, H. (1995). *The War Against the Poor: The Underclass and Antipoverty Policy*. New York: Basic Books.

Garrett, L. (2000). *Betrayal of Trust: The Collapse of Global Public Health*. New York: Oxford University Press.

Gillen, M. (2005). Urban governance and vulnerability: exploring the tensions and contradictions in Sydney's response to bushfire threat. *Cities*, **22**, 55–64.

Goenjian, A. K., Molina, L., Steinberg, A. M. *et al.* (2001). Posttraumatic stress and depressive reactions among Nicaraguan adolescents after Hurricane Mitch. *American Journal of Psychiatry*, **158**, 788–794.

Grieger, T. A., Fullerton, C. S., Ursano, R. J. & Reeves, J. J. (2003). Acute stress disorder, alcohol use, and perception of safety among hospital staff after sniper attacks. *Psychiatric Service*, **54**, 1383–1387.

Guha-Sapir, D., Hargitt, D. & Hoyois, P. (2004). Center for Research on the Epidemiology of Disasters. *Thirty Years of Natural Disasters: 1974–2003: The Numbers*. Louvain-la-Neuve: Presses Universitaires de Louvain.

Haddon, W. Jr. (1972). A logical framework for organizing highway safety phenomena and activity. *Journal of Trauma*, **12**, 193–207.

Haddon, W. Jr. (1980). Advances in the epidemiology of injuries as a basis for public policy. *Public Health Reports*, **95**, 411–421.

Halpern R. (1995). *Rebuilding the Inner City. A History of Neighborhood Initiatives to Address Poverty in the United States*. New York: Columbia University Press.

Hatch, M., Ron, E., Bouville, L., Zablotska, L. & Howe, G. (2005). The Chernobyl disaster: cancer following the accident at the Chernobyl nuclear power plant. *Epidemiologic Reviews*, **27**, 56–66.

Henrich, J. & McElreath, R. (2003). The evolution of cultural evolution. *Evolutionary Anthropology*, **12**, 123–135.

International Federation of Red Cross and Red Crescent Societies (1996). *World Disasters Report 1996*. New York: Oxford University Press.

Jernigan, D. B., Raghunathan, P. L., Bell, B. P. *et al.* (2002). Investigation of bioterrorism-related anthrax, United States, 2001: epidemiologic findings. *Emerging Infectious Diseases*, **10**, 1019–1028.

Kaniasty, K. & Norris, F. (1993). A test of the support deterioration model in the context of natural disaster. *Journal of Personality and Social Psychology*, **64**, 395–408.

Kaplan, G. A. (1999). What is the role of the social environment in understanding inequalities in health? *Annals of the New York Academy of Sciences*, **896**, 116–119.

Kaplan, G. A. (2004). What's wrong with social epidemiology and how can we make it better? *Epidemiological Reviews*, **26**, 124–135.

Karpati, A., Galea, S., Awerbuch, T. & Levins, R. (2002). Variability and vulnerability at the ecological level: implications for understanding the social determinants of health. *American Journal of Public Health*, **92**, 1768–1772.

Katz, M. (1989). *The Undeserving Poor. From the War on Poverty to the War on Welfare*. New York: Pantheon.

Kawachi, I. & Berkman, L. F. (2001). Social ties and mental health. *Journal of Urban Health*, **78**, 458–467.

Kawachi, I., Kennedy, B. P., Lochner, K. & Prothrow-Stith, D. (1997). Social capital, income inequality, and mortality. *American Journal of Public Health*, **87**, 1491–1498.

Kennedy, B. P., Kawachi, I., Prothrow-Stith, D., Lochner, K. & Gupta, V. (1998). Social capital, income inequality, and firearm violent crime. *Social Science and Medicine*, **47**, 7–17.

Kious, J. W. & Tilling, R. I. (1996). This dynamic Earth: the story of plate tectonics. Available at the US Geological Survey site: http://pubs.usgs.gov/publications/text/dynamic.html. Accessed May 1, 2007.

Kirschenbaum, A. (2004). *Chaos Organization and Disaster Management*. New York: Marcel Dekker.

Krewski, D., Balbus, J., Butler-Jones, D. *et al.* (2002). Managing health risks from drinking water – a report to the Walkerton inquiry. *Journal of Toxicology and Environmental Health*, **65**, 1635–1823.

Krieger, N. (1994). Epidemiology and the web of causation: has anyone seen the spider? *Social Science and Medicine*, **39**, 887–903.

Krieger, N. (2001). Theories for social epidemiology in the 21st century: an ecosocial perspective. *International Journal of Epidemiology*, **30**, 668–677.

Kumar-Range, S. (2001). Environmental management and disaster risk reduction: a gender perspective. United Nations: Division for the Advancement of Women (DAW). Available at http://www.un.org/womenwatch/daw/csw/env_manage/documents/BP1-2001Nov04.pdf. Accessed May 1, 2007.

Lakoff, A. (2005). From disaster to catastrophe: the limits of preparedness. In: The Social Science Research Council website. *Understanding Katrina: Perspectives from the Social Sciences*. Available at http://understandingkatrina.ssrc.org/Lakoff/. Accessed May 1, 2007.

Landesman, L. Y. (2001). *Public Health Management of Disasters: The Practice Guide*. Washington, D.C.: American Public Health Association.

Last, J. M. (ed.) (2001). *A Dictionary of Epidemiology, 4th edn*. New York: Oxford University Press.

Lilienfeld, D. E. & Stolley, P. D. (1994). *Foundations of Epidemiology, 3rd edn*. New York: Oxford University Press.

Lincoln, C. E. & Mamiya, L. H. (1990). *The Black Church in the African American Experience*. Durham, N.C.: Duke University Press.

Logue, J. N., Melick, M. E. & Hansen, H. (1981). Research issues and directions in the epidemiology of health effects of disasters. *Epidemiologic Reviews*, **3**, 140–162.

Mackenbach, J. (1993). Public health epidemiology. *Journal of Epidemiology and Community Health*, **49**, 333–334.

Mahue-Giangreco, M., Mack, W., Seligson, H. & Bourque, L. B. (2001). Risk factors associated with moderate and serious injuries attributable to the 1994 Northridge earthquake, Los Angeles, California. *Annals of Epidemiology*, **11**, 347–357.

Mandelblatt, J. S., Yabroff, K. R. & Kerner, J. F. (1999). Equitable access to cancer services: a review of barriers to quality care. *Cancer*, **86**, 2378–2390.

Marsella, A. J. & Christopher, M. A. (2004). Ethnocultural considerations in disasters: an overview of research, issues, and directions. *Psychiatric Clinics of North America*, **27**, 521–539.

McLeod, L. & Kessler, R. (1990). Socioecological status differences in vulnerability to undesirable life events. *Journal of Health and Social Behavior*, **31**, 162–172.

McMichael, A. J. (1999). Prisoners of the proximate: loosening the constraints on epidemiology in an age of change. *American Journal of Epidemiology*, **149**, 887–897.

Morrow, B. H. (1997). Stretching the bonds: the families of Andrew. In *Hurricane Andrew: Ethnicity, Gender, and the Sociology of Disasters*, eds. W. G. Peacock, B. H. Morrow & H. Gladwin, pp. 141–170. London: Routledge.

Nates, J. L. & Moyer, V. A. (2005). Lessons from hurricane Katrina, tsunamis, and other disasters. *Lancet*, **366**, 1144–1146.

Noji, E. K. (ed.) (1997a). *The Public Health Consequences of Disasters*. New York: Oxford University Press.

Noji, E. K. (ed.) (1997b). Earthquakes. In *The Public Health Consequences of Disasters*, pp. 35–78. New York: Oxford University Press.

Norris, F. H. (2005). Psychosocial consequences of natural disasters in developing countries: what does past research tell us about the potential effects of the 2004 tsunami? Available at National Center for PTSD, US Department of Veteran's Affairs site: www.ncptsd.va.gov/ncmain/ncdocs/fact_shts/fs_tsunami_research.html?opm=1&rr=rr81&srt=d&echorr=true.

Norris, F. H. & Kaniasty, K. (1996). Received and perceived social support in times of stress: a test of the social support deterioration deterrence model. *Journal of Personality and Social Psychology*, **71**, 498–511.

Norris, F. H. & Kaniasty, K. (2004). Social support in the aftermath of disasters, catastrophes, and acts of terrorism. In *Bioterrorism: Psychological and Public Health Interventions*, eds. R. Ursano, A. Norwood & C. Fullerton, pp. 200–229. Cambridge: Cambridge University Press.

Norris, F., Friedman, M., Watson, P. *et al.* (2002a). 60 000 disaster victims speak, part 1: An empirical review of the empirical literature, 1981–2001. *Psychiatry*, **65**, 207–239.

Norris, F., Friedman, M. & Watson, P. (2002b). 60 000 disaster victims speak, part 2: Summary and implications of the disaster mental health research. *Psychiatry*, **65**, 204–260.

Oliver-Smith, A. (1996). Anthropological research on hazards and disasters. *Annual Review of Anthropology*, **25**, 303–328.

Pearce, N. (1996). Traditional epidemiology, modern epidemiology, and public health. *American Journal of Public Health*, **86**, 678–683.

Peek-Asa, C., Ramirez, M. R., Shoaf, K., Seligson, H. & Kraus, J. F. (2000). GIS mapping of earthquake-related deaths and hospital admissions from the 1994 Northridge, California, earthquake. *Annals of Epidemiology*, **10**, 5–13.

Peek-Asa, C., Ramirez, M., Seligson, H. & Shoaf, K. (2003). Seismic, structural, and individual factors associated with earthquake related injury. *Injury Prevention*, **9**, 62–66.

Pfefferbaum, B., Reissman, D. B., Pfefferbaum, R. L., Klomp, R. W. & Gurwitch, R. H. (2006). Building resilience to mass trauma events. In *Handbook of Injury and Violence Prevention.*, eds. L. Doll, S. Bonzo, J. Mercy & D. Sleet. New York: Kluwer Academic/Plenum Publishers.

Pickett, K. E. & Pearl, M. (2001). Multilevel analyses of neighborhood socioecological context and health outcomes: a critical review. *Journal of Epidemiology and Community Health*, **55**, 111–122.

Poundstone, K. E., Strathdee, S. A. & Celentano, D. D. (2004). The social epidemiology of human immunodeficiency virus/acquired immunodeficiency syndrome. *Epidemiologic Reviews*, **26**, 22–35.

Quarantelli, E. L. (1985). Social support systems: some behavioral patterns in the context of mass evacuation activities. In *Disasters and Mental Health: Selected Contemporary Perspectives*, ed. B. Sowder, pp. 122–136. Rockville, Md.: National Institute of Mental Health.

Quarantelli, E. L. (1995). What is a disaster? Six views of the problem. *International Journal of Mass Emergencies and Disasters*, **13**, 221–229.

Quarantelli, E. L. (ed.) (1998). *What is a Disaster? Perspectives on the Question*. London: Routledge.

Quarantelli, E. L. (2005). Catastrophes are different from disasters: some implications for crisis planning and managing drawn from Katrina. In: The Social Science Research Council website: *Understanding Katrina: Perspectives from the Social Sciences*. Available at http://understandingkatrina.ssrc.org/Quarantelli/. Accessed May 1, 2007.

Quarantelli, E. L. (2006). Emergencies, disasters, and catastrophes are different phenomena. Available at http://www.udel.edu/DRC/preliminary/pp304.pdf. Accessed May 1, 2007.

Ramirez, M. & Peek-Asa, C. (2005). Epidemiology of traumatic injuries from earthquakes. *Epidemiologic Reviews*, **27**, 47–55.

Raphael, B. (2000). *Disaster Mental Health Response Handbook: An Educational Resource for Mental Health Professionals Involved in Disaster Management*. Sydney: NSW Health.

Reissman, D. B., Spencer, S., Tannielian, T. & Stein, B. D. (2005). Integrating behavioral aspects into community preparedness and response systems. In *The Trauma of Terrorism: Sharing Knowledge and Shared Care, an International Handbook*, eds. Y. Danieli, D. Brom & J. Sills. New York: Haworth Maltreatment and Trauma Press. [Published simultaneously as the *Journal of Aggression, Maltreatment and Trauma*, **9**, nos. 1/2 and nos. 3/4.]

Ritchie, E. C., Watson, P. J. & Friedman, M. J. (eds.) (2005). *Interventions Following Mass Violence and Disasters: Strategies for Mental Health Practice*. New York: Guilford Press.

Rovai, E. L. (1994). The social geography of disaster recovery: differential community response to the north coast earthquakes. In *Yearbook of the Association of Pacific Coast Geographers*, vol. 56, ed. D. E. Turbeville. Oregon: Oregon State University Press.

Rundell, J. R. & Christopher, G. W. (2004). Differentiating manifestations of infection from psychiatric disorders and fears of having been exposed to bioterrorism. In *Bioterrorism: Psychological and Public Health Interventions*, eds. R. J. Ursano, A. E. Norwood & C. S. Fullerton, pp. 88–108. New York: Cambridge University Press.

Runyan, C. (1998). Using the Haddon Matrix: introducing the third dimension. *Injury Prevention*, **4**, 302–307.

Rutherford, W. H. & de Boer, J. (1983). The definition and classification of disasters. *Injury*, **15**, 10–12.

Sarewitz, D. & Pielke Jr. R. A. (2001). Extreme events: a research and policy framework for disasters in context. *International Geology Review* **43**, 406–418.

Science, (2005). Dealing with Disasters (special section of brief articles.). *Science*, **309**, 1029–1046. Available at: www.sciencemag.org/sciext/disasters. Accessed on May 1, 2007.

Shipton, P. (1990). African famines and food insecurity: anthropological perspectives. *Annual Review of Anthropology*, **19**, 353–394.

Shoaf, K. I., Sareen, H. R., Nguyen, L. H. & Bourque, L. B. (1998). Injuries as a result of California earthquakes in the past decade. *Disasters*, **22**, 218–235.

Shultz, J. M., Russell, J. & Espinel, Z. (2005). Epidemiology of tropical cyclones: the dynamics of disaster, disease, and development. *Epidemiologic Reviews*, **27**, 21–35.

Shultz, J. M., Espinel, Z., Flynn, B. W., Cohen, R. E. & Hoffman, Y. (2007). *DEEP PREP: All Hazards Disaster Behavioral Health Training*. Tampa, FL: Disaster Life Support Publishing.

Simkin, T., Unger, J. D. & Tilling, R. I. *et al.* (2004). The dynamic planet: world map of volcanoes, earthquakes, impact craters, and plate tectonics. Available at US Geological Survey site: http://pubs.usgs.gov/pdf/planet. html. Accessed May 1, 2007.

Skrabski, A., Kobb, M. & Kawachi, I. (2004). Social capital and collective efficacy in Hungary: cross sectional associations with middle aged female and male mortality rates. *Journal of Epidemiology and Community Health*, **58**, 340–345.

Solomon, Z. (1985). Stress, social support and affective disorders in mothers of pre-school children: a test of the stress-buffering effect of social support. *Social Psychiatry*, **20**, 100–105.

Somasundaram, D., Norris, F. H., Asukai, N. & Murthy, R. S. (2003). Natural and technological disasters. In *Trauma Interventions in War and Peace: Prevention, Practice, and Policy*, eds. B. L. Green, M. J. Friedman, J. de Jong, *et al.*, pp. 291–318. New York: Kluwer Academic/Plenum Publishers.

Sooman, A., Macintyre, S. & Anderson, A. (1993). Scotland's health – a more difficult challenge for some? The price and allocation of healthy foods in social contrasting localities in the west of Scotland. *Health Bulletin*, **51**, 276–284.

Staab, J. P., Grieger, T. A., Fullerton, C. S. & Ursano, R. J. (1996). Acute stress disorder, subsequent posttraumatic stress disorder, and depression after a series of typhoons. *Anxiety*, **2**, 219–225.

Subramanian, S. V., Kim, D. J. & Kawachi, I. (2002). Social trust and self-rated health in U.S. communities: a multilevel analysis. *Journal of Urban Health*, **79**, S21–S34.

Susser, M. (1994). The logic of ecological. 1: The logic of analysis. *American Journal of Public Health*, **84**, 825–829.

Susser, M. (1998). Does risk factor epidemiology put epidemiology at risk? Peering into the future. *Journal of Epidemiology and Community Health*, **52**, 608–611.

Susser, M. & Susser, E. (1996). Choosing a future for epidemiology. II. From black boxes to Chinese boxes and eco-epidemiology. *American Journal of Public Health*, **86**, 674–677.

Thomas, S. B., Quinn, S. C., Billingley, A. & Caldwell, C. (1994). The characteristics of northern black churches with community health outreach programs. *American Journal of Public Health*, **84**, 575–579.

Torry, W. I. (1986). Economic development, drought, and famine: some limitations of dependency explanations. *Geojournal*, **12**, 5–18.

United Nations Development Program (2004). *Reducing Disaster Risk: A Challenge for Development*. Available at United Nations Development Program, Bureau for Crisis Prevention and Recovery site: www.undp.org/bcpr. Accessed May 1, 2007.

Ursano, R. J. (2002). Terrorism and mental health: public health and primary care. Presentation at the Eighteenth Annual Rosalyn Carter Symposium on Mental Health Policy. Status Report: Meeting the Mental Health Needs of the Country in the Wake of September 11, 2001. November 6–7, 2002. Atlanta, GA.: The Carter Center.

Ursano, R. J., Fullerton, C. S. & McGaughey, B. G. (1994). Trauma and disaster. In *Individual and Community Responses to Trauma and Disaster: The Structure of Human Chaos*, eds. R. J. Ursano, B. G. McGaughey & C. S. Fullerton, pp. 3–27. Cambridge: Cambridge University Press.

Williams, D. R. & Collins, C. (2002). Racial residential segregation: a fundamental cause of racial disparities in health. In: *Race, Ethnicity and Health: A Public Health Reader*, ed. T. A. LaVeist, pp. 369–390. San Francisco, Calif.: Jossey Bass.

Williams, D. R., Lavizzo-Mourey, R. & Warren, R. C. (1994). The concept of race and health status in America. *Public Health Reports*, **109**, 26–41.

Woodward, A. (1996). What makes populations vulnerable to ill health? *New Zealand Medical Journal*, **109**, 265–267.

World Bank (2005). *Natural Disaster Hotspots: A Global Risk Analysis*. Washington, D.C.: World Bank Group.

World Health Organization/EHA/EHTP (1999). *Emergency Health Training Programme for Africa. Training Modules.* Geneva: World Health Organization.

World Health Organization (2002). Gender and health in disasters. Available at http://www.who.int/gender/other_health/en/genderdisasters.pdf. Accessed May 1, 2007.

World Health Organization (2005). Health action in relation to crises and emergencies. WHO Fifty-Eighth World Health Assembly, Provisional Agenda Item 13.3. Geneva: World Health Organization.

Zhao, C., Wang, X., Gao, L. *et al.* (2000). Longitudinal study of earthquake-related PTSD in North China. *Chinese Mental Health Journal*, **14**, 361–363.

5

Neurobiology of disaster exposure: fear, anxiety, trauma, and resilience

Rebecca P. Smith, Craig L. Katz, Dennis S. Charney, &
Steven M. Southwick

Introduction

To date, clinical and research approaches to disaster mental health have focused primarily on the psychological experience of disaster survivors, and the development and effectiveness of psychological treatments. While these studies have contributed greatly to our understanding of the human response to disaster, it has become clear in recent years that, in addition to psychological approaches, neurobiological approaches to disaster-related psychopathology and resilience are also potentially informative.

Multiple neurobiological systems are involved in the human response to threat. Simultaneous activation of various brain regions and neurotransmitter systems allows the organism to assess and appropriately respond to potential dangers. This dynamic process contributes to the development of anxiety, fear, and the "fight or flight" response that allows the organism to protect itself by either fleeing from, or actively confronting, danger. Fear triggers the familiar "fight or flight" response, characterized by acute increased heart rate, breathing, and muscle tension, which facilitate escape from danger or defense against danger (e.g., predator). Based on a complex process of recognition and appraisal of internal and external stimuli, the brain regulates the strength and duration of this coping mechanism, and generally turns it off when it is appropriate to do so. Malfunction of regulatory systems, however, can lead to excessive fear, anxiety disorders such as post-traumatic stress disorder (PTSD) and significant impairment and disability in vulnerable individuals.

Most neurobiological research in PTSD as well as in the neurobiology of resilience has been concentrated on two systems that are critical for survival: the sympathetic nervous system (SNS) and the hypothalamic–pituitary–adrenal (HPA) axis. In this chapter, we will begin by reviewing the findings of human and animal studies which have characterized normal function in the SNS and the HPA axis, and then briefly describe PTSD-associated abnormalities seen in each system. We will then present several evolving models of PTSD, which attempt to explain abnormalities in these two systems. Next, we will review three key neuroanatomic structures/regions involved in the fear response: the amygdala, the hippocampus, and the prefrontal cortex. We will then describe neuroimaging findings associated with PTSD-related changes in structure and function in these three areas. Data on the genetics of risk for PTSD will also be discussed briefly. Finally, the focus on pathology will be supplemented by a brief review of recent findings, elucidating some of the key neural circuits and neurochemical systems that may underlie human resilience in the face of uncontrollable stress.

Although the current review focuses on the noradrenergic system and the HPA axis, it is important to emphasize that numerous neurobiological systems, such as the serotonin system, the opiate

Table 5.1 Sympathetic nervous system
and hypothalamic–pituitary–adrenal (HPA) axis

- Psychophysiologic reactivity
- Increased epinephrine and norepinephrine
- Propranolol
- Sensitization
- Fear conditioning

system, and sex steroidal systems, are also involved in pathological and protective responses to stress, although less is known about their involvement in the genesis of PTSD and other disaster-related psychopathology. While a full discussion of these systems is beyond the scope of this chapter, several other relevant neurotransmitters, neuropeptides, and neurohormones will also be mentioned.

The sympathetic nervous system

Within the central nervous system, noradrenergic neural circuitry serves as one of the brain's principal general alarm systems (Gold & Chrousos, 2002) (see Table 5.1). The highest concentration of noradrenergic cell bodies in the brain is found in the locus ceruleus (LC), located in the mid pons. A single LC neuron can have as many as 100 000 nerve terminals and can innervate cells in multiple structures in the brain (Gold & Chrousos, 2002). The LC is activated by a host of different stressors, both intrinsic (decreased blood volume, hypoglycemia, decreased blood pressure, distension of the colon or bladder) and extrinsic (fear, threat, environmental stress). It has been suggested that the LC is critical in determining the organism's overall state of arousal and attention (Abercrombie & Zigmond, 1995; Robbins & Everitt, 1995). Under conditions of extreme stress, the LC–*norepinephrine* (NE) system operates to privilege instinctual responses, such as the "fight or flight" response, by dampening the functioning of the prefrontal cortex, the seat of higher order complex functioning. During the "fight or flight" response, the SNS increases blood flow to

muscles and vital organs, limits blood loss, and mobilizes energy for use by large muscle groups.

Norepinephrine is also involved in the organism's ability to focus, and to selectively attend to meaningful stimuli. By selectively enhancing strong excitatory or inhibitory input, NE facilitates the processing of relevant stimuli. In related work by Waterhouse and others, NE has been shown to "gate" postsynaptic activity in target neurons (Waterhouse *et al.*, 1988). Thus, target neurons that fail to respond to a particular stimulus become responsive to that same stimulus if sufficient NE is present. Norepinephrine-enhanced responsivity to both excitatory and inhibitory inputs has been reported to occur in the same neocortical cells.

Stressful stimuli of many types produce significant increases in brain noradrenergic activity. Stress produces regional increases in NE turnover in the LC, limbic regions (hypothalamus, hippocampus, and amygdala), and the cerebral cortex. These changes can be produced in animals by subjecting them to immobilization stress, foot shock, or conditioned fear. Repeated exposure to stressors from which the animal cannot escape results in behavioral deficits described as learned helplessness. The learned helplessness state is associated with depletion of NE, probably reflecting the point at which synthesis cannot keep up with demand.

Sympathetic nervous system alterations in PTSD

Findings from clinical physiological, receptor binding, and pharmacologic challenge studies have provided evidence for noradrenergic hyper-reactivity in traumatized individuals with PTSD (Orr *et al.*, 1990; Southwick & Friedman, 2001; Southwick *et al.*, 1999). This exaggerated activity is generally not present under baseline or resting conditions but instead is evident during stress, especially stress associated with traumatic reminders.

Numerous psychophysiological studies have documented heightened SNS arousal in combat veterans who suffer from PTSD (Orr *et al.*, 1990;

Prins *et al.*, 1995). Psychophysiological studies typically measure biological parameters such as heart rate, blood pressure, skin conductance, and electromyographic activity of facial muscles at baseline and in response to various trauma-relevant stimuli, generic stressors, and neutral stimuli.

Script-driven imagery of personally experienced traumas as well as generic visual or auditory reminders of traumas similar to the one experienced by the participant are examples of potential trauma-related stimuli.

Trauma victims with PTSD respond with greater psychophysiological reactivity (particularly heart rate) to trauma-relevant stimuli than do comparison groups such as trauma victims without PTSD and nontraumatized controls. Although some studies have reported a higher baseline resting heart rate in PTSD compared with control groups, most studies have found no differences (Orr *et al.*, 1990; Prins *et al.*, 1995). In addition, response to generic stressors has typically been the same in groups with and without PTSD (Pitman *et al.*, 1990). In summary, trauma survivors with PTSD appear to have normal resting SNS activity as reflected by heart rate and blood pressure that becomes abnormally reactive in response to specific reminders of a personally experienced trauma but not in response to generic stressors (Murburg, 1994; Prins *et al.*, 1995).

Biochemical correlates of this heightened SNS activation in veterans and civilians with PTSD include increased excretion of epinephrine and NE in urine collected over a 24-h period (Davidson & Baum, 1986; Kosten *et al.*, 1987; Yehuda *et al.*, 1992), and decreased numbers of alpha-2 adrenergic receptors on the surface of platelets (Perry, 1994; Perry *et al.*, 1987). Laboratory research suggests that chronically elevated levels of circulating epinephrine and NE may lead to a decrease in the number of adrenergic receptors. In a study designed to assess dynamic functioning of alpha-2 receptors, Perry (1994) incubated intact platelets with high levels of epinephrine and found a greater and more rapid loss in receptor number among subjects with PTSD as compared to controls, suggesting that alpha-2

adrenergic receptors in subjects with PTSD were particularly sensitive to stimulation by the agonist epinephrine (Perry, 1994).

These increases in epinephrine and NE may not be present during resting states. However, compared with healthy controls, it appears that PTSD subjects, as a group, respond to a variety of stressors with exaggerated increases in catecholamines (McFall *et al.*, 1990; Murburg, 1994; Southwick *et al.*, 1995). For example, greater increases in epinephrine have been observed in veterans with war-related PTSD compared with controls during and after viewing a combat film, but not in response to a film of an automobile accident (McFall *et al.*, 1990). Auditory reminders of trauma have also been used as in vivo nonpharmacologic probes of noradrenergic responsivity in combat veterans with PTSD. In a study of 15 combat veterans with PTSD compared to 6 combat veterans without a mental disorder, Blanchard *et al.* (1991) sampled plasma NE before and after exposure to combat-related auditory stimuli. The PTSD group showed a 30% increase in plasma NE compared to no change in the combat control comparison group. The PTSD group also showed a concomitant increase in heart rate (Blanchard *et al.*, 1991).

Pharmacologic provocation studies have also revealed exaggerated catecholamine responses in patients with PTSD as compared to healthy controls without PTSD. To more directly assess adrenergic responsivity of both the peripheral and central nervous system, one study administered intravenous yohimbine to 20 Vietnam combat veterans with PTSD and 18 healthy controls (Southwick *et al.*, 1993). Yohimbine is an alpha-2 adrenergic receptor antagonist that activates noradrenergic neurons by blocking the alpha-2 adrenergic autoreceptor, thereby increasing the release of endogenous NE. Yohimbine caused a marked increase in anxiety and PTSD-specific symptoms, as 70% of combat veterans with PTSD experienced yohimbine-induced panic attacks, and 40% had flashbacks. There were no panic attacks and one flashback in response to placebo. Subjects with PTSD also had significantly greater increases in heart rate and a greater than two fold increase in plasma 3-methoxy-4-hydroxy phenylglycol (MHPG), which is a breakdown product of NE. In the above-cited study, the yohimbine-induced increase in catecholamine activity may have produced a biological context that resembled the biological state at the time of traumatic memory encoding, which then facilitated the retrieval of traumatic memories, a phenomenon known as "state-dependent recall."

To date, interventions designed to suppress noradrenergic hyper-reactivity directly in trauma survivors with PTSD have been limited to open pharmacologic trials with the antiadrenergic agents clonidine (Kinzie & Leung, 1989), guanfacine (Horrigan, 1996), prazosin (Raskind *et al.*, 2002), and propranolol (Pitman *et al.*, 2002). In a randomized double-blind study, Pitman *et al.* administered propranolol 40 mg four times daily vs. placebo to survivors of car accidents within 6 h of the accident. Treatment lasted for 10 days. The study's ability to detect a difference between treatment and control was diminished by bias in loss to follow-up. Although PTSD symptom scores at 1 and 3 months post trauma did not differ significantly between the two groups, at 3 months the propranolol group demonstrated significantly less psychophysiologic reactivity (heart rate, skin conductance, corrugator electromyogram) to mental imagery that symbolized or resembled the index trauma. Positive results with propranolol have also been reported in accident victims presenting to an emergency room with tachycardia (Vaiva *et al.*, 2003). In a recent case report of a woman with PTSD in remission, Taylor and Cahill (2002) described the successful use of propranolol (within 48 h of a new trauma) to treat re-emergent symptoms of PTSD. Those reports are consistent with data in healthy humans, where Southwick *et al.* (1995) found a positive association between enhanced noradrenergic activity and enhanced long-term memory, and Cahill and colleagues reported that propranolol blocked enhanced memory for an arousing story (Cahill *et al.*, 1994). However, it is important to note that preclinical evidence has shown that propranolol can block extinction of fear-related memories (Cain *et al.*, 2004).

Taken together, the above evidence suggests that at least a subgroup of individuals with PTSD has increased responsivity of the SNS that is most clearly evident when the individual is re-stressed (Southwick *et al.*, 1995).

Hypothalamic–pituitary–adrenal (HPA) axis

Whereas the SNS prepares the organism to react to stressful stimuli, the HPA axis appears to serve a catabolic, restorative role (Yehuda, 1997b). When an organism is stressed, the hypothalamus releases corticotropin-releasing hormone (CRH) which then stimulates the release of adrenocorticotropic hormone (ACTH) from the pituitary gland. ACTH in turn stimulates the adrenal gland to release cortisol. Cortisol serves to mobilize and replenish energy stores, and contributes to increased arousal, vigilance, focused attention and memory formation, as well as inhibition of the growth and reproductive systems and containment of the immune response. It also helps to terminate a variety of neurobiological reactions that have been set in motion by stressful stimuli.

Stress-related HPA activation results in transient elevation of plasma cortisol during and shortly after the cessation of the stressful stimulus. It is key, however, that the stress-induced increase in cortisol ultimately be constrained through an elaborate negative feedback system involving glucocorticoid (GC) and mineralocorticoid (MR) receptors. Excessive sustained cortisol secretion can have adverse effects, including hypertension, osteoporosis, immunosuppression, insulin resistance, dyslipidemia, dyscoagulation, and, ultimately, atherosclerosis and cardiovascular disease.

CRH cell bodies and receptors are found in high concentrations in the hypothalamus and throughout the brain, including the prefrontal and cingulate cortices, the central nucleus of the amygdala, as well as the LC. CRH is one of the most important mediators of the stress response, coordinating the adaptive behavioral and physiological changes that occur during stress (Grammatopoulos & Chrousos, 2002). Moreover, intraventricular administration of CRH can produce a variety of behavioral effects that show a striking similarity to those seen following a natural stressor. Given the important role of the amygdala in fear and anxiety it is not surprising that many effects of CRH given intraventricularly may result from actions in the amygdala or closely related structures. In general, these effects are not eliminated by adrenalectomy or hypophysectomy, indicating that they result from direct actions in the brain.

HPA axis alterations in PTSD

The facts that cortisol levels are increased during stress and that the magnitude of the stress response is associated with the magnitude of increases in cortisol led to the hypothesis that cortisol should be increased in PTSD. However, 20 years ago, the first report of cortisol in PTSD yielded counterintuitive results: the mean 24-h urinary excretion of cortisol was lower in patients with PTSD when compared with other psychiatric patients (Mason et al., 1986). Ambiguity has persisted in the literature regarding the direction of any PTSD-associated change in cortisol levels, as some investigators have reported increased urinary cortisol excretion in PTSD. Yehuda (2002) noted that PTSD is associated with a dysregulation of the cortisol response, rather than a clear-cut directional response (cortisol levels that are "too low" or "too high") as would be found in an endocrinopathy.

Present evidence supports the hypothesis that pre-existing low cortisol is associated with increased risk for PTSD. Several recent studies have found that trauma victims who develop PTSD have lower initial cortisol responses to a traumatic event than trauma victims who do not develop PTSD (McFarlane et al., 1997; Resnick et al., 1997). And in combat veterans with chronic PTSD, low plasma levels of cortisol have been recorded throughout the day and night, especially in the early morning and late evening (Yehuda, 2002). Finally, in a randomized double-blind placebo-controlled study, Schelling et al. (2001) assessed the effect of hydrocortisone versus placebo

administered during septic shock. Physiologic stress doses of hydrocortisone did have a moderate protective effect against PTSD (Schelling et al., 2001).

Receptor binding studies have found an increased number of GC receptors in subjects with PTSD compared with controls without PTSD (Yehuda, 1997a; Yehuda et al., 1995a). An increased number of receptors would enhance sensitivity by providing more binding sites for cortisol. Consistent with increased receptor number and sensitivity is the finding that subjects with PTSD hyper-respond to administration of dexamethasone, a synthetic GC that acts like cortisol (Yehuda, 1997a; Yehuda et al., 2004). Normally, when dexamethasone is administered to healthy individuals, it engages GC receptors that serve as part of a negative feedback mechanism. When engaged, these receptors signal the hypothalamus and pituitary to decrease the release of CRH and ACTH, which in turn results in decreased stimulation of the adrenal gland and diminished release of endogenous cortisol. In several different populations of trauma survivors with PTSD, dexamethasone has had an exaggerated effect, with the result that endogenous cortisol release is reduced to a greater degree than in normal controls. These HPA axis findings in PTSD differ markedly from findings in studies of major depressive disorder, where cortisol tends to be elevated, and the cortisol response to dexamethasone administration is reduced.

Additional findings in subjects with PTSD include elevated CRH levels in cerebrospinal fluid (Baker et al., 1997; Bremner et al., 1997), blunted ACTH response to CRH infusion (Smith et al., 1989), and increased ACTH response to metyrapone (Yehuda et al., 2004). These findings are consistent with pre-clinical studies in primates that have experienced early life stress (Coplan et al., 1996). Animal data assessing the effects of a nonpeptide CRH receptor 1 antagonist (antalarmin) that penetrates the blood–brain barrier has found that it blocks the development, consolidation, and expression of conditioned fear (Deak et al., 1999). Recent studies in rhesus macaques also show that oral administration of antalarmin significantly inhibits stress-induced increases in plasma NE, cortisol and anxiety-related behaviors (Habib *et al.*, 2000). If applicable to humans, these data suggest that a CRH antagonist could be helpful after an acute traumatic event, or in preventing harmful CNS changes that occur during chronic stress (Gold *et al.*, 2005).

In summary, most PTSD studies demonstrate alterations consistent with enhanced feedback inhibition of the HPA axis and increased HPA reactivity. The degree to which these abnormalities represent predisposing neurobiological risk factors for the development of PTSD versus consequences of trauma and/or living with PTSD is not yet clear (Yehuda, 2002).

It is also important to note that stressors experienced within critical periods of neurodevelopment may exert long-term effects on HPA axis function. Early postnatal experiences such as maternal separation are associated with long-term alterations in basal concentrations of hypothalamic CRH mRNA, hippocampal glucocorticoid mRNA and the magnitude of the stress-induced release of CRH, corticosterone, and ACTH (Heim & Nemeroff, 2001). Thus, early stress experiences can have long-term consequences on HPA axis responsivity to future stressors.

Stress sensitization

The alterations in both the SNS and the HPA axis that are found in patients with PTSD suggest that sensitization of both systems may contribute to PTSD. Sensitization refers to a stressor-induced increase in behavioral or physiological responsiveness following exposure to subsequent stressors of the same or lesser magnitude (Post, 1992; Post *et al.*, 1995; Prasad *et al.*, 1995). When a neurobiological system becomes sensitized, its behavioral, physiological, and biochemical responses to a given stressor gradually increase in intensity over time. The time interval between the initial stressors appears to be an important factor in the development of sensitization. In some cases, a single stressful stimulus may be capable of initiating behavior sensitization if sufficient time has passed between the initial

stressor and subsequent stressors. Because the organism may be better prepared for future dangers, the capacity to respond more readily to stressors may be adaptive and increase the possibility of survival (Post *et al.*, 1995; Prasad *et al.*, 1995). However, sensitization might also leave the organism in a hyper-responsive state, where it may exhibit exaggerated responses to minor stressors. The organism may become hypervigilant and continue to act biologically as if a danger exists when, in fact, minimal or no threat is present (Southwick *et al.*, 1995).

Evidence characterizing the neurochemical and neuroanatomic systems mediating sensitization is as yet incomplete. The most extensively studied systems in the development and maintenance of stress-induced sensitization in mammals have been catecholamine systems (especially dopamine and NE). Evidence for sensitization of catecholamine systems in humans comes from an earlier cited study where equivalent doses of yohimbine caused significantly greater increases in heart rate, plasma MHPG, anxiety, vigilance, and intrusive memories in combat veterans with PTSD, compared with health controls. Recent genetic studies also suggest that alpha-2 adrenoreceptor gene polymorphisms play a role in baseline catecholamine levels, intensity of stress-induced SNS activation, and rate of catecholamine return to baseline after stress. In a study of healthy subjects, homozygous carriers for the alpha-2 cDel322–325-AR polymorphism had exaggerated total-body noradrenergic spillover at baseline, exaggerated yohimbine-induced increases in anxiety and total-body noradrenergic spillover, and a slower than normal return of total body noradrenergic spillover to baseline after yohimbine infusion (Neumeister *et al.*, 2005). It is possible that such individuals may be more vulnerable to stress-related psychiatric disorders such as PTSD and depression.

The HPA axis may also be sensitized in patients with PTSD. As noted above, in subjects with PTSD compared to controls, researchers have reported elevated levels of CSF CRH, exaggerated suppression of cortisol in response to dexamethasone, and greater CRF-induced increases in ACTH and cortisol. Further, in a study using a personalized trauma script in abused women with and without PTSD, Elzinga *et al.* (2003) reported increased cortisol levels in patients with PTSD as compared with controls.

Fear conditioning

Several investigators have noted that the behavioral and physiological responses of veterans with war neuroses or PTSD (Kardiner & Spiegel, 1947; Kolb, 1987) are similar to the effects of fear conditioning in animals. "Fear conditioning" refers to the process through which a previously innocuous stimulus (unconditioned stimulus or US) is paired with a fear-provoking stimulus and as a result transformed into a fear-conditioned stimulus (CS) that is capable of evoking fear, and related responses, in its own right (Blair *et al.*, 2001).

Fear conditioning can be adaptive. The individual who can predict a threat by responding to conditioned contextual cues can rapidly engage in appropriate defensive behaviors. Clinically, specific environmental stimuli (CS) may be linked to a traumatic event, a spontaneous panic attack, or an embarrassing social situation (US), such that exposure to a similar cue produces a recurrence of symptoms of anxiety and fear. For example, to survivors of the terrorist attacks on the World Trade Center, the sound of an airplane flying overhead may no longer be a neutral stimulus, and, instead, may now serve as a CS that is capable of evoking fear and fear-based behaviors.

Fear conditioning occurs outside of conscious awareness (LeDoux, 1996). A traumatized disaster survivor may not be consciously aware that a formerly neutral stimulus has become frightening because it has been transformed into a fear-conditioned stimulus. Clinically, this means that a traumatized individual, when exposed to a fear-conditioned cue, may become frightened, anxious or irritable for reasons that he or she does not understand.

Fear-conditioned responses, once they are established, can persist for long periods. Theoretically, once a conditioned-fear stimulus is no longer associated with an aversive outcome, the conditioned-fear response should extinguish. However, recent evidence suggests that extinction is an active process that may involve new learning, and that the old fear-conditioned association may persist indefinitely and under the right circumstances become reactivated (Bouton & Nelson, 1994).

While the neurobiological underpinnings of fear conditioning are not completely understood, it is clear that the amygdala plays a pivotal role in both unconditioned and conditioned fear (Aggleton, 1992; Blanchard & Blanchard, 1972).

The amygdala and the hippocampus: key neuroanatomic structures involved in fear and anxiety states

The amygdala, a small almond-shaped structure in the anterior temporal lobe, is a crucial node in a neural network that mediates both conditioned and unconditioned fear (see Table 5.2). Ledoux proposed a cellular-molecular model to explain how the lateral amygdala mobilizes long-term potentiation (LTP), such as changes that permit long-term storage of memories during fear conditioning. The formation of short-term memories requires calcium entry through the N-methyl-D-aspartate (NMDA) receptor (LeDoux, 1996). However, in order to consolidate synaptic changes into long-term memory, in addition to the calcium entry through NMDA receptors, an influx of calcium through voltage-gated calcium channels is required (Blair *et al.*, 2001). In addition to its role in threat and fear conditioning, recent research demonstrates that the amygdala is involved in both the encoding of reward learning (Gottfried *et al.*, 2003) and translating the perception of potential benefit as well as potential harm.

Table 5.2 Neuroanatomy

- Amygdala
- Hippocampus
- Medial prefrontal cortex
- Locus ceruleus

The amygdala is comprised of several separately functioning clusters of cell bodies or nuclei. Key among these nuclei are the basolateral complex and the central nucleus. The basolateral complex receives input from sensory systems and is necessary for acquisition of fear conditioning. The central nucleus is the main output for the basolateral complex and is involved in emotional arousal. Projections from the basolateral complex activate the hypothalamus, the SNS, the reticular nucleus for increased reflexes, the trigeminal nerve and facial nerve for facial expressions of fear, and the ventral tegmental area, LC, and laterodorsal tegmental nucleus for activation of dopamine, NE, and epinephrine systems. The amygdala reacts to dangerous situations by erring on the side of excessive safety – "false positives" and "false alarms."

The amygdala influences the focusing of cortical attention on stimuli that may be associated with threat, even if those stimuli are outside of conscious awareness. In return, these higher cortical structures and associated cortico-striato-thalamic circuits facilitate gating, organizing and bringing into awareness the information conveyed via the senses about the perceived threat. They also provide critical top-down control of the amygdala fear response, suppressing the response once danger has passed or when critical new information has changed the meaning of a potentially threatening situation. This capacity for modulating the "fight or flight" response in response to changes in the perceived meaning of a threat underlies the capacity for cognitive reframing. The ability to reframe threats as challenges or as opportunities for growth is a key component of resilience.

Stress, plasticity and the hippocampus

The hippocampus is instrumental in assessing the context of a threat. Dysfunction of the hippocampus may result in poor contextual stimulus discrimination and overgeneralization of fear responses, which are a cardinal feature of the anxiety disorders (Charney et al., 1993).

Acute stress can suppress neurogenesis in the dentate gyrus (Cameron & Gould, 1996) and in the CA3 region of the hippocampus. Stress-induced increases in adrenal stress hormones and excitatory amino acid neurotransmitters can cause atrophy of dendrites and possibly cognitive impairment in short-term memory and visual-spatial ideational tasks (McEwen, 2002). When stress is severe and prolonged, it can result in actual neuronal loss. Because the hippocampus also exerts inhibitory control over ACTH, damage to the hippocampus can result in even greater increases in glucocorticoids, which in turn cause additional damage to the hippocampus.

Investigations of the hippocampus, using a combination of behavioral, morphological, molecular, and pharmacological approaches, have yielded evidence contrary to the historic view that the adult brain is unable to generate new neurons once they are damaged or lost. Evidence suggests that structural plasticity and neurogenesis in the hippocampus includes structural plasticity, neuronal replacement, remodeling of dendrites, and turnover of synapses. For example, one recent study involving post mortem brains of cancer patients found that the hippocampus retains the capacity for neurogenesis throughout human life (Eriksson et al., 1998). Investigators found that post mortem brains of cancer patients, who had been given the nucleoside analog bromodeoxyuridine (BrdU) for diagnostic studies, still contained the BrdU even though the BrdU had been administered before death. Only dividing cells could have incorporated the BrdU and maintained it in the brain. This suggests that neurogenesis occurred in the hippocampus prior to the death.

Treatment with the serotonin releasing drug D-fenfluramine has been associated with the finding of increased neurogenesis (Gould, 1999) in the adult dentate gyrus. Blockade of serotonergic 5HT1A receptors had the opposite effect, and prevented the effect of D-fenfluramine treatment. Similarly, aerobic exercise has been shown to increase brain-derived neurotrophic factor (BDNF) in the hippocampus and to serve a protective role by buffering against reductions in stress-associated reductions in BDNF.

Cortex and neural circuits

Of the many subcortical brain regions which are active in the stress and fear response, the amygdala and hippocampus have been the most widely studied, but they clearly operate in the context of multiple controls and inputs. One of the most important of these involves cortical circuitry particularly the medial frontal cortex, which provides higher order control over the stress- and fear-related responses of the amygdala and hippocampus.

Under normal conditions, the prefrontal cortex modulates the behavioral, affective, cognitive, and physiological responses typically set in motion by the amygdala during responses to stress. The prefrontal cortex plays key roles in complex problem solving, in part by sequentially switching attention between tasks (Smith & Jonides, 1999). The subgenual prefrontal cortex is involved in cognitively assessing whether a given situation is likely to produce punishment or reward, and in linking affect to changes in the environment (Gold & Chrousos, 2002). The ventral, prefrontal, and subgenual cortex also exert inhibition on the SNS and the HPA axis. Humans with lesions of the subgenual prefrontal cortex show exaggerated autonomic and endocrine responses to stress (Smith & Jonides, 1999).

In contrast to noradrenergic effects mediated by alpha-1 and beta-1 adrenergic receptors, stimulation of alpha-2 adrenoreceptors protects prefrontal cortex cognitive function during stress. Animal research in rodents and primates suggests that prefrontal cortical cognitive functioning is improved by moderate basal release of NE, through its preferential binding to postsynaptic alpha-2 receptors. Psychopharmacologic agents which act on the alpha-2 receptor have been shown to improve cortical functioning in monkeys whose NE has been depleted naturally or experimentally. For example, clonidine and guanfacine have been shown to improve performance on tasks that assess prefrontal

function, whereas the alpha-2 adrenergic receptor antagonist yohimbine impairs performance. The alpha-2 agonist guanfacine is even more potent than clonidine in protecting against stress-induced prefrontal cortex dysfunction (Birnbaum et al., 2000). However, under stressful conditions (particularly uncontrollable stress), when NE release is increased above basal levels in the prefrontal cortex, postsynaptic alpha-1 receptors become activated, resulting in a decline in prefrontal cortex functioning. It has been proposed that this inhibition of prefrontal cortex functioning during stressful or dangerous situations has value for survival by allowing the organism to employ rapid habitual subcortical modes of response (Arnsten & Goldman-Rakic, 1998; Birnbaum et al., 1999). In this way, NE can act as a chemical switch, determining which brain structures have control over behavior. The intracellular signaling initiated by high levels of NE in the prefrontal cortex is the focus of intensive study.

Additionally, the medial prefrontal cortex is involved in fear extinction. In the short term, fear extinction is not just a forgetting or an erasure, but rather an inhibition of an autonomic nervous system response to a conditioned stimulus (Morgan et al., 1993). The ability of firefighters to run into burning buildings demonstrates how cortical inputs can override the autonomic "fight or flight" responses normally associated with an aversive stimulus.

We now briefly review PTSD-related neuroimaging research findings which further characterize the normal structure and function of the amygdala, hippocampus and relevant cortical regions, as well as the abnormalities associated with PTSD.

Neuroimaging in fear and anxiety: focus on PTSD

Neurobiological models of the structure, function and neurochemistry of the brain have evolved significantly as a result of recent input from findings of neuroimaging studies. In humans, neuroimaging studies of PTSD have primarily focused on the amygdala, the hippocampus, medial prefrontal cortex, and anterior cingulate cortex.

PTSD: findings from structural neuroimaging studies

Quantitative magnetic resonance imaging (MRI) studies allow visualization of gross structural abnormalities and provide a method for estimating brain structure volumes. Reduced hippocampal volume has been reported in a diverse population of adults with PTSD, both those with a history of childhood trauma and those who suffered trauma as adults. However, not all published studies report smaller hippocampal findings in subjects with PTSD (Bonne et al., 2001). Possible explanations for discrepant findings of hippocampal volume in PTSD include variability in intensity and duration of trauma exposure, presence of comorbid psychiatric disorders, and differences in imaging methodology (Vythilingam et al., 2005). There is also controversy about how long it may take volume-related changes to occur in trauma survivors with PTSD. Bonne and colleagues found that early after a traumatic event, at 1 week or at 6 months, subjects with PTSD did not have smaller hippocampal volume than subjects without PTSD, nor was there a reduction in hippocampal volume between 1 week and 6 months in these subjects (Bonne et al., 2001). However, more recently, Wignall and colleagues (2004) evaluated 15 patients with PTSD on average 5 months after the trauma, finding significantly reduced right-sided hippocampal volume when compared to controls, after correcting for effects of age and whole-brain volume. Patients also had lower whole-brain volume.

There is also ambiguity in the literature about whether PTSD is associated with reduced hippocampal volume in children (De Bellis et al., 2001). Recent studies suggest that traumatic stress in early development may have more diffuse effects on total brain volume, rather than only effects on hippocampal volume (De Bellis et al., 2002a, 2002b). Additionally, hippocampal volume has been reported to be reduced in burns patients compared to controls. However, hippocampal volume did not differ between burns patients with and without PTSD, suggesting that the trauma associated with being severely burned, as opposed to PTSD per se, was most likely associated with smaller hippocampal volume (Winter & Irle, 2004).

The first study showing decreased hippocampal volume in adults with PTSD was conducted by Bremner and associates (1995), who found that among 26 combat veterans with PTSD, right mean hippocampal volumes were 8% smaller than in healthy combat veterans without PTSD. Those veterans with PTSD and reduced right hippocampal volume also had short-term verbal memory deficits that correlated with hippocampal volume (Bremner et al., 1995). However, in a study of 21 women with histories of severe childhood sexual abuse, 15 of whom had PTSD, significant reductions in left hippocampal volumes were observed in those with abuse histories, but not in controls without abuse histories (Stein et al., 1997). Generalized white matter atrophy as well as bilateral reductions in hippocampal volume were found in another study, with depression and PTSD symptom scores negatively correlated with left hippocampal volume (Villarreal et al., 2002).

Whether the apparent unilaterality of the structural differences reported in these studies is a measurement artifact due to insufficient sample size is not known. The fact that these changes in hippocampal volume may not occur in the first 6 months after a traumatic experience, and that they have not been found in children may indicate that decreased hippocampal volume may take time to develop and/or that it is associated with comorbid mental disorders, or alcohol/substance use. Further, a recent neuroimaging study conducted among identical twins raises the possibility that small hippocampal volume may be a risk factor for developing PTSD. Identical twins of veterans with reduced hippocampal volume and PTSD themselves had reduced hippocampal volume, despite having had no exposure to combat and no history of PTSD. In some individuals, smaller hippocampal volumes may pre-date their trauma exposure and PTSD, and may represent a risk factor for PTSD, rather than a consequence of PTSD (Gilbertson *et al.*, 2002).

PTSD: findings from functional neuroimaging studies

Functional imaging studies using cognitive activation models, script-driven imagery, or other methods of provoking the experience of symptoms have generally found exaggerated activation of the amygdala and/or reduced activation of the prefrontal cortex, to revealing that an overactive amygdala may be receiving insufficient negative feedback from the anterior cingulate gyrus and the medial prefrontal cortex.

To date, most functional imaging studies have examined responses to threat or trauma-relevant stimuli. However, the nature and anatomical bases of attentional and working memory deficits in PTSD are also becoming the focus of intense study in functional neuroimaging. Using positron emission tomography (PET), working memory deficits in PTSD have been found to be associated with reduced left dorsolateral prefrontal cortical (DLPFC) activity (Clark *et al.*, 2003). However, it is also important to sort out how neural networks function in PTSD in the absence of threat-related stimuli. A recent study explored PTSD responses to a selective attention task that engages anterior cingulate cortex networks, but in response to a non-threatening stimulus. Bryant and colleagues (2005) investigated whether anterior cingulate-amygdala dysregulation in PTSD was specific to processing threat-related stimuli, or generalized to more generic, nonthreatening stimuli. They believe that their findings of enhanced anterior cingulate responses, as well as activation in the left amygdala and posterior parietal networks, in response to nonthreatening stimuli, may reflect generalized hypervigilance.

In the first ligand binding neuroimaging study in PTSD, Bremner and colleagues (2000) used ^{123}I iomazenil and single positron emission computer tomography (SPECT) to measure changes in benzodiazepine neuroreceptor binding in combat veterans and matched healthy controls. In the prefrontal cortex, benzodiazepine receptor binding was 41% lower in PTSD (Bremner *et al.*, 2000). It may be that this decrease in receptor binding is associated with chronic PTSD, as Fujita and colleagues (2004) did not replicate this finding in more recently traumatized Desert Storm veterans.

In summary, in PTSD, numerous but not all structural MRI studies have found that decreased hippocampal volume is associated with PTSD in adults. In general, functional neuroimaging studies in trauma survivors with PTSD have reported exaggerated rCBF in the amygdala and other paralimbic regions, as well as relative decreases in prefrontal cortical rCBF. Increased stress-induced activation of the amygdala in combination with reduced inhibition by the prefrontal cortex might leave the trauma survivor with an exaggerated and relatively unchecked amygdala-driven "fight or flight" response.

Genetic risk of stress-related psychopathology

There is mounting evidence that genetic factors influence vulnerability to stress-related psychopathology such as PTSD. In an investigation of twin pairs from the Viet Nam twin Registry, True and colleagues (1993) found that genetic factors accounted for approximately one-third of the variance with regard to PTSD symptoms and exceeded the contributions made by trauma severity. With regard to specific genes, recent studies have failed to confirm an association between a dopamine receptor polymorphism and PTSD (Gelernter *et al.*, 1999).

A recent epidemiologic investigation found that adults possessing a common functional allele (the "s" allele) of a variant of the serotonin transporter gene (5-HTTLPR), which is associated with reduced transcription and functional capacity of the serotonin transporter, were at increased risk for developing depression if they had a history of childhood maltreatment or recent stressful events. Having the "s" allele was not associated with depression in adults who did not have a history of childhood maltreatment or recent stressful events. In contrast, having two "l" alleles appeared to confer relative protection from stress-induced depression (Caspi *et al.*, 2003).

Multidisciplinary studies that use neurochemical, neuroimaging, genetic, and psychosocial approaches may in the future clarify the complex relationships between genotype, phenotype, and psychobiological responses to stress. For example, recent studies have begun to assess gene and environment interactions in the response to extreme stress. In a recent study examining social-support-maltreated children, Kaufman *et al.* (2004) found a moderating effect of social support on the risk of trauma-related depression even in children with the "s" allele of the 5-HTTLPR.

Neurobiology of resilience

While postdisaster psychopathology is relatively common, it is important to note that it is the exception rather than the rule. Even after significant exposures to trauma, most survivors do not develop lasting psychopathology. Increasing interest in stress resilience has led to research on the neurobiological basis of protective factors as well as risk factors for post-traumatic psychopathology. We will briefly review preliminary results of studies characterizing neurochemical, neuroanatomic and genetic factors which may contribute to resilience in the face of stress (see Table 5.3).

Neurochemistry of resilience

In recent years several neurochemicals have been associated with resilience. Undoubtedly the neurochemistry of stress resilience is extremely complex

Table 5.3 Neurobiology of resilience

- Neuropeptide Y
- Galanin
- Neurosteroids
- Neurobiology of social support and attachment
- Neurobiology of trust

---

and the following discussion only touches briefly on a few potential neurochemical candidates.

Neuropeptide Y

Neuropeptide Y (NPY) is a highly conserved 36-amino-acid peptide, and is one of the most abundant peptides found in the mammalian brain. It is also found in the autonomic nervous system, and is colocalized and released with neurons containing NE. In addition to its actions in the modulation of appetite and vascular tone, NPY has anxiolytic properties and has been implicated in the regulation of energy balance, memory, and learning. Neuropeptide Y is released along with NE when the SNS is strongly activated (Southwick *et al.*, 1999). One of its actions is to inhibit the continued release of NE, maintaining SNS activity within an optimum window of activity.

In rats exposed to anxiety-inducing laboratory tests, NPY agonists act as an anxiolytic: microinjection of NPY into the central nucleus of the amygdala reduces anxious behaviors; NPY mRNA becomes upregulated after chronic stress, suggesting that NPY may be involved in adaptation to stress exposure (Thorsell *et al.*, 1999); and NPY opposes the actions of CRH (which is known to increase anxiety-related behaviors).

Preliminary studies in highly resilient special operations soldiers (Special Forces) have shown that during extreme training, robust NPY responses are associated with better performance (Morgan *et al.*, 2000a, 2000b). These robust increases in NPY may constrain the parallel stress-related increases in NE. In contrast, resting and yohimbine-induced levels of NPY have been found to be low in combat veterans with PTSD when compared with controls (Rasmusson *et al.*, 2000). The exaggerated yohimbine-induced increases in heart rate, blood pressure, respiratory rate, anxiety, panic, vigilance, and intrusive combat-related memories observed in combat veterans with PTSD may have resulted from excess release of NE and/or insufficient release of NPY to appropriately contain the robust noradrenergic response (Southwick *et al.*, 1999).

Taken together, these results suggest that the ability to mount a vigorous NPY response in the face of extreme stress may serve as a neurochemical resilience factor.

Galanin

Approximately 80% of noradrenergic cells in the LC co-express the neuropeptide galanin. A dense galanin fiber system originating in the LC innervates the hippocampus, amygdala, and prefrontal cortex, as well as other structures (Gentleman et al., 1989; Perez et al., 2001). Galanin is involved in diverse physiological and behavioral functions, including learning, memory, pain control, and cardiovascular regulation. It is preferentially released under conditions of high NE activity, and, like NPY, reduces the firing rate of neurons in the LC. In animal studies involving rodents, galanin inhibits the firing of rodent NE, serotonin and dopaminergic neurons and reduces their release in forebrain target regions, possibly through a galanin 1 receptor, which acts as an autoreceptor (Sevcik et al., 1993; Xu et al., 2001). Intracerebral administration of galanin reduces fear- and anxiety-related behaviours. Thus, like NPY, galanin appears to modulate the behavioral effects of NE hyperactivity.

Neurosteroids

Dehydroepiandrosterone (DHEA) is a steroid hormone that is synthesized de novo from cholesterol in the central nervous system (Pisu & Serra, 2004). Neurosteroids have heterogeneous effects on fear and anxiety. Some are associated with increases in anxiety and anxiety disorders, while others are associated with anxiolysis. In humans, data support DHEA as a potential neurobiological resilience and stress protective factor. In response to the administration of ACTH, Rasmusson and colleagues (2000) found a negative correlation between DHEA reactivity and severity of PTSD symptoms. Additionally, a positive correlation between the DHEA/cortisol ratio and performance has been observed in Special Forces soldiers undergoing intense survival school training (Morgan et al., 2004).

Neuroanatomic basis of resilience

Neural pathways involved in fear conditioning, consolidation of memory, reconsolidation of memory, and extinction are potentially involved in resilience. These neural circuits have all been implicated in the pathophysiology of PTSD (Bremner et al., 1999). It has been hypothesized that when compared to people who are vulnerable to stress, stress-resilient individuals are less likely to over-consolidate emotional memories, and may have an enhanced ability to reorganize existing emotional memories and extinguish traumatic memories (Charney, 2004b). Such individuals may also be less likely to over-generalize specific conditioned stimuli to a larger context.

In recent years, significant advances have also been made in delineating brain neurocircuitry involved in the regulation of reward and motivation. The mesolimbic dopamine system plays a central role in motivation and reward. In nonhuman primates, the firing patterns of dopamine neurons in the ventral tegmental area are sensitive indices of reward expectations. These neurons increase their firing relative to the predictability of reward, and decrease activity when rewards are omitted or less than expected. They do not change their rate of firing if rewards are consistent with expectations (Yun et al., 2004).

The neural mechanisms that mediate these functions may be relevant to understanding the role that reward plays in some individuals during and in response to a disaster. During acute stress, reward neurocircuitry is activated (Piazza et al., 1996) and it may be that some individuals have exceptionally active reward and motivation neural circuits, enabling them to experience rewards even under extreme uncontrollable stress. It is possible that the capacity for acts of heroism, altruism, and teamwork often reported after a disaster result from enhanced activity in the neural circuitry of motivation and reward. Similarly, optimal functioning in these neural pathways may enhance other resilience-enhancing characteristics, such as the ability to maintain hopefulness, optimism, and a positive outlook when exposed to chronic stress, abuse, and an unrewarding environment (Charney, 2004a). The ability to maintain a positive self concept and hopefulness could lead to an enhanced ability to seek out support and perhaps to bond with other supportive individuals.

Neurobiology of social support and attachment

Among psychological sources of resilience, high levels of perceived psychosocial support have repeatedly been identified as protective. In a study of 2490 Viet Nam veterans, Boscarino and colleagues found that after controlling for level of combat exposure, veterans with low social support had approximately 180% greater risk for PTSD than those with higher levels of social support (Boscarino, 1995). Strong social support has also been associated with better psychological outcomes after a trauma in survivors of a cruise ship disaster (Joseph *et al.*, 1992).

A number of animal studies have implicated the opiate system, oxytocin, and vasopressin in the central mediation of numerous complex social behaviors related to support, including affiliation and parental care. In nonhuman primates, the role of the neuropeptide oxytocin is well established in social interactions, as well as in the initiation of maternal behavior and pair bonding. Recent data from Insel and Winslow demonstrate that a genetically engineered mouse lacking oxytocin emitted few isolation calls and was socially withdrawn (Winslow *et al.*, 2000).

Research on a monogamous rodent, the prairie vole (*Microtus ochrogaster*), and a closely related species, the montane vole (*Microtus montanus*), suggests that oxytocin and vasopressin are also involved in the control of behaviors associated with monogamy, including pair bonding, paternal care, and mate guarding. Prairie and montane voles are similar genetically but vary greatly in their social behavior. The prairie vole is highly social and forms long-lasting attachments (Carter & Getz, 1993; Shapiro & Dewsbury, 1990). Comparative studies in voles have identified species-specific patterns of oxytocin- and vasopressin-receptor expression in the brain that appear to be associated with a monogamous versus nonmonogamous social structure (Young *et al.*, 1998). Molecular studies suggest that differences in the regulation of oxytocin- and vasopressin-receptor gene expression underlie these species differences in receptor distribution. In particular, the more social prairie voles have high levels of oxytocin receptors in the nucleus accumbens and basolateral amygdala relative to the less social montane voles. Similarly, prairie voles have higher densities of the vasopressin 1A receptor on the ventral pallidum and medial amygdala than montane voles (Young *et al.*, 1997). Infusion of vasopressin produced dramatically different effects in the two voles. Prairie voles increased social interaction, whereas montane voles increased nonsocial behaviors such as grooming themselves. The neural mechanisms responsible for the effects of oxytocin and vasopressin on social behavior are thought to involve some of the same circuitry (the nucleus accumbens and ventral pallidum) involved in reward-related behavior.

Neurobiology of trust

In addition to preclinical evidence of oxytocin's involvement in the regulation of social attachment-related behaviors, recent clinical studies in humans suggest a role for oxytocin in promoting trust-associated behaviors. If given intranasally, oxytocin crosses the blood–brain barrier and enters the central nervous system. In a placebo-controlled double-blind study, 37 healthy men were exposed to experimentally produced social stress and randomized to receive intranasal oxytocin or placebo as well as either psychosocial support from a friend during the preparation period or no support. The results showed that oxytocin enhanced the buffering effects of social support on stress responsiveness (Heinrichs *et al.*, 2003), as salivary cortisol responses to stress were reduced.

In another recent study, subjects participated in a game involving the actual exchange of money, and assessed whether the administration of oxytocin to the central nervous system before the game would affect the amount of trusting behavior displayed in the game. Before playing, each individual in the experiment was randomized to receive either an intranasal dose of oxytocin, or an intranasal dose of placebo, and then assigned the role of investor or trustee. In the game, the risk is taken by the investor, and it is based on the uncertainty about how the trustee will behave, i.e., the risk is embedded in a social interaction. Of the 29 subjects, 13 (45%) in the oxytocin group displayed increased trust behavior, compared to only 6 of the 29 (21%) in the placebo group ($p < 0.05$) (Kosfeld et al., 2005).

Concluding remarks

It is anticipated that within disaster mental health, increasing focus on neurobiological as well as psychosocial studies of risk and resilience in the face of uncontrollable stress will lead to the development of new approaches to the prevention and treatment of disaster-related mental distress and mental disorders such as PTSD. Interventions designed to bolster resilience and prevent the development of disaster-related psychopathology will most likely focus on a number of neurobiological processes including stress sensitization, memory consolidation, memory retrieval, fear conditioning, fear extinction, modulation of excessive arousal and limbic reactivity, cortical and executive function, attachment, and relevant gene–environment interactions. Efforts to enhance prevention will require a better understanding of genetic, developmental, and environmental factors that either increase or reduce the risk for developing postdisaster psychopathology. The importance of these factors will differ from one person to the next and require a sophisticated understanding of gene–environment interactions as they relate to trauma exposure and its aftermath. The effect of social support, training and preparedness and stress inoculation on psychosocial and neurobiological resilience is

an emerging and important area of study. In addition to research on prevention, scientists have begun to study the efficacy of early interventions for disaster survivors who become symptomatic. These efforts are challenging since a high percentage of disaster survivors experience some stress-related symptoms immediately after the disaster but only a minority of survivors go on to develop long-standing psychopathology. Accurately predicting which disaster survivors are most likely to develop long-standing psychopathology is of critical importance, since it is well known that repeated bouts of excessive arousal may increase the likelihood that stress-related neurobiological systems (e.g., noradrenergic system and HPA axis) become sensitized and that once these systems are sensitized, treatment is more difficult and probably less successful (Morgan et al., 2003). Currently, psychological and pharmacological interventions are being targeted at survivors who experience excessive peritraumatic arousal (Brewin et al., 1999), dissociation (Bremner et al., 1992; Koopman et al., 1994), and depression (Shalev et al., 1998) because these responses are known to predict later PTSD.

Pharmacological intervention aimed at treating early severe symptoms which are known to be predictive of later PTSD, such as excessive arousal, is one possible avenue of study. One rational pharmacologic approach to treating excess arousal involves the short-term use of hypnotics and benzodiazepine anxiolytics to treat pronounced insomnia and anxiety. Other potential avenues for decreasing arousal in highly symptomatic individuals might include short-term use of anti-adrenergic agents such as propranolol, which may prevent the overconsolidation of fear-related memories and thus prevent PTSD (Morgan et al., 2003; Pitman et al., 2002). As with benzodiazepines, the use of beta-blockers for the treatment of trauma survivors remains controversial, since in addition to potential effects on overconsolidation of emotional memory, beta-blockers have been shown to interfere with extinction of fear-related memories. Another approach might target trauma-induced depressive symptoms. Freedman et al. (1999) found that high levels of depressive symptoms 1 and 5 weeks after a trauma predict the development of PTSD. Already shown to be effective in the treatment of PTSD, selective serotonin reuptake inhibitors (SSRIs) might also be shown in future studies to be effective in the immediate postdisaster period in the prevention of PTSD among at-risk trauma survivors. Other pharmacologic approaches to prevention of PTSD might include the administration of NPY, particularly in people who do not naturally release sufficient amounts. The development of new CRH antagonists such as antalarmin show potential promise in the treatment and prevention of PTSD as well. Randomized trials of pharmacological agents such as these, as well as other interventions aimed at prevention of PTSD in the acute aftermath of trauma are clearly indicated.

REFERENCES

Abercrombie, E. D. & Zigmond, M. J. (1995). Modification of central catecholaminergic systems by stress and injury. In *Psychopharmacology: The Fourth Generation of Progress*, eds. F. E. Bloom & D. J. Kupfer, pp. 355–361. New York: Raven Press.

Aggleton, J. (1992). *The Amygdala: Neurobiological Aspects of Emotion, Memory and Mental Dysfunction*. New York: Wiley-Liss.

Arnsten, A. F. & Goldman-Rakic, P. S. (1998). Noise stress impairs prefrontal cortical cognitive function in monkeys: evidence for a hyperdopaminergic mechanism. *Archives of General Psychiatry*, **55**, 362–368.

Baker, D. G., West, S. A., Orth, D. N. *et al.* (1997). Cerebrospinal fluid and plasma beta-endorphin in combat veterans with post-traumatic stress disorder. *Psychoneuroendocrinology*, **22**, 517–529.

Birnbaum, S., Gobeske, K. T., Auerbach, J., Taylor, J. R. & Arnsten, A. F. (1999). A role for norepinephrine in stress-induced cognitive deficits: alpha-1-adrenoceptor mediation in the prefrontal cortex. *Biological Psychiatry*, **46**, 1266–1274.

Birnbaum, S. G., Podell, D. M. & Arnsten, A. F. (2000). Noradrenergic alpha-2 receptor agonists reverse working memory deficits induced by the anxiogenic drug, FG7142, in rats. *Pharmacology, Biochemistry, and Behavior*, **67**, 397–403.

Blair, H. T., Schafe, G. E., Bauer, E. P., Rodrigues, S. M. & LeDoux, J. E. (2001). Synaptic plasticity in the lateral amygdala: a cellular hypothesis of fear conditioning. *Learning and Memory*, **8**, 229–242.

Blanchard, D. C. & Blanchard, R. J. (1972). Innate and conditioned reactions to threat in rats with amygdaloid lesions. *Journal of Comparative and Physiological Psychology*, **81**, 281–290.

Blanchard, E. B., Kolb, L. C., Prins, A., Gates, S. & McCoy, G. C. (1991). Changes in plasma norepinephrine to combat-related stimuli among Vietnam veterans with posttraumatic stress disorder. *Journal of Nervous and Mental Disease*, **179**, 371–373.

Bonne, O., Brandes, D., Gilboa, A. *et al.* (2001). Longitudinal MRI study of hippocampal volume in trauma survivors with PTSD. *The American Journal of Psychiatry*, **158**, 1248–1251.

Boscarino, J. A. (1995). Post-traumatic stress and associated disorders among Vietnam veterans: the significance of combat exposure and social support. *Journal of Traumatic Stress*, **8**, 317–336.

Bouton, M. E. & Nelson, J. B. (1994). Context-specificity of target versus feature inhibition in a feature-negative discrimination. *Journal of Experimental Psychology Animal Behavior Processes*, **20**, 51–65.

Bremner, J. D., Southwick, S., Brett, E. *et al.* (1992). Dissociation and posttraumatic stress disorder in Vietnam combat veterans. *The American Journal of Psychiatry*, **149**, 328–332.

Bremner, J. D., Krystal, J. H., Southwick, S. M. & Charney, D. S. (1995). Functional neuroanatomical correlates of the effects of stress on memory. *Journal of Traumatic Stress*, **8**, 527–553.

Bremner, J. D., Licinio, J., Darnell, A. *et al.* (1997). Elevated CSF corticotropin-releasing factor concentrations in posttraumatic stress disorder. *The American Journal of Psychiatry*, **154**, 624–629.

Bremner, J. D., Narayan, M., Staib, L. H. *et al.* (1999). Neural correlates of memories of childhood sexual abuse in women with and without posttraumatic stress disorder. *The American Journal of Psychiatry*, **156**, 1787–1795.

Bremner, J. D., Innis, R. B., Southwick, S. M. *et al.* (2000). Decreased benzodiazepine receptor binding in prefrontal cortex in combat-related posttraumatic stress disorder. *The American Journal of Psychiatry*, **157**, 1120–1126.

Brewin, C. R., Andrews, B., Rose, S. & Kirk, M. (1999). Acute stress disorder and posttraumatic stress disorder in victims of violent crime. *The American Journal of Psychiatry*, **156**, 360–366.

Bryant, R. A., Felmingham, K. L., Kemp, A. H. *et al.* (2005). Neural networks of information processing in post-traumatic stress disorder: a functional magnetic resonance imaging study. *Biological Psychiatry*, **58**, 111–118.

Cahill, L., Prins, B., Weber, M. & McGaugh, J. L. (1994). Beta-adrenergic activation and memory for emotional events. *Nature*, **371**, 702–704.

Cain, C. K., Blouin, A. M. & Barad, M. (2004). Adrenergic transmission facilitates extinction of conditional fear in mice. *Learning and Memory*, **11**, 179–187.

Cameron, H. A. & Gould, E. (1996). Distinct populations of cells in the adult dentate gyrus undergo mitosis or apoptosis in response to adrenalectomy. *The Journal of Comparative Neurology*, **369**, 56–63.

Carter, C. S. & Getz, L. L. (1993). Monogamy and the prairie vole. *Scientific American*, **268**, 100–106.

Caspi, A., Sugden, K., Moffitt, T. E. *et al.* (2003). Influence of life stress on depression: moderation by a poly-morphism in the 5-HTT gene. *Science*, **301**, 386–389.

Charney, D. S. (2004a). The neurobiology of anxiety dis-orders. In *Neurobiology of Mental Illness*, eds. D. S. Charney & E. J. Nestler. Oxford: Oxford University Press.

Charney, D. S. (2004b). Psychobiological mechanisms of resilience and vulnerability: implications for successful adaptation to extreme stress. *The American Journal of Psychiatry*, **161**, 195–216.

Charney, D. S., Deutch, A. Y., Krystal, J. H., Southwick, S. M. & Davis, M. (1993). Psychobiologic mechanisms of posttraumatic stress disorder. *Archives of General Psy-chiatry*, **50**, 295–305.

Clark, C. R., McFarlane, A. C., Morris, P. *et al.* (2003). Cerebral function in posttraumatic stress disorder during verbal working memory updating: a positron emission tomography study. *Biological Psychiatry*, **53**, 474–481.

Coplan, J. D., Andrews, M. W., Rosenblum, L. A. *et al.* (1996). Persistent elevations of cerebrospinal fluid concentrations of corticotropin-releasing factor in adult nonhuman primates exposed to early-life stressors: implications for the pathophysiology of mood and anxiety disorders. *Proceedings of the National Acad-emy of Sciences of the United States of America*, **93**, 1619–1623.

Davidson, L. M. & Baum, A. (1986). Chronic stress and posttraumatic stress disorders. *Journal of Consulting and Clinical Psychology*, **54**, 303–308.

De Bellis, M. D., Hall, J., Boring, A. M., Frustaci, K. & Moritz, G. (2001). A pilot longitudinal study of hippo-campal volumes in pediatric maltreatment-related posttraumatic stress disorder. *Biological Psychiatry*, **50**, 305–309.

De Bellis, M. D., Keshavan, M. S., Frustaci, K. *et al.* (2002a). Superior temporal gyrus volumes in maltreated children and adolescents with PTSD. *Biological Psychiatry*, **51**, 544–552.

De Bellis, M. D., Keshavan, M. S., Shifflett, H. *et al.* (2002b). Brain structures in pediatric maltreatment-related posttraumatic stress disorder: a sociodemo-graphically matched study. *Biological Psychiatry*, **52**, 1066–1078.

Deak, T., Nguyen, K. T., Ehrlich, A. L. *et al.* (1999). The impact of the nonpeptide corticotropin-releasing hor-mone antagonist antalarmin on behavioral and endo-crine responses to stress. *Endocrinology*, **140**, 79–86.

Elzinga, B. M., Schmahl, C. G., Vermetten, E., van Dyck, R. & Bremner, J. D. (2003). Higher cortisol levels following exposure to traumatic reminders in abuse-related PTSD. *Neuropsychopharmacology*, **28**, 1656–1665.

Eriksson, P. S., Perfilieva, E., Bjork-Eriksson, T. *et al.* (1998). Neurogenesis in the adult human hippocampus. *Nature Medicine*, **4**, 1313–1317.

Freedman, S. A., Brandes, D., Peri, T. & Shalev, A. (1999). Predictors of chronic post-traumatic stress disorder. A prospective study. *The British Journal of Psychiatry*, **174**, 353–359.

Fujita, M., Southwick, S. M., Denucci, C. C. *et al.* (2004). Central type benzodiazepine receptors in Gulf War veterans with posttraumatic stress disorder. *Biological Psychiatry*, **56**, 95–100.

Gelernter, J., Southwick, S., Goodson, S. *et al.* (1999). No association between D2 dopamine receptor (DRD2) "A" system alleles. *Biological Psychiatry*, **45**, 620–625.

Gentleman, S. M., Falkai, P., Bogerts, B. *et al.* (1989). Dis-tribution of galanin-like immunoreactivity in the human brain. *Brain Research*, **505**, 311–315.

Gilbertson, M. W., Shenton, M. E., Ciszewski, A. *et al.* (2002). Smaller hippocampal volume predicts patholo-gic vulnerability to psychological trauma. *Nature Neuroscience*, **5**, 1242–1247.

Gold, P. W. & Chrousos, G. P. (2002). Organization of the stress system and its dysregulation in melancholic and atypical depression: high vs. low CRH/NE states. *Molecular Psychiatry*, **7**, 254–275.

Gold, P. W., Wong, M. L., Goldstein, D. S. *et al.* (2005). Cardiac implications of increased arterial entry and reversible 24-h central and peripheral norepinephrine levels in melancholia. *Proceedings of the National Academy of Sciences of the United States of America*, **102**, 8303–8308.

Gottfried, J. A., O'Doherty, J. & Dolan, R. J. (2003). Encoding predictive reward value in human amygdala and orbitofrontal cortex. *Science*, **301**, 1104–1107.

Gould, E. (1999). Serotonin and hippocampal neurogenesis. *Neuropsychopharmacology*, **21(2 Suppl)**, 46S–51S.

Grammatopoulos, D. K. & Chrousos, G. P. (2002). Functional characteristics of CRH receptors and potential clinical applications of CRH-receptor antagonists. *Trends in Endocrinology and Metabolism*, **13**, 436–444.

Habib, K. E., Weld, K. P., Rice, K. C. *et al.* (2000). Oral administration of a corticotropin-releasing hormone receptor antagonist significantly attenuates behavioral, neuroendocrine, and autonomic responses to stress in primates. *Proceedings of the National Academy of Sciences of the United States of America*, **97**, 6079–6084.

Heim, C. & Nemeroff, C. B. (2001). The role of childhood trauma in the neurobiology of mood and anxiety disorders: preclinical and clinical studies. *Biological Psychiatry*, **49**, 1023–1039.

Heinrichs, M., Baumgartner, T., Kirschbaum, C. & Ehlert, U. (2003). Social support and oxytocin interact to suppress cortisol and subjective responses to psychosocial stress. *Biological Psychiatry*, **54**, 1389–1398.

Horrigan, J. P. (1996). Guanfacine for PTSD nightmares. *Journal of the American Academy of Child and Adolescent Psychiatry*, **35**, 975–976.

Joseph, S., Andrews, B., Williams, R. & Yule, W. (1992). Crisis support and psychiatric symptomatology in adult survivors of the Jupiter cruise ship disaster. *The British Journal of Clinical Psychology*, **31**, 63–73.

Kardiner, A. & Spiegel, H. (1947). *War, Stress, and Neurotic Illness*. New York: Hoeber.

Kaufman, J., Yang, B. Z., Douglas-Palumberi, H. *et al.* (2004). Social supports and serotonin transporter gene moderate depression in maltreated children. *Proceedings of the National Academy of Sciences of the United States of America*, **101**, 17316–17321.

Kinzie, J. D. & Leung, P. (1989). Clonidine in Cambodian patients with posttraumatic stress disorder. *The Journal of Nervous and Mental Disease*, **177**, 546–550.

Kolb, L. C. (1987). A neuropsychological hypothesis explaining posttraumatic stress disorders. *The American Journal of Psychiatry*, **144**, 989–995.

Koopman, C., Classen, C. & Spiegel, D. (1994). Predictors of posttraumatic stress symptoms among survivors of the Oakland/Berkeley, Calif., firestorm. *The American Journal of Psychiatry*, **151**, 888–894.

Kosfeld, M., Heinrichs, M., Zak, P. J., Fischbacher, U. & Fehr, E. (2005). Oxytocin increases trust in humans. *Nature*, **435**, 673–676.

Kosten, T. R., Mason, J. W., Giller, E. L., Ostroff, R. B. & Harkness, L. (1987). Sustained urinary norepinephrine and epinephrine elevation in post-traumatic stress disorder. *Psychoneuroendocrinology*, **12**, 13–20.

LeDoux, J. (1996). *The Emotional Brain*. New York: Simon and Schuster.

Mason, J. W., Giller, E. L., Kosten, T. R., Ostroff, R. B. & Podd, L. (1986). Urinary free-cortisol levels in post-traumatic stress disorder patients. *The Journal of Nervous and Mental Disease*, **174**, 145–149.

McEwen, B. S. (2002). The neurobiology and neuroendocrinology of stress. Implications for post-traumatic stress disorder from a basic science perspective. *The Psychiatric Clinics of North America*, **25**, 469–494, ix.

McFall, M. E., Murburg, M. M., Ko, G. N. & Veith, R. C. (1990). Autonomic responses to stress in Vietnam combat veterans with posttraumatic stress disorder. *Biological Psychiatry*, **27**, 1165–1175.

McFarlane, A. C., Atchison, M. & Yehuda, R. (1997). The acute stress response following motor vehicle accidents and its relation to PTSD. *Annals of the New York Academy of Sciences*, **821**, 437–441.

Morgan, C. A. 3rd, Wang, S., Mason, J. *et al.* (2000a). Hormone profiles in humans experiencing military survival training. *Biological Psychiatry*, **47**, 891–901.

Morgan, C. A. 3rd, Wang, S., Southwick, S. M. *et al.* (2000b). Plasma neuropeptide-Y concentrations in humans exposed to military survival training. *Biological Psychiatry*, **47**, 902–909.

Morgan, C. A. 3rd, Krystal, J. H. & Southwick, S. M. (2003). Toward early pharmacological posttraumatic stress intervention. *Biological Psychiatry*, **53**, 834–843.

Morgan, C. A. 3rd, Southwick, S., Hazlett, G. *et al.* (2004). Relationships among plasma dehydroepiandrosterone sulfate and cortisol levels, symptoms of dissociation, and objective performance in humans exposed to acute stress. *Archives of General Psychiatry*, **61**, 819–825.

Morgan, M. A., Romanski, L. M. & LeDoux, J. E. (1993). Extinction of emotional learning: contribution of medial prefrontal cortex. *Neuroscience Letters*, **163**, 109–113.

Murburg, M. M. (1994). *Catecholamine Function in Post-Traumatic Stress Disorder: Emerging Concepts.* Washington, D.C.: American Psychiatric Press.

Neumeister, A., Charney, D. S., Belfer, I. *et al.* (2005). Sympathoneural and adrenomedullary functional effects of alpha2C-adrenoreceptor gene polymorphism in healthy humans. *Pharmacogenetics and Genomics*, **15**, 143–149.

Orr, S. P., Claiborn, J. M., Altman, B. *et al.* (1990). Psychometric profile of posttraumatic stress disorder, anxious, and healthy Vietnam veterans: correlations with psychophysiologic responses. *Journal of Consulting and Clinical Psychology*, **58**, 329–335.

Perez, S. E., Wynick, D., Steiner, R. A. & Mufson, E. J. (2001). Distribution of galaninergic immunoreactivity in the brain of the mouse. *The Journal of Comparative Neurology*, **434**, 158–185.

Perry, B. D. (1994). Neurobiological sequelae of childhood trauma; PTSD in children. In *Catecholamine Function in Post-Traumatic Stress Disorders: Emerging Concepts, Progress in Psychiatry*, ed. M. Murburg, pp. 233–255. Washington, D.C.: American Psychiatric Press.

Perry, B. D., Giller, E. L. Jr. & Southwick, S. M. (1987). Altered platelet alpha 2-adrenergic binding sites in posttraumatic stress disorder. *The American Journal of Psychiatry*, **144**, 1511–1512.

Piazza, P. V., Rouge-Pont, F., Deroche, V. *et al.* (1996). Glucocorticoids have state-dependent stimulant effects on the mesencephalic dopaminergic transmission. *Proceedings of the National Academy of Sciences of the United States of America*, **93**, 8716–8720.

Pisu, M. G. & Serra, M. (2004). Neurosteroids and neuroactive drugs in mental disorders. *Life Sciences*, **74**, 3181–3197.

Pitman, R. K., Orr, S. P., Forgue, D. F. *et al.* (1990). Psychophysiologic responses to combat imagery of Vietnam veterans with posttraumatic stress disorder versus other anxiety disorders. *Journal of Abnormal Psychology*, **99**, 49–54.

Pitman, R. K., Sanders, K. M., Zusman, R. M. *et al.* (2002). Pilot study of secondary prevention of posttraumatic stress disorder with propranolol. *Biological Psychiatry*, **51**, 189–192.

Post, R. M. (1992). Transduction of psychosocial stress into the neurobiology of recurrent affective disorder. *The American Journal of Psychiatry*, **149**, 999–1010.

Post, R. M., Weiss, S. R., Smith, M., Rosen, J. & Frye, M. (1995). Stress, conditioning, and the temporal aspects of affective disorders. *Annals of the New York Academy of Sciences*, **771**, 677–696.

Prasad, B. M., Sorg, B. A., Ulibarri, C. & Kalivas, P. W. (1995). Sensitization to stress and psychostimulants. Involvement of dopamine transmission versus the HPA axis. *Annals of the New York Academy of Sciences*, **771**, 617–625.

Prins, A., Kaloupek, D. G. & Keane, T. M. (1995). Psychophysiological evidence for autonomic arousal and startle in traumatized adult populations. In *Neurobiological and Clinical Consequences of Stress: From Normal Adaptation to Post-Traumatic Stress Disorder*, eds. M. J. Friedman, D. S. Charney & A. Y. Deutch, pp. 291–314. Philadelphia: Lippincott-Raven.

Raskind, M. A., Thompson, C., Petrie, E. C. *et al.* (2002). Prazosin reduces nightmares in combat veterans with posttraumatic stress disorder. *The Journal of Clinical Psychiatry*, **63**, 565–568.

Rasmusson, A. M., Hauger, R. L., Morgan, C. A. *et al.* (2000). Low baseline and yohimbine-stimulated plasma neuropeptide Y (NPY) levels in combat-related PTSD. *Biological Psychiatry*, **47**, 526–539.

Resnick, H. S., Yehuda, R. & Acierno, R. (1997). Acute post-rape plasma cortisol, alcohol use, and PTSD symptom profile among recent rape victims. *Annals of the New York Academy of Sciences*, **821**, 433–436.

Robbins, T. & Everitt, B. J. (1995). Central norepinephrine neurons and behavior. In *Psychopharmacology: The Fourth Generation of Progress*, eds. F. E. Bloom & D. J. Kupfer, pp. 363–372. New York: Raven Press.

Schelling, G., Briegel, J., Roozendaal, B. *et al.* (2001). The effect of stress doses of hydrocortisone during septic shock on posttraumatic stress disorder in survivors. *Biological Psychiatry*, **50**, 978–985.

Sevcik, J., Finta, E. P. & Illes, P. (1993). Galanin receptors inhibit the spontaneous firing of locus coeruleus neurones and interact with mu-opioid receptors. *European Journal of Pharmacology*, **230**, 223–230.

Shalev, A. Y., Freedman, S., Peri, T. *et al.* (1998). Prospective study of posttraumatic stress disorder and depression following trauma. *The American Journal of Psychiatry*, **155**, 630–637.

Shapiro, L. E. & Dewsbury, D. A. (1990). Differences in affiliative behavior, pair bonding, and vaginal cytology in two species of vole (*Microtus ochrogaster* and *M. montanus*). *Journal of Comparative Psychology*, **104**, 268–274.

Smith, E. E. & Jonides, J. (1999). Storage and executive processes in the frontal lobes. *Science*, **283**, 1657–1661.

Smith, M. A., Davidson, J. & Ritchie, J. C. (1989). The corticotropin-releasing hormone test in patients with post-traumatic stress disorder. *Biological Psychiatry*, **26**, 349–355.

Southwick, S. M. & Friedman, M. J. (2001). Neurobiological models of posttraumatic stress disorder. In *The Mental Health Consequences of Torture*, eds. E. Gerrity, T. M. Keane & F. Tuma, pp. 73–87. New York: Kluwer Academic/Plenum Publishers.

Southwick, S. M., Krystal, J. H., Morgan, C. A. *et al.* (1993). Abnormal noradrenergic function in posttraumatic stress disorder. *Archives of General Psychiatry*, **50**, 266–274.

Southwick, S. M., Yehuda, R. & Morgan, C. A. (1995). Clinical studies of neurotransmitter alterations in posttraumatic stress disorder. In *Neurobiological and Clinical Consequences of Stress: From Normal Adaptation to Post-Traumatic Stress Disorder*, eds. M. J. Friedman, D. S. Charney & A. Y. Deutch, pp. 335–349. Philadelphia: Lippincott-Raven.

Southwick, S. M., Bremner, J. D., Rasmusson, A., Morgan, C. A. 3rd, Arnsten, A. & Charney, D. S. (1999). Role of norepinephrine in the pathophysiology and treatment of posttraumatic stress disorder. *Biological Psychiatry*, **46**, 1192–1204.

Stein, M. B., Koverola, C., Hanna, C., Torchia, M. G. & McClarty, B. (1997). Hippocampal volume in women victimized by childhood sexual abuse. *Psychological Medicine*, **27**, 951–959.

Taylor, F. & Cahill, L. (2002). Propranolol for reemergent posttraumatic stress disorder following an event of retraumatization: a case study. *Journal of Traumatic Stress*, **15**, 433–437.

Thorsell, A., Carlsson, K., Ekman, R. & Heilig, M. (1999). Behavioral and endocrine adaptation, and up-regulation of NPY expression in rat amygdala following repeated restraint stress. *Neuroreport*, **10**, 3003–3007.

True, W. R., Rice, J., Eisen, S. A. *et al.* (1993). A twin study of genetic and environmental contributions to liability for posttraumatic stress symptoms. *Archives of General Psychiatry*, **50**, 257–264.

Vaiva, G., Ducrocq, F., Jezequel, K. *et al.* (2003). Immediate treatment with propranolol decreases posttraumatic stress disorder two months after trauma. *Biological Psychiatry*, **54**, 947–949.

Villarreal, G., Hamilton, D. A., Petropoulos, H. *et al.* (2002). Reduced hippocampal volume and total white matter volume in posttraumatic stress disorder. *Biological Psychiatry*, **52**, 119–125.

Vythilingam, M., Luckenbaugh, D. A., Lam, T. *et al.* (2005). Smaller head of the hippocampus in Gulf War-related posttraumatic stress disorder. *Psychiatry Research*, **139**, 89–99.

Waterhouse, B. D., Sessler, F. M., Cheng, J. T. *et al.* (1988). New evidence for a gating action of norepinephrine in central neuronal circuits of mammalian brain. *Brain Research Bulletin*, **21**, 425–432.

Wignall, E. L., Dickson, J. M., Vaughan, P. *et al.* (2004). Smaller hippocampal volume in patients with recent-onset posttraumatic stress disorder. *Biological Psychiatry*, **56**, 832–836.

Winslow, J. T., Hearn, E. F., Ferguson, J. *et al.* (2000). Infant vocalization, adult aggression, and fear behavior of an oxytocin null mutant mouse. *Hormones and Behavior*, **37**, 145–155.

Winter, H. & Irle, E. (2004). Hippocampal volume in adult burn patients with and without posttraumatic stress disorder. *The American Journal of Psychiatry*, **161**, 2194–2200.

Xu, Z. Q., Tong, Y. G. & Hokfelt, T. (2001). Galanin enhances noradrenaline-induced outward current on locus coeruleus noradrenergic neurons. *Neuroreport*, **12**, 1779–1782.

Yehuda, R. (1997a). Sensitization of the hypothalamic–pituitary–adrenal axis in posttraumatic stress disorder. *Annals of the New York Academy of Sciences*, **821**, 57–75.

Yehuda, R. (1997b). Stress and glucocorticoid. *Science*, **275**, 1662–1663.

Yehuda, R., Southwick, S., Giller, E. L., Ma, X. & Mason, J. W. (1992). Urinary catecholamine excretion and severity of PTSD symptoms in Vietnam combat veterans. *The Journal of Nervous and Mental Disease*, **180**, 321–325.

Yehuda, R., Boisoneau, D., Lowy, M. T. & Giller, E. L. Jr. (1995a). Dose–response changes in plasma cortisol and lymphocyte glucocorticoid receptors following dexamethasone administration in combat veterans with and without posttraumatic stress disorder. *Archives of General Psychiatry*, **52**, 583–593.

Yehuda, R., Kahana, B., Binder-Brynes, K. *et al.* (1995b). Low urinary cortisol excretion in Holocaust survivors with posttraumatic stress disorder. *The American Journal of Psychiatry*, **152**, 982–986.

Yehuda, R., Golier, J. A., Halligan, S. L., Meaney, M. & Bierer, L. M. (2004). The ACTH response to dexamethasone in PTSD. *The American Journal of Psychiatry*, **161**, 1397–1403.

Young, L. J., Winslow, J. T., Nilsen, R. & Insel, T. R. (1997). Species differences in V1a receptor gene expression in monogamous and nonmonogamous voles: behavioral consequences. *Behavioral Neuroscience*, **111**, 599–605.

Young, L. J., Wang, Z. & Insel, T. R. (1998). Neuroendocrine bases of monogamy. *Trends in Neurosciences*, **21**, 71–75.

Yun, I. A., Wakabayashi, K. T., Fields, H. L. & Nicola, S. M. (2004). The ventral tegmental area is required for the behavioral and nucleus accumbens neuronal firing responses to incentive cues. *The Journal of Neuroscience*, **24**, 2923–2933.

PART III

Clinical care and interventions

6

Early intervention for trauma-related problems following mass trauma

Patricia J. Watson

Over the last decade, the field of post-traumatic early intervention has made a concerted effort to evaluate and recommend interventions that have the potential to attenuate suffering and/or facilitate recovery trajectories following mass traumatic events. Progress in this field has been beset by difficulties in obtaining empirical support, as well as lack of a conceptual framework in which to organize clinical, consensus, and research recommendations. Interventions in the immediate aftermath of mass traumatic events have received very little solid research support, and, in the absence of a theoretically derived organizing framework, interventionists often perceive two contradictory recommendations from "experts": an "intervention for all" (e.g., group debriefing) strategy, and a "wait and see" strategy (i.e., do nothing before the passage of time reveals those in need of formal treatment from those who recover on their own). There are no comparative studies of the two different intervention strategies at this time, and limited data to support either strategy.

While other chapters in the volume have focused on long-term intervention strategies following disaster, this chapter addresses public mental health interventions in the immediate phase following disasters and mass violence. In most literature related to mass violence interventions (Shalev & Ursano, 2004), the immediate phase has been identified as 0–14 days postincident; intermediate phase, 14 days to 3 months; and the later phase, 3 months onward.

While interventions may be similar across phases, this differentiation takes into account the expected trajectory of recovery from trauma, as well as the changing needs of survivors across time. Disasters, terrorism, and mass violence situations do not always have clearly defined time boundaries, such as in situations of ongoing threat. The empirical literature is therefore examined in light of these phases, while taking into account the somewhat arbitrary nature of their boundaries.

Due to the dearth of empirical studies examining immediate postdisaster interventions, discussion and recommendations that follow draw heavily from theoretical conceptualizations, extrapolations from individual trauma interventions, and consensus recommendations evolving from expert panel discussions and consensus conferences. Necessary next steps regarding the further development and refinement of acute public mental health interventions for mass violence and disaster will be addressed at the end of the chapter.

Empirical literature base

Studies of the impact of disasters

Researchers wishing to conduct methodologically sound studies on acute interventions following disaster face many methodological challenges. Early interventions typically take place in chaotic and uncontrolled settings, with little preplanning, funding or coordination between researchers and interventionists, a focus on action and assistance rather than research, and cross-community barriers between local responders and external researchers. Additionally, there has been a lack of empirical support or clear theoretical guidance on which to build potential interventions. These dilemmas are troubling given that randomized, controlled trials are particularly needed in the acute time frame where symptoms are labile and varied, the majority of responses cannot be clearly defined into prescriptive diagnostic categories, and most individuals naturally experience a rapid decline in symptoms (Brewin & Saunders, 2001; Valentiner et al., 1996). Random assignment to experimental or control groups maximizes the chances that improved functioning and symptom reduction are due to the research intervention rather than to a natural, expected change over time or to self-referral for the intervention.

Therefore, in the absence of well-controlled intervention studies, an initial examination of the effects of disasters, as well as risk and protective factors, has often been the basis for developing interventions that foster identified protective factors and ameliorate vulnerability factors. While a full review of this literature is covered elsewhere in this volume, a recent review of the effects of disasters by Norris and Elrod (2006) indicated that seeking to reduce the long-term impact of disasters is a valid pursuit based purely on the findings on magnitude of events. While the majority (50%) of disaster studies reviewed showed moderate effects, indicative of increased or prolonged stress but little enduring psychopathology, a significant proportion of studies showed severe (24%) or very severe (17%) effects, indicative of a high (25%–49%) or very high (50% +) prevalence of clinically significant distress or psychological disorder. However, in general, symptoms and effects were most likely exhibited in the first year postdisaster, with 70% of the samples showing improvement as time passed. In many studies, levels of symptoms in the early phases of disaster recovery were good predictors of symptom levels in later phases of recovery, consistent with literature on trauma in general (Brewin et al., 2002).

Rates of traumatic stress disorders and functional impairment in the general population may be somewhat low over time, as evidenced by recent epidemiological studies following the September 11 terrorism attack in New York (Galea et al., 2002). Galea found a sharp decline in post-traumatic stress disorder (PTSD) symptoms in New York over the course of 6 months, from 7.5% to 0.6%. However, of those with strong exposure to the incident, such as those in the buildings or injured, rates were 37% and 30%, respectively. Therefore, not everyone will require early interventions, particularly in the immediate aftermath of disaster, and some level of screening for predictors of continued distress is recommended, although other than symptom severity at 1–2 weeks post-trauma, no algorithm for predictive factors has been created as yet (McNally et al., 2003).

The question of normal reactivity versus pathognomonic status is noteworthy. Many researchers are attempting to address the question of when distress ceases to be a "sign" of exposure and becomes instead a "symptom" of dysfunction. Galea's work gives the basis for understanding normal refractory curves in this circumstance, and Bonanno's work related to grief and resilience indicates that there are many possible "trajectories of reactivity" following traumatic insult, including increased adaptive functioning (Bonanno, 2004). It remains to be seen whether introducing early interventions in the immediate phase postevent is a necessary or even desired strategy for significantly facilitating an accelerated or enhanced recovery for the majority of affected individuals.

Of those individuals exhibiting a negative recovery trajectory following disasters, the effects most commonly observed in research samples were: PTSD (with intrusion and arousal more often prevalent and avoidance less so), dissociative responses, acute stress disorder, depression, anxiety, demoralization, perceived stress, negative affect, physical health problems and/or somatic concerns, high physiological indicators of stress, poor sleep quality, and increases in the use of alcohol, and drugs (which generally are more persistent in nature than mental health effects; Schlenger *et al.*, 2002). Declines in psychosocial resources (particularly declines in social embeddedness and perceived social support) as well as chronic problems in living (interpersonal, familial, financial, and ecological changes and stress) have sometimes been defined as mediating factors that intervene between acute exposure and chronic psychological effects (Norris & Elrod, 2006). The breadth of the outcomes observed indicated that researchers should not focus too narrowly on any one aspect of mental health, and that interventions aimed at those suffering from lasting negative impacts should seek to address the multitude of possible effects of disasters, and to foster the protective mediating factors and reduce vulnerability factors.

Of the factors commonly influencing the likelihood of serious or lasting psychological problems following disasters (Norris & Elrod, 2006), severity of exposure has been one of the strongest, defined differentially as number of stressors, bereavement, injury to self or family member, life threat, panic during the disaster, property damage or financial loss and relocation. Other factors include: female gender, middle-age range, specific minority ethnic group membership, lower socioeconomic status, spouse's symptom severity, parenthood, parental distress (predicts child distress), predisaster psychological symptoms (one of the best predictors of postdisaster symptoms), avoidance coping, and assignment of blame.

Protective factors following disasters include active outreach, informed pragmatism, reconciliation, coping self-efficacy (the perception that one is capable of managing the specific demands related to the disaster), higher perceived control, self-esteem, trait hopefulness, future temporal orientation, optimism, and hardiness, social embeddedness (the size, activeness, and closeness of the network), received support, and perceived support (the general sense of belongingness and belief in the availability of support). The effects of certain variables are mediated by other variables; e.g., acute stressors increase the likelihood of chronic stressors, which in turn increase the likelihood of psychological distress. Reviews of the literature call for research to aim for a more fully integrated understanding of how factors interact and increase or decrease postdisaster vulnerability (Norris & Elrod, 2006; Layne *et al.*, in press).

Theoretical models of stress, trauma, and disasters

The dearth of empirical literature to support interventions in the immediate phase postincident is compounded by a lack of a systematic conceptual framework for defining, investigating, and utilizing information relating to mediating variables such as risk, protective, and vulnerability factors, and the mechanisms, processes, and pathways of influence through which they exert their influence (Layne *et al.*, in press). The theories reviewed here are offered as an introduction to conceptual approaches.

Research on postdisaster mental health belongs to the broader field of stress research. Specific theories of the stress process differ in their relative attention to the different components of the model, be they stressor characteristics, appraisals, or vulnerabilities/resources. Stress theory generally assumes that external *demands* (e.g., the traumatic event as primary stressor) evoke *responses* that draw on inner and external *resources*. Loss of resources, either concrete (social, financial) or symbolic (beliefs, expectations) may, as secondary stressors, significantly impact the recovery trajectory (Raphael & Wilson, 2000). Survivors' own responses (e.g., anxiety, insomnia, depression) may additionally tax overall resources, becoming tertiary stressors (Bryant *et al.*, 1998). With sufficient infusion of resources and the passage of time, recovery is the expected outcome of time-limited exposure to a stressor (with great variation depending on the intensity and duration of the stressor) (Hobfall, 1989; Shalev, in preparation). Stress management therefore typically involves identifying and ameliorating those factors that interfere with recovery (e.g., lack of supportive others, ongoing stressors, maladaptive beliefs), and providing the resources that help to support, organize, and help make a plan for survivors (Norris *et al.*, 2002a, b, c).

Studies on the relative contribution of early arousal to subsequent PTSD, and the possible pharmacological strategies to reduce expressed adrenergic activity, suggest that the initial "stress response" is a necessary but insufficient cause of traumatic stress disorders (Ozer *et al.*, 2003; Shalev, unpublished manuscript). Within stress theory, four observable indicators of successful coping are: (1) sustained task performance, (2) controllability of emotion, (3) sustained capacity to enjoy rewarding human contacts, and (4) a sustained sense of personal worth (Shalev, 2002). Accordingly a failure to cope will be expressed in reduced task performance, overwhelming emotions, inability to relate to others and self-blame (or self-denigrating rumination). The expected outcome of stress management is better coping, as expressed by improved task performance, better interpersonal interactions, controllable emotion, and sustained self-esteem. Early interventions for those who have suffered severe stress may facilitate this outcome by providing interventions designed to reduce excessive, uncontrollable distress, correct negative appraisal, facilitate social connectedness, and provide pragmatic resources. For instance, solution-focused methods assist survivors to identify and utilize their strengths in the recovery process by helping them to define concerns, imagine and set goals, identify strategies to achieve the goals, and develop an action plan.

Studies on the relative contribution of early arousal to subsequent PTSD, and the possible pharmacological strategies to reduce expressed adrenergic activity, suggest that the initial "stress response" is a necessary but not sufficient cause of traumatic stress disorders (Ozer *et al.*, 2003; Shalev, unpublished manuscript). Traumatic stress theories often draw on psychobiological research that has identified and mapped biological processes distinctly reactive to traumatic stress (Greene *et al.*, 2000; Pearlin & Schooler, 1978). These findings support the proposition that when traumatic responses are overwhelming, uncontrollable, and involve extreme physiological arousal they may consolidate the link between fear and traumatic recall, leading to avoidance, repeated recall, and ultimately to PTSD. Additional adversity, such as often seen in the aftermath of major disaster, can create a chain of mutually reinforcing reactions, the memory of which may be etched forever in a person's brain.

Ehlers and Clark's (2000) cognitive model of trauma provides the most detailed account of the maintenance and treatment of PTSD, with support from research findings. This model suggests that individuals are at higher risk for persistent PTSD when they make excessively negative appraisals of the trauma and exhibit disturbed memory processes such as poor elaboration and contextualization, strong associative memory, and strong perceptual priming. In the acute period, certain styles of peri-traumatic cognitive processing contribute to the development of disorganized or problematic memories that, in turn, increased risk for subsequent PTSD (Halligan *et al.*, 2003). Because a central process in PTSD response is an inability to distinguish past trauma associations of threat with current conditions, these researchers advocate interventions that assist with contextual discrimination of past and present circumstances.

Therefore, in those at significant risk for developing PTSD, efforts to reduce stress alone are not sufficient to prevent PTSD. Intrusive recollections do not abate when the stressor ends, and are not amenable to "stress management." They challenge rules, expectations and assumptions, as well as the worldview and the ability to discriminate between past and present cues, and therefore pose a different challenge. Shalev therefore proposes the necessity of processing incongruous, intrusive, distressing, and unremitting recollections, as well as the cognitive and behavioral response to them, that are the unique factors that should be addressed by trauma interventions above and beyond stress management (Watson & Shalev, 2005).

Dual representation theories of trauma such as the Brewin's cognitive model (Brewin *et al.*, 1996; Brewin & Holmes, 2003) and the Schematic,

Propositional, Analogue, and Associative Representational Systems (SPAARS) model of emotional experiences, suggest that traumatic information and memories are encoded at multiple levels: (1) *propositionally*, in readily accessible verbal form, and (2) *analogically* as visual, olfactory, auditory, gustatory, body state, and proprioceptive "images," which are not amenable to voluntary control, do not decay with time, and must be further "processed" in order to become normal autobiographic recollections (that is, amenable to voluntary recall and forgetfulness) (Dalgleish, 2004). Finally, memory and information is encoded *schematically*, as abstract, generic knowledge that integrates information from the prepositional and analog representations. Information is proposed to be organized via dominant (supraordinate) schematic representations of the world, self, and others, such as "self as competent." New information streams are filtered in favor of those congruent to the supraordinate schema, and individuals differ as to how inhibitory versus integrative they are of information that does not conform with existing schemas. These proposed responses show that pre-existing life events, defensive styles, and schematic representations of the world and self may affect how an individual reacts to and recovers from trauma.

There are many implications for acute interventions derived from this model. First, the model hypothesizes that the body's response to threat remains active until physical safety is restored. Survivors cannot begin to integrate a threatening experience in the context of ongoing fear activation in the body. Greater exposure, pain, injury, and life threat will clearly increase the need for establishing safety as the first step in recovery. When physical safety is restored, the environment can then begin to act as a proxy for restoring world schemas of safety, predictability, and controllability. Providers can additionally help early on by encouraging self-schemas of competence and control regarding survival, recovery, self-care, and care of others.

Second, the model accounts for differential reactions to post-trauma interventions. For instance, in individuals whose pretrauma schemata are characterized by viewing the world or self in a negative way, exposure to the trauma memory may become potentially overwhelming, as any buffering effects of pretrauma world schemata are absent. While individuals with balanced prior-life schemata may recover with social support and resources, vulnerabilities in some individuals may require additional assistance from mental health providers.

Third, the model posits that different predominant emotions may require different intervention foci. Because fear is a prospective emotion, in individuals with sufficiently positive pretrauma schemas, exposure to the traumatic memory via self-paced retelling of the incident is apt to reduce fear as the memory becomes integrated with a positive recovery environment. However, emotions such as anger, shame, and guilt are retrospective. If these emotions are the predominant response to the trauma, recounting of the trauma memory is likely to accentuate them, and therefore reframing and redirection (from past to future perspective) techniques may be more appropriate interventions.

Finally, the information and memories about the trauma may be represented differently in the prepositional (verbal) and analog (visual, bodily, sensory) systems, so that access via one system may not sufficiently allow for full integration of the trauma information in another system. Evidence suggests that information can move interchangeably between analog, prepositional, and schematic representations in most individuals, but it may be that pretrauma factors impede the interchangeability of information across systems for some individuals. For those individuals resistant or unresponsive to cognitive interventions, there may be a need to work directly with imagery/bodily/sensory processes to access the analog system. Additionally, there is evidence that a tapping task in the immediate aftermath of a traumatic event may prevent encoding of trauma information in the analog system, resulting in a reduction in intrusions, while not precluding the encoding of trauma information in the prepositional system (Brewin & Saunders, 2001). More research stimulated by this multi-representational cognitive model may provide impetus for the development of new treatment methods in the immediate phase post-trauma.

Social cognitive theory places the individual as an active contributor to the adaptive process, suggesting that communities have a proactive role in the recovery process including planning and constructing environmental conditions to promote successful resolution (Bandura, 1997, 2001). Within this framework, a variety of environmental factors have been identified that protect or buffer individuals from the effects of stressors (Cassel, 1976). In the Conservation of Resources theory (Hobfoll, 1989), stress occurs when critical resources (e.g., food, housing, shelter) as well as psychological resources (e.g., self-esteem and mastery) are threatened or lost, and loss spirals result when those with depleted resources lose ever more critical resources as they attempt to cope. A number of disaster studies have provided strong support that resource loss is highly predictive of psychological outcomes (Benight et al., 2004). Intervention implications from this theory suggest an important intervention component is physical and psychological/social resource investment over the recovery period, and with those who are more at risk for loss spirals.

Social resources, such as social support, socio-economic status, and access to services, have shown strong effects on mental health and played a variety of roles in the stress process (Norris & Murrell, 1984). Social cognitive theorists have speculated that this can come about for a number of reasons (Benight et al., 2004). For example, supportive actions of fellow disaster survivors model effective coping responses, and provide encouragement and reinforcement for healthy adaptation. These positive effects of social support serve then to elevate perceptions of one's own coping self-efficacy, an important individual factor in predicting disaster outcomes (Benight & Bandura, 2004). Mediational analyses support this hypothesis and show that social support provides its benefits to the extent that it raises perceived self-efficacy to manage environmental demands (Benight et al., 1999).

However, beyond receiving positive social support, a number of research studies on social support indicate that it is not positive, but negative social support that impacts recovery. For example, in a study of 41 adult Outward Bound participants, it was found that the amount of social support strongly predicted changes in participants' "psychological resilience" (Neill & Dias, 2001). In this study, there were four measures of social support – overall group support, instructor support, support from the most supportive group member, and support from the least supportive group member. Interestingly, it was the support received from the least supportive person that best predicted gains in resilience. Dunmore et al. (2001) report that it is the perception of negative social interactions rather than perceived positive support that predicts chronic PTSD. These research findings point to the need for introducing programs that reinforce social support and modeling, reinforce a sense of coping self-efficacy, and provide feedback and education to family and friends about the effects of providing low or negative support, as well as providing support to those individuals who are perceiving that they are receiving low support.

The "Social Support Deterioration Model" posits that declines in perceived support and social embeddedness are critical mediators of the adverse effects of disaster exposure on mental health (Kaniasty & Norris, 1993). The model cautions that deterioration of social support may be deterred when sufficient resources are received after the event, but that various social, political, and cultural dynamics interfere with the adequacy and equity of resource distribution. Implications for intervention include cross-community collaboration regarding attention to social, political, and cultural dynamics that may interfere with the perception of resource adequacy and equity.

Intervention studies

To date, there are few published randomized controlled trials (RCTs) of interventions initiated in the first 14 days following mass violence. As a number of reviews of the literature have concluded, Critical Incident Stress Debriefing (CISD), a structured

group model designed to explore facts, thoughts, reactions, and coping strategies following trauma, has not yielded any evidence that it prevents long-term negative outcomes. Additionally, there have been two RCTs of CISD that reported a higher incidence of negative outcomes in those who received CISD compared with those who did not receive an intervention (Bisson, 2003; Litz et al., 2002; McNally et al., 2003; Watson et al., 2002). In a recent large-scale RCT of a group debriefing intervention with active duty personnel, Litz and colleagues (2004) found no differences among the CISD, stress education, and survey-only conditions on any behavioral health outcome, including PTSD, depression, general well-being, aggressive behavior, marital satisfaction, perceived organizational support, or morale. Heart rate and blood pressure readings before and after the sessions did not indicate a change in physiological stress; subjective ratings of distress did not change pre to post-session; soldiers rated their satisfaction with CISD as high; and mental health outcomes at follow-up did not worsen as a result of CISD. Similar studies with civilian populations will clarify whether these findings can generalize to disaster settings.

While many of the CISD studies, particularly those showing negative outcomes, have methodological flaws, theoretically there are many possible explanations for both neutral and negative findings. For example, it is possible that CISD interventions with primary civilian survivors of disaster are too brief to allow for adequate emotional processing, that they increase arousal and anxiety levels, or that they inadvertently decrease the likelihood that individuals will pursue more intensive interventions. It is possible that future research will demonstrate that CISD may be useful for some populations, or has more subtle positive effects, such as perceived social support. In the meantime, numerous reviews of the best-controlled studies conclude that it cannot be endorsed as an intervention which prevents long-term distress or psychopathology, given the current state of the research (Gray et al., 2004; McNally et al., 2003; Rose & Bisson, 2004). Given the negative findings associated with CISD, as

well as preliminary evidence that increased arousal in the immediate phases post-trauma is linked to long-term pathology, there is concern that any intervention that focuses on emotional processing during this period may be contraindicated. It has therefore been recommended that any interventions involving one-session interventions that require emotional processing be more fully researched prior to recommending their routine practice postdisaster (Watson, 2004).

There has been only one RCT published to date on the use of psychopharmacological interventions for acute stress responses. Pitman and colleagues (2002) conducted a randomized, double-blind pilot study in which they administered propranolol within 6 h of a traumatic event (hypothesizing that the medication might interfere with fear conditioning). While the propranolol group did not appear to exhibit decreased PTSD symptoms 3 months later, it did exhibit reduced physiological reactivity. More work is needed with a larger sample size to better understand these findings, particularly with at least three corroborative studies on the correlation between increased heart rate in the acute phase post-trauma and the development of PTSD (Bryant et al., 2000; Shalev et al., 1998; Zatzick et al., 2005).

Other studies of psychopharmacological interventions in the acute stages after trauma suffer from serious methodological weaknesses that limit their interpretability and generalizability. Given the lack of evidence with pharmacological agents in the acute phases post-trauma, experts recommend use of pharmacology for symptomatic relief only, particularly when individuals are exhibiting intense psychiatric symptoms that are impairing functioning (i.e., prolonged insomnia, suicidality, psychosis, intense anxiety, mania, etc.) (Simon & Gorman, 2004).

As indicated elsewhere in this volume (Chapter 7), at this time short-term (four to five sessions) cognitive-behavioral interventions (i.e., education, anxiety management training, imaginal exposure therapy, in vivo exposure, and cognitive restructuring) delivered within a month of trauma currently have the most empirical support for prevention of psychopathology and distress, having been tested in RCTs with individual survivors of motor vehicle accidents (including those with acute injuries), industrial accidents, and nonsexual assault who have been diagnosed with acute stress disorder (Bisson *et al.*, 2004; Bryant *et al.*, 1998, 1999; Ehlers *et al.*, 2003; Zatzik *et al.*, 2004). This model results in prevention of PTSD and in decreased depressive symptoms when compared to repeated assessment, self-help, education and support, and benefits in psychological functioning are maintained 9 months to 4 years later (Bryant *et al.*, 2003; Ehlers *et al.*, 2003). In trials with individual traumas, neither cognitive-behavioral therapy (CBT) nor eye movement desensitization and reprocessing (EMDR) has been empirically examined in the immediate aftermath (0–14 days) of trauma.

Recent work with injury and accident victims, as discussed in Chapter 9, has sought to evaluate services in the acute phases postincident, but generally occurs greater than 14 days post-trauma (Bisson *et al.*, 2004; Bryant *et al.*, 2003; Zatzick, 2003; Zatzick *et al.*, 2004). Bisson's randomized early intervention study with injured individuals included a four-session CBT treatment at 5–10 weeks post-trauma, with findings not as robust as in previous studies with acute stress disorder (ASD) patients. Possible next steps to Bisson's intervention would be implementation in mass violence settings, traumatically bereaved populations, and different timeframes following trauma. Zatzick and colleagues (2004) conducted an RCT to test the effectiveness of a multifaceted collaborative care (CC) intervention, which included continuous postinjury case management, motivational interviews targeting alcohol abuse/dependence, and evidence-based pharmacotherapy and/or CBT for patients with persistent PTSD at 3 months after injury. CC patients were significantly less symptomatic with regard to PTSD and alcohol abuse/dependence than the control group, with no difference in PTSD symptoms from baseline to 12 months, whereas the control group had a 6% increase during the year.

Victims of accidents do not experience the disruption in the physical and social environment that is typical of mass trauma. The nature, frequency, and controllability of the initiating event are critical factors that require more investigation as determinants of differential patterns of long-term adjustment. Therefore, further research is needed to determine whether the early provision of CBT-influenced interventions following mass violence or disaster is indicated earlier than 2 weeks post-trauma. Members of recent consensus efforts (Watson, 2004; Watson *et al.*, manuscript in preparation) agreed that the chaotic and stressful postevent environment precludes the energy and effort needed to show progress in CBT-informed treatments (i.e., homework, emotional, and time investment), and for reasons indicated above, emotional processing in this immediate phase is often contraindicated. They suggest that structured cognitive-behavioral interventions are not to be implemented until secondary stressors in the environment are under sufficient control to allow the individual to focus on the intervention (usually not sooner than 3 weeks postincident) (Watson, 2004).

Recent efforts in acute intervention following disasters are based on utilizing cognitive-behavioral principles in community-based interventions, such as the program of post-traumatic stress management (PTSM) implemented following community stressors (i.e., suicide cluster, bus accident). The model is put into place within 24 h, and involves a series of individual and group interventions designed to help people orient, stabilize, and improve coping skills (i.e, identification of access to support and resources, nonverbal and verbal processing of the trauma narrative, psychoeducation regarding the neurophysiology of traumatic stress and its impact on psychosocial functioning, and planning, problem-solving, and self-care). While this model has not been studied in an RCT, survey information indicates that the most useful parts of the program were providing direction to help communities heal and helping the communities come together to handle the crisis. Program creators recommend that this program can be overlaid on existing human services programs until a trained resource network is in place and stable (Macy *et al.*, 2004).

In one of the few RCTs conducted following mass violence, the community-based implementation (CBI) program was offered in the West Bank and Gaza in 2003 in the largest scale psychosocial support program known to date (over 100 000 children completed the full 15-session program). The CBI program, designed by creators of PTSM, is a psychosocial integration and recovery program for children, adolescents and their adult caregivers who are exposed to psychological trauma. The CBI is a 5-week, 15-session classroom- or camp-based group intervention, involving a series of structured activities, which aims to identify existing coping resources among children and youth facing difficult circumstances, and to sustain the utilization of those resources in the service of psychological and psychosocial recovery over time. Outcome measures of a randomized and controlled impact study (involving 664 children) revealed that CBI helped children feel better, happier, and more confident. Families reported that they found their children more optimistic and more cooperative at home. Teachers reported that students were more focused after CBI, more ready to learn, and less aggressive overall. The CBI program produced a number of distinctive positive psychological changes in young Palestinian boys and girls (aged 6–11 years) as well as in adolescent girls (aged 12–16 years) participating in the study, including enhanced communication, decreased self-blame, decreased emotional and behavioral difficulties such as hyperactivity, emotional arousal symptoms, and disruptive behaviors, increased pro-social behavior, increased hope and self-efficacy, negotiation skills, self-reliance, and positive self-esteem and satisfaction with self. These positive psychological changes contributed to an increase in the children's sense of psychosocial re-integration, allowing them to function "normally" with respect to family, school, and play. In other words, CBI succeeded in maintaining coping strengths and resiliency.

Creative implementation strategies for CBT-based interventions include brief telephone (Greist et al., 2000; Mohr et al., 2000; Somer et al., 2005) and internet interventions (Gega et al., 2004), which have proven helpful with a variety of mental health problems. One study employing a cognitive-behavioral telephone hotline intervention (e.g., relaxation breathing and challenging maladaptive thoughts) in Israel before the most recent American invasion of Iraq (Somer et al., in press) indicated decreased anxiety on several measures post-intervention. A study by Gidron et al. (2001) reported reductions in PTSD symptoms at 3- to 4-month follow-up utilizing a CBT-based telephone intervention within the first 48 h postincident. Litz et al. (2004) have conducted an RCT on a cognitive-behavioral therapist-assisted, internet-based, self-help intervention that uses an 8-week structured form of stress inoculation training for both secondary prevention of PTSD and treatment of the chronic disorder with survivors of the attack on the Pentagon on September 11. While outcomes are pending, preliminary results indicate that no symptom exacerbation or treatment drop-outs occurred.

Expert consensus recommendations

Experts from several consensus conferences (National Institutes of Mental Health, 2002; Watson, 2004; Watson et al., in preparation) have attempted to incorporate empirical findings into more coordinated guidance regarding overall systems of post-disaster care. Consensus findings indicate that the foundation for an effective public mental health disaster response is an integrated local, state, and federal emergency preparedness response community (emergency management associations, public health offices, hospitals, faith-based community, law enforcement, etc.), with recognition among community leaders and planners that each aspect of the disaster response can impact on community mental health. Central tenets include prior training of relevant responders (i.e., mental health professionals, media, government, public agencies, and educational institutions), limitation of inappropriate interventions, initiation of Psychological First Aid (PFA) to those who need it, identification of the needs of at-risk individuals who may require

Table 6.1 Key components of disaster behavioral interventions

I. Systems issues/program management process
  - Prepare/foster capacity and resilience
  - Conduct needs assessments
  - Monitor the rescue and recovery environment
  - Foster recovery
  - Evaluate outcomes

II. Interventions/direct survivor care
  - Provide for basic needs
  - Triage
  - Psychological First Aid
  - Outreach and information dissemination
  - Technical assistance, consultation, and training
  - Treatment

Table 6.2 Factors assessed in the acute phase

- Basic needs (food, housing, medical, information)
- Immediate risk to life/suicidality
- Functional capacity/impairment
  - Factors which prevent recovery
  - Continuation of adversity
  - Secondary stressors (loss of resources)
  - Uncontrolled reactions
  - Major risk factors (i.e., past trauma, bereavement, exposure level)
- Strengths/resources (social support, coping skills, finances, etc.)
- Information availability (TV, newspapers, Internet access, transportation)
- Patient – focused self-report of what they think they need to further recovery
- Current need

additional surveillance and evidence-based intervention over time, provision of pragmatic and culturally competent programs that enhance natural resilience in as many individuals and communities as possible, periodic monitoring of at-risk individuals, and evaluation of services. Primary goals are to increase the evidence-informed principles of safety, efficacy, hope, connectedness, and calming (see Table 6.1).

The key components overlap in time, are provided by a range of individuals, organizations, and professionals, and create an overall framework within which recovery from mass violence can be maximized. Experts have recommended a stepped care approach with these components, such that some early deliveries may help most people in early adaptation but, as time progresses, more individualized and time-consuming interventions are reserved for a minority of people who require it (Zatzick *et al.*, 2004). In the immediate phase, the components of meeting basic needs, triage, PFA, and outreach/information dissemination are most salient, and therefore the following discussion will be limited to these components, acknowledging that they should always be placed within an overall system of care (see Table 6.2).

Provide for basic needs

Consensus recommendations suggest that during the immediate response period, all responders (including mental health providers) should focus primarily on helping survivors to meet their basic needs (e.g., safety, shelter, food, rest), as well as on providing soothing human contact and information necessary to meet basic needs. This is supported by theory and evidence that the process of post-traumatic recovery can best proceed in a safe, comforting environment (Shalev, 2002). Traditional "treatment" is neither the appropriate intervention nor the goal at this point.

Triage

The primary goals of triage in the immediate aftermath of mass violence are to screen for those who may need emergency hospitalization or immediate mental health referral. Another goal of assessment should be to identify individuals and groups at elevated risk for development of problems over time. The "Screen and Treat" model proposes that immediate intervention be restricted to providing information, support, and education, but that survivors be followed up to detect individuals with persistent symptoms, who can then be treated with empirically supported interventions (Brewin, unpublished manuscript). As stated above (McNally *et al.*, 2003), research indicates that levels of symptoms assessed very soon after an event do not predict the future course of disorder well. Therefore, it is not appropriate to screen for symptoms in the immediate aftermath (days) of mass violence. In the immediate aftermath, assessing functioning and pragmatic needs is most important for knowing how and when to provide assistance.

Panelists also recommended being responsive to the experience of the person who is traumatized to maximize acceptability of screening and engage for further follow-up. Additionally, developmental and cultural issues must be addressed in setting up screening protocols. All assessment should be practical, achievable, and implementable at the local level, and informed by an entire system of care. It is therefore best to put systems in place prior to an incident, with planning coordinated at federal, regional, state, and local levels.

Psychological First Aid (PFA)

Early response, beginning immediately at the scene of an incident and continuing for several days or weeks, is increasingly being organized around a set of actions collectively labeled as "Psychological First Aid" (PFA). Many of these actions are not specifically psychological in nature but are essentially for improving function and mental health response, related to the meeting of basic needs for physical safety, connectedness, security, and survival. PFA also involves orienting survivors to the disaster response site, helping them navigate services, or allowing them the opportunity to share their thoughts and feelings or experiences (if desired). PFA allows room for those who do not wish to discuss the trauma to avoid doing so. In this way, PFA is noninterventionist.

A recent national expert group developing PFA modules has designed PFA to be consistent with research evidence, applicable in field settings, tailored to the full developmental spectrum, and culturally informed (Steinberg *et al.*, in preparation). Different components of PFA can be delivered by either mental health or nonmental health responders, who provide acute assistance following trauma in a variety of settings (shelters, schools, workplace, etc.). Later phase interventions (from 1 to 8 weeks postevent) are also included which will overlap with the longer term recovery interventions. The following goals of PFA drive the interventions listed below.

Immediate goals of PFA

1. *Engagement.* Initiating contact in a nonintrusive and helpful manner. Listening and responding to immediate needs and concerns. Enhancing adaptive coping.
2. *Safety and orientation.* Ensuring immediate safety, comfort, orientation, and access to resources. Protecting affected persons from unnecessary exposure to stressors.
3. *Stabilization and Self-Regulation.* Helping affected persons to recognize, understand, and modulate changes in emotional reactivity.
4. *Connectedness.* Promoting a feeling that other people care and can help, and that one can care about and help others.

These goals are achieved through the following components of PFA:

- Engagement (i.e., acknowledging and being respectful, listening empathically, refraining from making assumptions.)
- Identifying needs [i.e., determining what basic needs have not been met and who needs to go where, the nature of information received, whether there are injuries, if there are children involved, if there has been contact with emergency services, if there are referral needs, identifying support systems (family, etc.), mental status when indicated, resource status.]
- Relaying accurate information (i.e., to parents on the psychological effects on children, information

transfer to incident command system and Red Cross.)

- Providing instrumental aid (knowing the situation, having accurate information, creating predictability.)
- Offering practical assistance (insulating and removing from unnecessary exposure to reminders/triggers, providing a safer location, locating and reconnecting to families/community services, helping to implement surrogate caregiver procedures, helping survivors access the resource network.)
- Promoting connectedness (empowering/mobilizing natural support systems, for instance by bringing people together who can support each other.)
- Giving comfort (attenuating distress, fostering perseverance, containing emotional responses, rather than encouraging catharting, refraining from disabling coping styles or telling people "it will be okay".)
- Making available collaborative services (facilitating stepped care, creating an atmosphere of predictability, being clear about handoff procedures/information transfer, knowing available resources, fostering an implied sense of hope, i.e., for assistance/resources, advocating for needs.)

Longer term goals of PFA, which has been tentatively labeled Psychological Secondary Aid (PSA), are more apt to include CBT-based strategies for reducing factors related to development of PTSD and increasing positive coping strategies. These include:

1. *Triage and screening.* Gathering and using information to identify individuals at risk for post-trauma problems. Collaboratively establishing goals to assist individuals in seeking services tailored to their needs.
2. *Restoration of functioning.* Helping to maintain or restore adaptive functioning and routines.
3. *Coping and self-regulation.* Providing the knowledge and skills needed to understand and effectively manage distress reactions.
4. *Problem-solving.* Promoting effective problem-solving in relation to immediate needs, concerns, and goals.

5. *Risk reduction.* Promoting understanding and the effective use of postdisaster/terrorism risk-related information.
6. *Resilence and recovery.* Promoting adaptive youth, family, and adult developmental progression. Mitigating disruptions to development (Steinberg *et al.*, in preparation).

These longer term goals are accomplished with many of the same actions listed above, with a different time-appropriate focus:

- Engagement (circulation and outreach, acknowledge, respect, listen empathically, don't make assumptions.)
- Triage/identification (engage in longer conversations than in the immediate phase, gather information about coping since event and risk factors, ask to contact at later date, get a resource status exam.)
- Giving and receiving accurate information (i.e., to parents on the psychological affects on children, transfer information across "care teams," offer information at regular times, provide information on managing post-trauma reactions and reminders.) Move to or expand to group and public education meetings to provide information on disaster responses, stress management, talking to children, etc.
- Providing instrumental aid (know the situation, avoid giving misinformation, have accurate information, create predictability.)
- Offering practical assistance (assist in getting basic needs met, remove from unnecessary exposure to reminders/triggers, provide safe location, locate and reconnect to social support and community resources, help to implement surrogate caregiver procedures, help survivor access the resource network, provide assistance in problem-solving, establishing proxies for familiar routines, health factors, managing reminders and reactions, and sleep hygiene, i.e., connect to physician/medication/alternative medicine, information on nightmares, problems based on realities of shelter, etc.)
- Promoting connectedness [empower/mobilize natural support systems, facilitate simple task

groups, as much as possible design the milieu for natural support, make phone lines available (casework line, mental health line, information line of services available)]

- Giving comforting care (help people tolerate the unknown and ever-changing, comfort, don't disable coping styles, "contain don't cathart," attenuate distress, never tell people it will be OK, foster perseverence, give information about reactions, help with information on reactions, reduce distress, provide resilience-based group techniques, get "care team" pyramid structures assembled for stepped care, provide scheduled day of activities.) The focus is still on normalizing, but includes the introduction of recovery tools, including cognitive restructuring principles such as thought insertion, thought stopping, stress management, positive coping, reframing of negative cognitions, dealing with reminders and triggers, coping with varied recovery trajectories in families, and anxiety management to deal with avoidance and replaying and intrusive thoughts.

- Making available collaborative services [make every effort to ensure continuum of care, create coordinated services, give context of role and limits of the contact, advocate (through pre-existing relationship to incident command structure), make spiritual support available, begin to think about making connections with providers in community, system advocacy, system assessment, start to structure and organize stepped care in more detail, consultation to people who will be delivering messages, be clear on what local resources can provide.]

Psychological First Aid components are increasingly endorsed for universal application after mass violence or disaster, in part because they are considered to hold little potential for harm, and they do not contain elements (such as systematic emotional processing) hypothesized to be potentially harmful for some in the immediate aftermath of trauma. While a small proportion of survivors may need immediate triage to more formal psychiatric or psychological interventions, epidemiological studies and anecdotal evidence suggest that most individuals are capable of recovering from traumatic stress with appropriate education, information, and social and practical support in the very early phase following exposure to disaster or mass violence. Observations from the field suggest that most individuals are not interested in receiving formalized mental health interventions in this very early stage after mass violence or disaster, and because resilience is considered to be the norm following trauma exposure, compulsory procedures that impose a particular model or timeline of recovery on all survivors of mass violence have been discouraged.

While PFA has not yet been systematically studied, experience in the field suggests that it is generally acceptable to and well received by consumers. Experts generally concur that PFA practices are evidence-consistent, if not evidence-based, in that they are extrapolated from the research on the protective and risk factors associated with post-traumatic recovery, as well as theoretical formulations and interventions for individual traumatic stress (Steinberg *et al.*, manuscript in preparation).

Outreach and information dissemination

Many of those affected by terrorist attacks or other disasters do not seek mental health care or use available services (DeLisi *et al.*, 2003; North *et al.*, 2002; Luce & Firth-Cozens, 2002). For instance, after the World Trade Center attacks in New York City, there was only a 3% increase (from 16.9% to 19.4%) in general health service utilization, from the month prior to the month following the attacks, only a 10% reported increased mental health service visits after the attacks compared to prior use, and a 5% reported decreased use (Boscarino *et al.*, 2002). Three to six months later, only 27% of those reporting severe psychiatric symptoms had obtained mental health treatment (DeLisi *et al.*, 2003). Generally, relatively little is known about how survivors make decisions about self-referral, how to encourage use of services, or how to increase acceptance of referral for more intensive counseling.

Because many trauma survivors are reluctant to use mental health services, accessibility of services may maximize engagement in the helping process and utilization of services for those individuals who may benefit from intervention. The FEMA-funded Crisis Counseling Program (CCP) is a frequently initiated American model of crisis intervention delivered within the first month (usually initiated from 14 to 30 days postevent) postdisaster. The program is oriented toward resilience, respect for individual recovery trajectories, community-based intervention, education, counseling, and outreach, and is offered free of charge to any community member impacted by a federally declared disaster. The program has not to date been subject to rigorous program evaluation or research, but is in the initial phases of program evaluation toolkit development. As part of that process, Norris and colleagues conducted a 5-year retrospective survey of crisis counseling programs. Results indicated that program directors and providers strongly endorsed the CCP model as superior to traditional mental health care in that it is acceptable (de-stigmatizing), accessible, and proactive. The use of indigenous workers in outreach activities is an important aspect of this approach.

Active outreach includes media activities and mobilization of face-to-face outreach. Specific outreach strategies may differ, depending on the pre-existing mental health infrastructure and the areas and individuals affected. A key tenet of outreach is respect for individual variation in recovery from trauma. In the acute phases postevent, this is particularly sailient, in that the fluctuating course of trauma response (from avoidance to processing) may render an individual incapable or unwilling to discuss their experiences or responses, and may indeed be an adaptive response (Raphael *et al.*, 1996; Watson & Shalev, 2005). Brewin (2001) cautions against interfering with natural recovery processes within the acute phases post-trauma.

Education is an important component of many individual, group, and community interventions offered in the aftermath of disasters. As a relatively brief, nonstigmatizing, low-cost form of care, post-disaster education is generally designed to be tailored to cover any number of the following points: (1) help survivors better understand a range of post-trauma responses; (2) view their post-trauma reactions as expectable and understandable (not as reactions to be feared, signs of personal failure or weakness, or signs of mental illness); (3) recognize the circumstances under which they should consider seeking further counseling; (4) know how and where to access additional help, including mental health counseling; (5) increase use of social supports and other adaptive ways of coping with the trauma and its effects; (6) decrease use of problematic forms of coping (e.g., excessive alcohol consumption, extreme social isolation); and (7) increase ability to help family members cope (e.g., information about how to talk to children about what happened). Accurate and timely information regarding the nature of the unfolding disaster situation is also an important part of education. Care should be taken when providing education, as its use is still being tested, and one study (Ehlers *et al.*, 2003) indicated that those who received a self-help manual as compared to repeated assessments or a more formal cognitive-behavioral intervention following traumatic stress did not fare as well at follow-up as either of the other groups. The researchers recommend that self-help advice be modified to take into account the conditions under which self-exposure to traumatic material is helpful, and to give more concrete advice regarding how to go through traumatic memories, how to address problematic appraisals, and how to change them (Ehlers *et al.*, 2003). Clearly this application following disasters is in need of study, as other cognitive-behavioral self-help interventions have been found to be effective for treatment of nontrauma-related anxiety problems in a number of controlled treatment outcome studies (Gould & Clum, 1995; Lidren *et al.*, 1994).

Conclusions

As can be seen in this review of the empirical literature on immediate interventions following mass violence, there are few well-controlled studies related to any particular intervention in this context. Rather, consensus based on both empirical literature and experiential practice endorses a multi-faceted approach to the management of traumatic stress following disasters and mass violence. Experts in this field are currently attempting to bring their expertise to bear in a number of mass violence situations and contexts, including situations of ongoing threat, ethnocultural contexts, and situations of infectious disease. Consensus guidelines offer the following basic recommendations for acute behavioral interventions following mass trauma:

1. Provide early interventions designed to reduce excessive, uncontrollable distress, correct negative appraisal, facilitate social connectedness, and provide pragmatic resources with the goal of improved task performance, better interpersonal interactions, controllable emotion, and sustained self-esteem.

2. Understand that, for most, the natural recovery process is an opportunity to integrate self-strength and social network strength in rallying towards recovery. Interventions should seek to assess, support, and facilitate natural strengths, and promote those factors that are contributive to recovery, such as social support and self-efficacy.

3. Assess for protective and vulnerability factors that may affect how an individual reacts to and recovers from trauma.

4. For those with higher exposure levels, assist in processing traumatic recollections at the survivor's preferred pace, which requires time, reiteration, good companions, and possibly evidence-based treatment.

5. Strive to make interventions culturally sensitive, developmentally appropriate, and related to the local formulation of problems and ways of coping.

6. Lack of distress and/or complete recovery may not be a desired outcome. Ethnic, political, and economic factors may contribute to differing goals for functioning and identity, and providers should be sensitive to the particular motivations of each survivor.

7. Strive to empirically determine whether these practices are effective in ameliorating specific outcomes, or whether new interventions should be designed to accomplish such objectives.

As we consider the many specific components of intervention, identification of key mechanisms of change and adaptational variables that predict functional changes or maladaptive trajectories across time. It is apparent that there is a great need for both program evaluation and RCTs that will evaluate the effectiveness of PFA principles in a number of contexts, and eventually rigorously evaluate the effectiveness of each separate component, especially with respect to the optimal post-traumatic timing of such interventions. This research should include a range of outcomes, including not only PTSD, but also substance abuse, depression, anger and violence, interpersonal and role functioning, and physical health. In addition to such individual outcomes, research is needed that focuses on group, organizational, and community outcomes, such as the behavioral, emotional, and functional consequences most likely to be expressed in the school or workplace (staff turnover, organizational cohesion, morale, absenteeism, performance deficits, or medical symptoms).

Questions remain regarding which survivors should be targeted for early treatment, and when such treatment should be offered. While offering CBT-based trauma-focused interventions may be helpful for some disaster survivors in the first month after the trauma, it may be lower on the hierarchy of needs for survivors faced with complex and chronic stressors. Further research into the needs of disaster-affected populations will help guide the timing of interventions, of both early and later-stage interventions after disasters. Research is also needed regarding the most appropriate interventions across a diversity of populations, such as individuals who suffer traumatic bereavement, children, and adolescents.

In addition to continued efforts to conduct intervention research, it is important to remain cautious in our overstatement of what early interventions can accomplish towards prevention of long-term functional and symptomatic impact. For instance, the provision of PFA principles may be more feasible than structured clinical interventions, but it is unknown whether such interventions are associated with significant improvements in functioning. As can be seen with the debriefing literature, overstating the proposed effects of an intervention prior to evidence of its impact can result in programs being implemented at the expense of careful consideration of more viable alternatives. Additionally, care should be taken to include the preferences of recipients as a disaster response is planned. The NIMH/SAMSHA expert panel on interventions following mass violence agreed that universal interventions should have a higher standard of care. That is, they warrant a low level of interference, and a high level of choice to prevent any possible negative effects. Research on service utilization indicates that the majority of individuals exposed to a traumatic event will not choose to seek mental health services, and, therefore, a careful study of what interventions are acceptable and supportive of natural recovery trajectories may be called for prior to strong recommendations for any mental health intervention. For instance, in keeping with social support research (Kaniasty & Norris, 1999), a more acceptable intervention than an individual crisis response might be to provide family and friends with the tools necessary for helping loved ones more effectively process traumatic stress, as distinct from severe stress.

Additionally, economic modeling and cost–benefit analyses may be helpful in determining which outlay of resources produces the most significant impact, whether it be interventions for the majority affected, or more intensive support for the most significantly impacted. For instance, Basoglu and colleagues (2005), in an RCT attempting to develop a brief treatment for disaster survivors, found that a single session of modified behavioral treatment in earthquake-related PTSD produced significant treatment effects on all measures at posttreatment. They concluded that brief behavioral treatment has promise as a cost-effective intervention for disaster.

Finally, international planning and coordination are needed when planning for the implementation of psychological interventions in different countries. Recent ethnocultural guidelines caution against applying Western standards to the different ethnocultural formulations of healing and recovery (Watson *et al.*, in preparation). As McNally and colleagues point out after an excellent review of the early intervention literature (2003), "the bottom line is that in the immediate aftermath of trauma, professionals should take their lead from the survivors and provide the help they want, rather than tell survivors how they will get better (p. 68)."

While the field of disaster behavioral health intervention is still in its infancy, it is hoped that continued examination of many of these factors and creative collaboration across disciplines will contribute to a realistic and informed approach to assisting in recovery from incidents of mass violence.

REFERENCES

Bandura, A. (1997). *Self-Efficacy: The Exercise of Control.* New York: Freeman.

Bandura, A. (2001). Social cognitive theory: an agentive perspective. *Annual Review of Psychology*, **52**, 1–26.

Basoglu, M., Salcioglu, E., Livanou, M., Kalender, D. & Acar, G. (2005). Single-session behavioral treatment of earthquake-related posttraumatic stress disorder: a randomized waiting list controlled trial. *Journal of Traumatic Stress*, **18**, 1–11.

Benight, C. C. (2004). Collective efficacy following a series of natural disasters. *Anxiety Stress and Coping*, **17**, 401–420.

Benight, C. C. & Bandura, A. (2004). Social cognitive theory of posttraumatic recovery: the role of perceived self-efficacy. *Behaviour Research and Therapy*, **42**, 1129–1148.

Benight, C. C., Swift, E., Sanger, J., Smith, A. & Zeppelin, D. (1999). Coping self-efficacy as a prime mediator of distress following a natural disaster. *Journal of Applied Social Psychology*, **29**, 2443–2464.

Bisson, J. I. (2003). Early interventions following traumatic events. *Psychiatric Annals*, **33**, 37–44.

Bisson, J. I., Shepherd, J. P., Joy, D., Probert, R. & Newcombe, R. G. (2004). Early cognitive-behavioural therapy for post-traumatic stress symptoms after physical injury: Randomised controlled trial. *British Journal Psychiatry*, **184**, 63–69.

Bonanno, G. A. (2004). Loss, trauma and human resilience: have we underestimated the human capacity to thrive after extremely adverse events? *American Psychologist*, **59**, 20–28.

Boscarino, J. A., Galea, S., Ahern, J., Resnick, H. & Vlahov, D. (2002). Utilization of mental health services following the September 11th terrorist attacks in Manhattan, New York City. *International Journal of Emergency Mental Health*, **4**, 143–155.

Brewin, C. R. (2001). A cognitive neuroscience account of posttraumatic stress disorder and its treatment. *Behaviour Research and Therapy*, **39**, 373–393.

Brewin, C. R. & Holmes, E. A. (2003). Psychological theories of posttraumatic stress disorder. *Clinical Psychology Review*, **23**, 339–376.

Brewin, C. R. & Saunders, J. (2001). The effect of dissociation at encoding on intrusive memories for a stressful film. *British Journal of Medical Psychology*, **74**, 467–472.

Brewin, C. R., Dalgleish, T. & Joseph, S. (1996). A dual representation theory of posttraumatic stress disorder. *Archives of General Psychiatry*, **50**, 294–305.

Brewin, C., Rose, S. & Andrews, B. (2002). Screening to identify individuals at risk after exposure to trauma. In *Early Intervention for Psychological Trauma*, ed. U. Schneider. Oxford: Oxford University Press.

Bryant, R. A. & Harvey, A. G. (2000). *Acute Stress Disorder: A Handbook of Theory, Assessment, and Treatment.* Washington, D.C.: American Psychological Association.

Bryant, R. A., Harvey, A. G., Dang, S. T., Sackville, T. & Basten, C. (1998). Treatment of acute stress disorder: a comparison of cognitive-behavioral therapy and supportive counseling. *Journal of Consulting and Clinical Psychology*, **66**, 862–866.

Bryant, R. A., Sackville, T., Dang, S. T., Moulds, M. & Guthrie, R. (1999). Treating acute stress disorder: an evaluation of cognitive behavioral therapy and supportive counseling techniques. *American Journal of Psychiatry*, **156**, 1780–1786.

Bryant, R. A., Moulds, M. L. & Nixon, R. V. (2003). Cognitive behaviour therapy of acute stress disorder: a four-year follow-up. *Behaviour Research and Therapy*, **41**, 489–494.

Cassel, J. (1976). The contribution of the social environment to host resistance. *American Journal of Epidemiology*, **104**, 107–123.

Dalgleish, T. (2004). Cognitive approaches to posttraumatic stress disorder: the evolution of multirepresentational theorizing. *Psychological Bulletin*, **130**, 228.

DeLisi, L. E., Maurizio, A., Yost, M. *et al.* (2003). A survey of New Yorkers after the Sept. 11, 2001, terrorist attacks. *American Journal of Psychiatry*, **160**, 780–783.

Dunmore, E., Clark, D. M. & Ehlers, A. (2001). A prospective investigation of the role of cognitive factors in persistent posttraumatic stress disorder (PTSD) after physical or sexual assault. *Behaviour Research and Therapy*, **39**, 1063–1084.

Ehlers, A. & Clark, D. M. (2000). A cognitive model of posttraumatic stress disorder. *Behaviour Research and Therapy*, **38**, 319–345.

Ehlers, A., Clark, D. M., Hackmann, A. *et al.* (2003). A randomized controlled trial of cognitive therapy, a self-help booklet, and repeated assessments as early interventions for posttraumatic stress disorder. *Archives of General Psychiatry*, **60**, 1024–1032.

Galea, S., Ahern, J., Resnick, H. *et al.* (2002). Psychological sequelae of the September 11 terrorist attacks in New York City. *New England Journal of Medicine*, **346**, 982–987.

Gega, L., Marks, I. & Mataix-Cols, D. (2004). Computer-aided CBT self-help for anxiety and depressive disorders: experience of a London clinic and future directions. *Journal of Clinical Psychology*, **60**, 147–157.

Gidron, Y., Gal, R., Freedman, S. A. *et al.* (2001). Translating research findings to PTSD prevention: results of a randomized-controlled pilot study. *Journal of Traumatic Stress*, **14**, 773–780.

Gould, R. A. & Clum, G. A. (1995). Self-help plus minimal therapist contact in the treatment of panic disorder: A replication and extension. *Behavior Therapy*, **26**, 533–546.

Gray, M. J., Maguen, S. & Litz, B. T. (2004). Acute psychological impact of disaster and large scale trauma: limitations of traditional interventions and future practice recommendations. *Prehospital and Disaster Medicine*, **19**, 64–72.

Greene, G. J., Lee, M. Y., Trask, R. & Rheinscheld, J. (2000). How to work with clients' strengths in crisis intervention. In *Crisis Intervention Handbook: Assessment, Treatment, and Research*, ed. A. Roberts. Oxford: Oxford University Press.

Greist, J. H., Osgood-Hynes, D. J., Baer, L. & Marks, I. M. (2000). Technology-based advances in the management of depression: focus on the COPE program. *Disease Management and Health Outcomes*, **4**, 193–200.

Halligan, S. L., Michael, T., Clark, D. M. & Ehlers, A. (2003). Posttraumatic stress disorder following assault: the role of cognitive processing, trauma memory, and appraisals. *Journal of Consulting and Clinical Psychology*, **71**, 419–431.

Hobfoll, S. E. (1989). Conservation of resources. A new attempt at conceptualizing stress. *American Psychologist*, **44**, 513–524.

Kaniasty, K. & Norris, F. H. (1993). A test of the social support deterioration model in the context of natural disaster. *Journal of Personality and Social Psychology*, **64**, 395–408.

Lidren, D. M., Watkins, P. L., Gould, R. A., Clum, G. A., Asterino, M. & Tulloch, H. L. (1994). A comparison of bibliotherapy and group therapy in the treatment of panic disorder. *Journal of Consulting and Clinical Psychology*, **62**, 865–869.

Litz, B. Implications for screening following mass trauma. Expert panel. Unpublished manuscript.

Litz, B. T., Gray, M. J., Bryant, R. A. & Adler, A. B. (2002). Early Intervention for Trauma: Current Status and Future Directions. *Clinical Psychology: Science and Practice*, **9**, 112–134.

Litz, B. T., Gray, M. J., Bryant, R. A. & Adler, A. B. (2004a). *Early intervention for trauma: current status and future directions*. Clinical Psychology: Science and Practice.

Litz, B. T., Williams, L., Wang, J., Bryant, R. & Engel, C. C. jr. (2004b). A therapist-assisted Internet Self-Help Program for Traumatic Stress. *Professional Psychology: Research and Practice*, **35**, 628–634.

Luce, A., Firth-Cozens, J., Midgley, S. & Burges, C. (2002). After the Omagh bomb: posttraumatic stress disorder in health service staff. *Journal of Traumatic Stress*, **25**, 27–30.

Macy, R. D., Behar, L., Paulson, R., Delman, J., Schmid, L. & Smith, S. F. (2004). Community-based, acute posttraumatic stress management: a description and evaluation of a psychosocial-intervention continuum. *Harvard Review of Psychiatry*, **12**, 217–228.

McNally, R. J., Bryant, R. A. & Ehlers, A. (2003). Does early psychological intervention promote recovery from posttraumatic stress? *Psychological Science in the Public Interest*, **4**, 45–79.

Mohr, D. C., Likosky, W., Bertagnolli, A. *et al.* (2000). Telephone-administered cognitive-behavioral therapy for the treatment of depressive symptoms in multiple sclerosis. *Journal of Consulting and Clinical Psychology*, **68**, 356–361.

National Institutes of Mental Health (2002). Mental Health and Mass Violence – Evidence Based Early Psychological Intervention for Victims/Survivors of Mass Violence: A Workshop to Reach Consensus on Best Practices. U.S. Department of Defense; U.S. Department of health and Human Services, the National Institute of Mental Health, the Substance Abuse and mental health Services Administration, Center for Mental Health Services; U.S. Department of Justice, Office for Victims of Crime; U.S. Department of Veterans Affairs, National Center for PTSD; and the American Red Cross. NIMH Report.

Neill, J. T. & Dias, K. L. (2001). Adventure education and resilience: the double-edged sword. *Journal of Adventure Education and Outdoor Learning*, **1**, 35–42.

Norris, F. H. & Elrod, C. L. (2006). Phychosocial consequences of disasters: A review of past research. In *Methods for Disaster Mental Health Research*, eds. F. H. Norris, S. Galea, M. J. Friedman & P. J. Watson. New York, NY: Guilford Press.

Norris, F. H. & Murrell, S. A. (1984). Protective function of resources related to life events, global stress, and depression in older adults. *Journal of Health and Social Behavior*, **25**, 424–437.

Norris, F. H., Friedman, M. & Watson, P. J. *et al.* (2002a). 60,000 disaster victims speak. Part II: Summary and implications of the disaster mental health research. *Psychiatry*, **65**, 240–260.

Norris, F. H., Friedman, M. J., Watson, P. J. (2002b). 60,000 disaster victims speak. Part I: An empirical review of the empirical literature, 1981–2001. *Psychiatry*, **65**, 207–239.

Norris, F., Kaniasty, K., Conrad, M. L., Inman, G. L. & Murphy, A. D. (2002c). Placing age differences in cultural context: a comparison of the effects of age on PTSD after disasters in the United States, Mexico, and Poland. *Journal of Clinical Geropsychology*, **8**, 153–173.

North, C. S. & Pfefferbaum, B. (2002). Research on the mental health effects of terrorism. *Journal of the American Medical Association*, **288**, 633–636.

Ozer, E., Best, S., Lipse, T. L. & Weiss, D. S. (2003). Predictors for posttraumatic stress disorder and symptoms in adults: a metaanalysis. *Psychological Bulletin*, **129**, 52–73.

Pearlin, L. I. & Schooler, C. (1978). The structure of coping. *Journal of Health and Social Behavior*, **22**, 337–356.

Pitman, R. K., Sanders, K. M., Zusman, R. M. *et al.* (2002). Pilot study of secondary prevention of post-traumatic stress disorder with propranolol. *Biological Psychiatry,* **51**, 189–192.

Raphael, B. & Wilson, J. P. (2000). *Psychological Debriefing: Theory, Practice, and Evidence.* Cambridge: Cambridge University Press.

Raphael, B., Wilson, J., Meldrum, L. & McFarlane, A. C. (1996). Acute preventive interventions. In *Traumatic Stress: The Effects of Overwhelming Experience on Mind, Body and Society,* ed. B. A. van der Kolk, A. C. McFarlane & L. Weisaeth pp. 463–447. New York: Guilford Press.

Robert, R., Blakeney, P. E., Villarreal, C., Rosenberg, L. & Meyer, W. J. (1999). Imipramine treatment in pediatric burn patients with symptoms of acute stress disorder: a pilot study. *Journal of the American Academy of Child and Adolescent Psychiatry,* **38**, 873–882.

Rose, S., Bisson, J. & Wesseley, S. (2001). *Psychological debriefing for preventing posttraumatic stress disorder.* Cochrane Library; Issue 3. Oxford, England: Update software; 2001.

Schlenger, W. E., Caddell, J. M., Ebert, L. *et al.* (2002). Psychological reactions to terrorist attacks: findings from the National Study of Americans' Reactions to September 11. *Journal of the American Medical Association,* **288**, 581–588.

Shalev, A. Y. Psycho-biological Perspectives on Early Reactions to Traumatic Events. Unpublished manuscript supported by a PHS research grant # NH-50379.

Shalev, A. Y. (2002). Treating survivors in the immediate aftermath of traumatic events. In *Treating Trauma Survivors with PTSD: Bridging the Gap Between Intervention Research and Practice,* ed. R. Yehuda. Washington, D.C.: American Psychiatric Press.

Shalev, A. Y. & Ursano, R. J. (1998). Mapping the multi-dimensional picture of acute responses to traumatic stress. In *Early Intervention for Psychological Trauma,* ed. U. Schneider. Oxford: Oxford University Press.

Simon, A. & Gorman, J. (2004). Psychopharmacological possibilities in the acute disaster setting. *Psychiatric Clinics of North America,* **27**, 425–458.

Somer, E., Tamir, E., Maguen, S. & Litz, B. T. (2005). Brief cognitive-behavioral phone-based intervention targeting anxiety about the threat of attack: a pilot study. *Behaviour Research and Therapy,* **43**, 669–679.

Valentiner, D. P., Foa, E. B., Riggs, D. S. & Gershuny, B. S. (1996). Coping strategies and posttraumatic stress disorder in female victims of sexual and nonsexual assault. *Journal of Abnormal Psychology,* **105**, 455–458.

Watson, P. (2004). Mental health interventions following mass violence. *Stresspoints,* **12**, 4–5.

Watson, P. J. & Shalev, A. Y. (2005). Assessment and treatment of adult acute responses to traumatic stress following mass traumatic events. *CNS Spectrums,* **10**, 123–131.

Watson, P. J., Friedman, M. J., Ruzek, J. I. & Norris, F. (2002). Managing acute stress response to major trauma. *Current Psychiatry Reports,* **4**, 247–253.

Zatzick, D. (2003). Posttraumatic stress, functional impairment, and service utilization after injury: a public health approach. *Seminars in Clinical Neuropsychiatry,* **8**, 149–157.

Zatzick, D. F., Roy-Byrne, P. P., Russo, J. E. *et al.* (2004). A randomized effectiveness trial of stepped collaborative care for acutely injured trauma survivors. *Archives of General Psychiatry,* **61**, 498–506.

Zatzick, D. F., Russo, J., Pitman, R. K., Rivara, F., Jurkovich, G. & Roy-Byrne, P. (2005). Reevaluating the association between emergency department heart rate and the development of posttraumatic stress disorder: a public health approach. *Biological Psychiatry,* **57**, 91–95.

7

Acute stress disorder and post-traumatic stress disorder in the disaster environment

David M. Benedek

Introduction

Post-traumatic stress disorder (PTSD) is an often severe, chronic, and disabling mental disorder that may develop after exposure to a traumatic event (or events) as may occur in disasters. Acute stress disorder (ASD) is characterized by similar – but transient – symptoms. Given their potential to result in widespread distress and dysfunction, PTSD and ASD deserve special consideration in disaster preparedness and response plans.

Beyond duration of symptoms, ASD is distinguished from PTSD by a diagnostic requirement for symptoms of peritraumatic dissociation. While ASD does not inevitably portend the later development of PTSD, dissociation may be the best predictor of the subsequent development of PTSD (Harvey & Bryant, 1998). Both PTSD and ASD are characterized by specific symptoms organized into core clusters of re-experience, hyperarousal, and avoidance/numbing. The common and distinguishing characteristics of the two disorders are described in the following section of this chapter, "Clinical presentation." Since other mental disorders (e.g., depression, substance abuse), stress reactions, and both acute and chronic distress-related behavioral changes not amounting to diagnosable disorders contribute greatly to the public health burden of disaster and often co-occur, the differential diagnosis and features associated with ASD and PTSD are also reviewed.

The atmosphere of chaos, disruption, unanticipated injury, loss, and death created by any disaster will establish a population meeting the traumatic exposure threshold criterion necessary – but not sufficient – for the development of ASD or PTSD. The section of this chapter entitled "Epidemiology" highlights the idea that many individuals exposed to significant trauma do not develop ASD or PTSD and describes subgroups that may be at greater risk for these conditions in the aftermath of disaster. The section of this chapter on "Neurobiology" reviews neurobiological mechanisms in normal and pathological traumatic stress responses. Abnormalities that may contribute to the development of ASD or PTSD and factors that may serve protective functions are described.

The remaining sections of this chapter review assessment and management considerations in the aftermath of disaster. After an outline of strategies and instruments used to assess for the presence of ASD and the emergence of PTSD over time, evidence-based psychopharmacologic, psychotherapeutic, and psychosocial approaches to the treatment of these illnesses are described. The role and limitations of published practice guidelines for the treatment of patients with ASD and PTSD are discussed, and research needs necessary to refine and improve assessment and treatment of these illnesses in disaster settings are summarized.

Clinical presentation

Core clinical features

ASD and PTSD are distinguished from other Axis I mental disorders by their requirement for exposure to an environmental stressor (such as a disaster) as part of their diagnostic criteria. Both ASD and PTSD are characterized by the onset of psychiatric symptoms temporally linked to exposure to an event that involves either witnessing or experiencing threatened death, injury, or threat to physical integrity. Both diagnoses also incorporate the individual's response to the event – which must involve intense fear or horror (American Psychiatric Association, 2000). Earlier conceptualizations of PTSD required that the traumatic event be "outside the range of normal human experience," (American Psychiatric Association, 1987) but this caveat was eliminated in DSM-IV. In both ASD and PTSD, establishing a diagnosis requires determination of the presence of at least one specified re-experiencing symptom from a list including recurring and distressing recollections or dreams of the event and acting or feeling as if the traumatic event were recurring. At least three specified avoidance symptoms (such as efforts to avoid thoughts, feelings, or conversations associated with the trauma, efforts to avoid activities, places, or people that evoke recollections of the trauma, feelings of detachment or estrangement from others) are also required for the diagnoses of either condition.

The diagnosis of PTSD requires at least two specified symptoms of increased arousal (such as difficulty falling or staying asleep or exaggerated startle) while the diagnostic criteria for ASD require only the presence of "symptoms of anxiety and increased arousal" without specifying a required number. ASD requires the presence of three or more dissociative symptoms during or after the traumatic event such as derealization, depersonalization, or a reduction in awareness of one's surroundings, e.g., "being in a daze." The diagnosis of ASD is made when symptoms occur within 4 weeks of a traumatic event and persist for a minimum of 2 days and a maximum of 4 weeks.

The diagnosis of PTSD is only made when symptoms persist for at least 1 month. *Acute* PTSD refers to an episode that lasts less than 3 months whereas *chronic* PTSD last 3 months or longer. PTSD *with delayed onset* refers to an episode that develops at least 6 months after the traumatic event (American Psychiatric Association, 2000). Table 7.1 lists the complete diagnostic criteria for ASD and PTSD; Table 7.2 offers a summarized comparison of the two disorders.

Associated clinical features

A number of additional features may be associated with PTSD. These include somatic complaints, shame, despair, hopelessness, impaired modulation of affect, social withdrawal, survivor guilt, anger, impulsive or self-destructive behavior, difficulties in interpersonal relationships, changed belief, or changed personality (American Psychiatric Association, 2000). Difficulty seeking or sustaining medical care has also been observed (Mellman, 1998). While clinical trials of either medications or psychotherapeutic interventions for the treatment of ASD or PTSD tend to target the core specific clinical features rather than associated symptoms, there can be little doubt that the latter group of less clearly quantifiable symptoms contributes greatly to the total burden of social and occupational dysfunction or impairment resulting from these disorders. Associated symptoms such as shame, inappropriate guilt, or hopelessness may also be indicative of depression, which is often co-morbid with PTSD. Depression also often occurs independently from PTSD in the aftermath of disaster and may require separate intervention (Jordan et al., 1991; Keane & Wolf, 1990). Somatic complaints without clear etiology are common phenomena among persons with histories of traumatic exposure and anxiety disorders including ASD and PTSD (Benedikt & Kolb, 1986; Drossman, 1995; Salmon & Calderbank, 1996). Symptoms of trauma-related dissociation are essential for the diagnosis of ASD, but are not necessary for the diagnosis of PTSD.

Table 7.1 Diagnostic criteria for ASD and PTSD

DSM-IV-TR diagnostic criteria for acute stress disorder (DSM-IV-TR code 308.3)	DSM-IV-TR diagnostic criteria for post-traumatic stress disorder (DSM-IV-TR code 309.81)

A. The person has been exposed to a traumatic event in which both of the following were present:
  1. the person experienced, witnessed, or was confronted with an event or events that involved actual or threatened death or serious injury, or a threat to the physical integrity of self or others
  2. the person's response involved intense fear, helplessness, or horror
B. Either while experiencing or after experiencing the distressing event, the individual has three (or more) of the following dissociative symptoms:
  1. a subjective sense of numbing, detachment, or absence of emotional responsiveness
  2. a reduction in awareness of his or her surroundings (e.g., "being in a daze")
  3. derealization
  4. depersonalization
  5. dissociative amnesia (i.e., inability to recall an important aspect of the trauma)
C. The traumatic event is persistently re-experienced in at least one of the following ways: recurrent images, thoughts, dreams, illusions, flashback episodes, or a sense of reliving the experience; or distress on exposure to reminders of the traumatic event
D. Marked avoidance of stimuli that arouse recollections of the trauma (e.g., thoughts, feelings, conversations, activities, places, people)
E. Marked symptoms of anxiety or increased arousal (e.g., difficulty sleeping, irritability, poor concentration, hypervigilance, exaggerated startle response, motor restlessness)
F. The disturbance causes clinically significant distress or impairment in social, occupational, or other important areas of functioning or impairs the individual's ability to pursue some necessary task such as obtaining necessary assistance or mobilizing personal resources by telling family members about the traumatic experience
G. The disturbance lasts for a minimum of 2 days and a maximum of 4 weeks and occurs within 4 weeks of the traumatic event
H. The disturbance is not due to the direct physiological effects of a substance (e.g., a drug of abuse, a medication) or a general medical condition, is not
	A. The person has been exposed to a traumatic event in which both of the following were present:
	  1. the person experienced, witnessed, or was confronted with an event or events that involved actual or threatened death or serious injury, or a threat to the physical integrity of self or others
	  2. the person's response involved intense fear, helplessness, or horror. Note: In children, this may be expressed instead by disorganized or agitated behavior
	B. The traumatic event is persistently re-experienced in one (or more) of the following ways:
	  1. recurrent and intrusive distressing recollections of the event, including images, thoughts, or perceptions. Note: In young children, repetitive play may occur in which themes or aspects of the trauma are expressed
	  2. recurrent distressing dreams of the event. Note: In children, there may be frightening dreams without recognizable content
	  3. acting or feeling as if the traumatic event were recurring (includes a sense of reliving the experience, illusions, hallucinations, and dissociative flashback episodes, including those that occur on awakening or when intoxicated). Note: In young children, trauma-specific re-enactment may occur
	  4. intense psychological distress at exposure to internal or external cues that symbolize or resemble an aspect of the traumatic event
	  5. physiological reactivity on exposure to internal or external cues that symbolize or resemble an aspect of the traumatic event
	C. Persistent avoidance of stimuli associated with the trauma and numbing of general responsiveness (not present before the trauma), as indicated by three (or more) of the following:
	  1. efforts to avoid thoughts, feelings, or conversations associated with the trauma
	  2. efforts to avoid activities, places, or people that arouse recollections of the trauma
	  3. inability to recall an important aspect of the trauma
	  4. markedly diminished interest or participation in significant activities

Table 7.1 (cont.)

DSM-IV-TR diagnostic criteria for acute stress disorder (DSM-IV-TR code 308.3)	DSM-IV-TR diagnostic criteria for post-traumatic stress disorder (DSM-IV-TR code 309.81)

better accounted for by Brief Psychotic Disorder, and is not merely an exacerbation of a pre-existing Axis I or Axis II disorder	5. feeling of detachment or estrangement from others
	6. restricted range of affect (e.g., unable to have loving feelings)
	7. sense of a foreshortened future (e.g., does not expect to have a career, marriage, children, or a normal life span)
	D. Persistent symptoms of increased arousal (not present before the trauma) as indicated by two (or more) of the following:
	  1. difficulty falling or staying asleep
	  2. irritability or outbursts of anger
	  3. difficulty concentrating
	  4. hypervigilance
	  5. exaggerated startle response
	E. Duration of the disturbance (symptoms in Criteria B, C, and D) is more than 1 month
	F. The disturbance causes clinically significant distress or impairment in social, occupational, or other important areas of functioning
	Specify if:
	Acute: if duration of symptoms is less than 3 months
	Chronic: if duration of symptoms is 3 months or more
	Specify if:
	With delayed onset: if onset of symptoms is at least 6 months after the stressor

Finally, trauma-exposed populations may experience co-morbid substance-related disorders (Galea *et al.*, 2002; Vlahov *et al.*, 2002). This relationship is complicated by the fact that substance intoxication may precede or precipitate traumatic experience (McFarlane, 1998).

Differential diagnosis

The differential diagnosis of ASD and PTSD encompasses a broad range of psychiatric and physical diagnoses as well as normative responses to extremely stressful events. Table 7.3 highlights disorders applicable to injured trauma survivors in the acute medical setting. As noted above, individuals exposed to events that fulfill exposure criteria for ASD or PTSD often experience transient symptoms that differ from ASD or PTSD only in duration or associated level of distress or functional impairment. In some professions – particularly those associated with disaster response (such as firefighters or policemen) – exposure to criterion 1 events is inevitable. To the extent to which symptoms persist, result in dysfunction or distress, but do not meet full diagnostic criteria for ASD or PTSD, a V code diagnosis (e.g., V 62.2 occupational problem) may be warranted. In others who do not experience the dissociative symptoms sufficient to meet criteria for ASD, but otherwise experience full or subthreshold PTSD symptoms for less than 1 month, the illness would be best

Table 7.2 Comparison of diagnostic criteria for ASD and PTSD

Description of criterion	ASD criterion	PTSD criterion
Characteristics of traumatic exposure Exposure to a traumatic event in which both of the following conditions were present: 1. the person experienced, witnessed, or was confronted with an event or events that involved actual or threatened death or serious injury, or a threat to the physical integrity of self or others 2. the person's response involved intense fear, helplessness, or horror	Criterion A	Criterion A
Dissociative symptom cluster Either while experiencing or after experiencing the distressing event, the individual has three (or more) of the following symptoms: 1. a subjective sense of numbing, detachment, or absence of emotional responsiveness 2. a reduction in awareness of his or her surroundings (e.g., being in a daze) 3. derealization 4. depersonalization 5. dissociative amnesia (i.e., inability to recall an important aspect of the trauma)	Criterion B	Not included in PTSD criteria
Re-experiencing cluster The traumatic event is persistently re-experienced in one (or more) of the following ways: 1. recurrent and intrusive distressing recollections of the event, including images, thoughts, or perceptions 2. recurrent distressing dreams of the event 3. acting or feeling as if the traumatic event were recurring (includes a sense of reliving the experience, illusions, hallucinations, and dissociative flashback episodes, including those that occur on awakening or when intoxicated) 4. intense psychological distress at exposure to internal or external cues that symbolize or resemble an aspect of the traumatic event 5. physiological reactivity on exposure to internal or external cues that symbolize or resemble an aspect of the traumatic event	Criterion C (except item 5)	Criterion B
Avoidance/numbing of response cluster Persistent avoidance of stimuli associated with the trauma and numbing of general responsiveness (not present before the trauma), as indicated by three (or more) of the following characteristics:	Criterion D (requires only marked avoidance of stimuli that arouse recollections of the trauma)	Criterion C

Table 7.2 (cont.)

Description of criterion	ASD criterion	PTSD criterion
1. efforts to avoid thoughts, feelings, or conversations associated with the trauma		
2. efforts to avoid activities, places, or people that arouse recollections of the trauma		
3. inability to recall an important aspect of the trauma		
4. markedly diminished interest or participation in significant activities		
5. feeling of detachment or estrangement from others		
6. restricted range of affect (e.g., unable to have loving feelings)		
7. sense of foreshortened future (e.g., does not expect to have a career, marriage, children, or a normal life span)		
Arousal cluster Persistent symptoms of increased arousal (not present before the trauma), as indicated by two (or more) of the following symptoms: 1. difficulty falling asleep or staying asleep 2. irritability or outbursts of anger 3. difficulty concentrating 4. hypervigilance 5. exaggerated startle response	Criterion E (requires only marked symptoms of anxiety or increased arousal)	Criterion D
Duration of disturbance	Minimum of 2 days, maximum of 4 weeks	Greater than 1 month (acute PTSD is diagnosed if duration is less than 3 months; chronic PTSD if duration is 3 months or greater)
Temporal relationship to traumatic event	Occurs within 4 weeks	Usually occurs within 3 months (if onset occurs more than 6 months after stressor, delayed onset is specified)
Distress or impairment in functioning: the disturbance causes clinically significant distress or impairment in social, occupational, or other important areas of functioning (or inability to pursue some necessary task in ASD)	Criterion F	Criterion F
Exclusion of other conditions 1. not due to the direct physiological effects of a substance (e.g., a drug of abuse, a medication) or a general medical condition 2. not better accounted for by a brief psychotic disorder 3. not an exacerbation of a pre-existing Axis I or Axis II disorder	Criterion H	Not included in PTSD criteria

Table 7.3 Differential diagnosis in the aftermath of disaster

Diagnosis	Symptomatic criteria	Functional criteria	Time course	Acute care considerations
Posttraumatic Stress Disorder (PTSD)	A. Exposure to a traumatic event in which the person experienced or witnessed a life-threatening event that was associated with intense emotions (e.g., physical injury) B. The event is persistently re-experienced C. Persistent avoidance of reminders of the event D. Persistent arousal symptoms	Symptoms are associated with clinically significant impairments in social, occupational, or physical function	Diagnosis must be made at least 1 month after the event	Patient's symptoms frequently appear before the 1-month point
Acute stress disorder (ASD)	A. Exposure to a traumatic event in which the person experienced witnessed a life-threatening event that was associated with intense emotions (e.g., physical injury) B. Either while experiencing the event or after, the person experiences three or more dissociative symptoms C. The event is re-experienced D. Avoidance of reminders of the event E. Symptoms of arousal	Symptoms are associated with clinically significant impairments in social, occupational, or physical function	Diagnosis can be made between 2 and 30 days after the event	Not all injured patients with immediate distress will experience these dissociative symptoms
Major depressive episode	Five or more of the following symptoms: depressed mood, diminished interest in pleasurable activities, weight loss or gain, insomnia or hypersomnia, agitation or retardation, fatigue or energy loss, feelings of worthlessness, poor concentration, and suicidal ideation	Symptoms are associated with clinically significant impairment in social, occupational, or physical function	Symptoms must be present for 2 weeks	Major depressive episode can be diagnosed in conjunction with ASD or PTSD. Injured trauma survivors frequently present with multiple symptoms of a depressive episode early on (i.e., before 2 weeks after the traumatic injury)

Traumatic grief	This evolving diagnostic category can be used when the events that lead to a patient's or relative's visit to the acute care setting involve sudden unanticipated loss. The symptoms of traumatic grief often involve distressing thoughts and experiences related to reunion, longing, and searching for the deceased loved one	The disturbance causes clinically significant impairment in social, occupational, or other important areas of functioning	Duration of disturbance is at least 2 months	Traumatic grief is applicable to patients who have experienced the death of a significant other
Adjustment disorder	A. Development of emotional or behavioral symptoms in response to an identifiable stressor. Symptoms can include depression, anxiety, conduct disturbance, or other emotional disturbance B. The symptoms or behaviors are clinically significant as evidenced by marked distress	Emotional or behavioral symptoms are associated with marked impairment in social, role, or physical function	Onset occurs within 3 months after the traumatic injury	DSM-IV suggests that the adjustment disorder diagnosis be used for patients who develop a symptom pattern that is not entirely consistent with the criteria for ASD/PTSD. Nonspecific symptomatic requirements make adjustment disorder a useful diagnosis for the many patients who experience post-traumatic behavioral and emotional disturbances that include symptoms that do not fit into other diagnostic rubrics (e.g., patients who present with marked somatic symptom amplification)

characterized as an adjustment disorder in DSM-IV terms. These persons would also meet criteria for acute stress reaction as defined by the ICD-10.

For a single discrete traumatic event, ASD and PTSD can be readily distinguished from one another based on the time interval that has passed since the event. However, for less discrete or recurring traumas as might be experienced in cases of domestic violence or a series of natural disasters such as might occur during the hurricane season in certain locations the distinction between ASD and PTSD may be less clear. No convention or consensus exists regarding the classification of symptom episodes lasting less than 1 month but recurring during the course of repetitive trauma over months to years. However, such symptom presentation may be better conceptualized as PTSD rather than recurrent ASD. Eliminating the source of threat (e.g., physical separation from violent partner or geographic relocation from dangerous environment) is essential to the resolution of symptoms regardless of classification.

A substantial proportion of trauma-exposed veterans, refugees, and civilians develop symptoms consistent with major depressive disorder (Kulka et al., 1990; North et al., 1999). Mood disorders may occur independently from PTSD, but they are also an established risk factor for the development of PTSD in newly exposed individuals (Bromet et al., 1998; North et al., 1999; Ursano et al., 1999). Symptoms of depression such as insomnia, poor concentration, and decreased interest in formerly enjoyable activities may also be present in ASD or PTSD. The restricted affect that accompanies emotional numbing in PTSD may resemble the diminished affect of depression. The DSM-IV permits the diagnosis of both major depressive disorder and PTSD (or ASD) when full symptom criteria for both are present.

Although the DSM-IV excluded *complicated grief* as a specific Axis I disorder (due to a lack of consensus on empirical evidence), investigators and clinicians involved in the development of DSM-V are considering such a diagnosis based on persistent, intense grief, intrusive recollections or images of the death, preoccupation with the loss, and avoid-ance of reminders. While the proposed symptoms overlap with those of PTSD and major depressive disorder, persons may experience grief symptoms without meeting full criteria for depression or PTSD (Horowitz et al., 1997). If preoccupation with the suddenness, violence, or catastrophic aspects of loss interferes with the normal bereavement process, the syndrome may represent a different (and pathological) bereavement process. "Traumatic grief" is another proposed diagnostic entity distinguished from complicated grief, by additional distress related to cognitive re-enactment of the death or loss, terror, and avoidance of reminders (Prigerson et al., 1999). Whether or not complicated or traumatic grief attains DSM-V classification, bereavement and grief-related syndromes should be considered in the differential diagnosis of persons who have experienced a traumatic loss.

Trauma-exposed populations and patients with PTSD may also engage in altered substance use patterns (alcohol, tobacco, or illicit substances) and may develop substance-related disorders. That ASD or PTSD often occurs in the wake of severe physical injury accounts to some degree for the increased somatic complaints associated with these disorders, but persistent somatic concerns in the absence of identifiable pathology may also suggest the presence of a somatoform disorder.

Finally, features of personality disorders and those associated with PTSD (e.g., impulsivity, irritability, difficulty with affect modulation, dissociative phenomena, and comorbid substance abuse) may overlap. Therefore, a PTSD diagnosis may be "hidden" by predominant personality disorder symptoms. Numerous studies identify a history of childhood trauma in adults with personality disorders, and still others describe childhood trauma as the underlying cause of adult PTSD symptoms. However, the extent to which symptoms may be misattributed to either personality disorder or PTSD has not been well studied. Regardless, personality disorders should be considered in the diagnosis of symptomatic persons in the aftermath of trauma either as the primary etiology of symptoms or as co-morbid illness.

Epidemiology

Multiple epidemiologic studies have revealed the fact that traumatic exposures (i.e., to an event that would meet DSM-IV Diagnostic Criterion 1A) are very common. The National Comorbidity Survey (Kessler *et al.*, 1995), a large-scale ($n = 5877$) nationally representative epidemiological study of psychiatric disorders in the United States, reported a lifetime history of at least one traumatic event for 60.7% of men and 51.2% of women, with many individuals (25%–50%) experiencing two or more such traumas. Other community-based samples have reported similar or even greater incidence figures (43%–92% of men and 37%–87% of women) for at least one traumatic exposure (Breslau *et al.*, 1991, 1998; Norris, 1992; Stein *et al.*, 1997). The most common types of trauma reported are witnessing someone being killed or injured, being involved in a natural disaster, and being involved in a life-threatening accident. Specific epidemiologic data regarding the percentage of persons who report traumatic exposure as a result of deliberate terrorist attacks are lacking, but such exposure would comprise a subset of those who reported witnessing the killing or injury of another.

The lifetime prevalence rate for ASD is unclear, but a number of community-based studies have examined the prevalence of PTSD. As with the studies of traumatic exposure, estimates vary with the diagnostic criteria applied (e.g., DSM III-R versus DSM-IV), the sample studied, and the assessment procedure used (e.g., telephone survey versus face-to-face interview, clinician versus lay interviewer, structured versus unstructured interview) (Brewin *et al.*, 2000). In a review of the data from 2985 participants in a central North Carolina community survey, Davidson and colleagues (1991) found a lifetime prevalence for DSM-III PTSD – which required symptom presence for at least 6 months – of 1.3%. A review of the St. Louis Epidemiologic Catchment Area sample found a lifetime prevalence of 1% (Helzer *et al.*, 1987). However, more recent United States population base estimates using DSM-III-R and DSM-IV criteria have

reported prevalence rates of 8%–9% (Breslau *et al.*, 1991; Kessler *et al.*, 1995). That PTSD may be precipitated by terrorist-attack-related disaster is evidenced by the fact that 7.5% of New York City residents living south of Canal Street developed PTSD within 5–8 weeks of the terrorist attacks on the World Trade Center Towers of September 11, 2001 (Galea *et al.*, 2002). Across community population studies the lifetime prevalence rate of PTSD in women has generally been twice that reported for men (Breslau, 2002; Breslau *et al.*, 1998; Kessler *et al.*, 1995).

Still, the relatively low rate of PTSD when compared with the substantially higher rate of traumatic exposure illustrates the point that while traumatic exposure is necessary for the development of PTSD, it is not sufficient. One major reason for this differentiation is that not all potentially traumatic events are equally associated with the development of PTSD. In fact some of the most commonly experienced traumatic events are least likely to be associated with PTSD. In the National Comorbidity Study, lifetime prevalence of being in a natural disaster or fire, and witnessing someone being badly injured or killed ranged from 14% to 36% (depending on specific event and gender). The prevalences of these exposures were all greater than the prevalence of being raped (less than 1% for men and approximately 9% for women). However, the prevalence of PTSD related to rape was 46% for men and 65% for women compared to less than 10% each for being in an accident, fire, or natural disaster, and witnessing someone badly injured or killed (Kessler *et al.*, 1995).

Also, reactions to traumatic events, even those most closely associated with the development of PTSD (such as rape), are often transient and may resolve within 4–12 weeks after the event. One study of rape victims evaluated weekly for the presence of PTSD symptoms found that while 94% met full symptom (but not duration) criteria 12 days after the assault, 64% met criteria 1 month after the assault at the point when PTSD could be first diagnosed. By 3 months 47% met criteria for chronic PTSD (Rothbaum *et al.*, 1992). Longitudinal studies of the cohort of New York City residents south of

Table 7.4 Risk factors for the development of mental disorders after traumatic events

Pre-event risk factors	Within-disaster risk factors	Postdisaster risk factors
Individual characteristics	**Severity of exposure**	**Environmental factors**
• Female gender	• Direct involvement in the event	• Resource depletion
• 40–60 years of age	• Witnessing the event	• Social support depletion
• Limited coping techniques	• Sustaining physical injury	• Social criticism
• Ethnic minority	• Reason to fear death or serious injury to self/loved ones	• Marital dysfunction
• Low socioeconomic status		• Loss of home/property or financial loss
• Prior psychiatric diagnosis	• Life threat	• Decline in perceived social support
• Prior trauma	• Panic	• Alienation and mistrust
• Below-average cognitive ability	• Horror	
• Neuroticism (proneness to experience irritability, depression, anxiety)	• Bereavement	**Peritraumatic reactions**
	• Relocation or displacement	• Derealization or time distortion (1-week post-trauma)
Family contex	• Extreme loss	• Emotional numbing, motor restlessness, or sense of reliving the trauma (within 1 month post-trauma)
• Being an adult with children	• Disrupted community	
• Being a female with a spouse		• Negative perceptions of other people's responses
• Being a child with a dysfunctional parent		• Negative perceptions of symptoms
• Instability in the family origin		• Exaggeration of future probability of trauma
Support and coping style		• Catastrophic attributions of responsibility
• Low belief in ability to control outcomes		• Avoidance coping
• Deteriorating social resources		**Postevent stressors and reactions**
		• Police interrogation
		• Media attention
		• Prolonged relocation
		• Continued separation and estrangement from family and friends
		• Bewilderment
		• Disorientation
		• Uncertainty about safety of self and significant others
		• Missing family members
		• Continued lack of control over what is happening

Adapted from: Watson & Shalev (2005).

Canal Street demonstrated a decline in PTSD from the 7.5% initially reported to 1.7% by 5 months (Galea *et al.*, 2003a) and 0.6% by 6–9 months after the attacks (Galea *et al.*, 2003b). Thus, the majority of persons exposed to traumatic events and who experience symptoms of PTSD experience natural recovery. A recent study of battle-injured American soldiers evacuated from Iraq showed that a considerable percentage of persons who failed to meet criteria at initial screening did so at the 3- or 6-months reassessment. This points to the potential for cross-sectional studies to underestimate the overall prevalence of this condition (Grieger *et al.*, 2006).

In addition to the type of trauma and the gender of the victim, several other risk factors have been identified as predictors of PTSD. In the National Women's Survey ($n = 4\,008$) fear of being killed or being injured (i.e., threat perception) as well as receipt of physical injury independently increased the likelihood of a lifetime diagnosis of PTSD (Resnick et al., 1993). Physical injury, regardless of gender, was associated with a considerably higher rate of PTSD in workers traumatically exposed to the Murrah Federal Building bombing (North et al., 1999). In a recent meta-analysis of risk factors, Brewin and colleagues found large effect sizes for severity of trauma, lack of social support following the trauma, and life stress following the trauma (Brewin et al., 2000). Other predictors included personal psychiatric history, family psychiatric history, and personal history of childhood abuse. Biological markers identified in recent preliminary investigations appear to include low cortisol in the acute aftermath of traumatic exposure and elevated resting heart rate (Delahanty et al., 2000; Shalev et al., 1998). Table 7.4 highlights identified risk factors for the development of mental disorders (including ASD and PTSD) in the aftermath of trauma.

Neurobiology

Neurobiology of the traumatic stress response

Advances in neuroimaging techniques, neurophysiology and molecular biology have led to a greater understanding of the effects of traumatic stress on the brain, the sympathetic nervous system and the endocrine system. The inter-relationship between genetics, developmental experience, and post-traumatic neural activity that leads to the development of ASD and PTSD in some, but not all, individuals exposed to similar trauma is beyond current understanding. However, advances over the last 10 years provide considerable insight into normative (adaptive) and pathological responses to extreme stressors and the processes related to intrusive memory development – which appear to drive the biological mechanisms and the behavioral responses to such stressors in disease progression (McFarlane et al., 2002).

Traumatic experience results in both immediate and long-term endocrine changes that affect metabolism and neurophysiology. The sympathetic nervous system is immediately activated by perceptions of danger and threat stimuli and, via the hypothalamus, signals the adrenal medulla to increase output of epinephrine and norepinephrine. These neurotransmitters act peripherally to affect the organ systems resulting in the increased heart rate, blood pressure, energy metabolism, and skin conductance that are characteristic of the "fight or flight" response. Acting through higher cognitive centers within the brain, noradrenergic activity results in heightened attention, and vigilance (plus altered sleep function) also characteristic of the stress response (see Figure 7.1). In addition, activation of the hypothalamic–pituitary–adrenal system leads to increased levels of cortisol. Chronically elevated cortisol levels (associated with chronic stress) has been associated with damage to the hippocampus and altered hippocampal function, which also plays a role in the development of PTSD symptoms (Charney, 2002; van der Kolk, 1997).

Neurobiology of post-traumatic symptoms

Noradrenergic cell bodies of the locus ceruleus (LC), through extensive branching, project to the medial prefrontal cortex (MPFC). The MPFC consists of orbitofrontal cortex, anterior cingulate, subcallosal gyrus, and prefrontal areas. Noradrenergic communication between the MPFC and other limbic structures (e.g., the amygdala, the hippocampus) mediate memory and learning in response to stressful or frightening stimuli. Since norepinephrine (NE) is also important in attention, memory and arousal it has been suggested that altered functioning of noradrenergic neurons may be particularly implicated in the hyperarousal and re-experiencing symptoms of PTSD (Southwick et al., 1999). The serotonergic

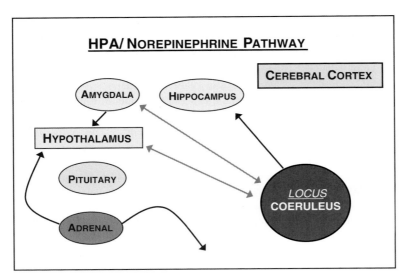

Figure 7.1 Noradrenergic circuitry in the traumatic stress response. Acute response: "fight or flight," fear, conditioning, memory consolidation, ASD/PTSD; associated symptoms: hypervigilence, arousal, fear, startle, flashbacks, intrusive recollections

inputs from the MPFC, cingulate, and hypothalamus influence noradrenergic activity in the LC, and are likely important to the as yet unelucidated mechanisms underlying efficacy of selective serotonin reuptake inhibitors (SSRIs) in the treatment of PTSD.

The circuitry described above is central to arousal, memory formation, and learning, and is important to current conceptualizations of PTSD as a failure of extinction learning (Pitman *et al.*, 2000). Memories of ordinary experience are temporarily "stored" within limbic circuitry as episodic memories – memories of personal experience and of events. Episodic memories include a sense of time and self – that is, they relate events to a person's life. While certain cognitive aspects of such memories appear to be stored in the hippocampus, emotions associated with particular life experiences appear to be stored in the amygdala. Processing or integrating emotional and semantic (factual) aspects of experience involves communication between these brainstem structures and the neocortex (e.g., the association areas of the frontal cortex). Thinking, talking, or dreaming about past experience involves the transfer of information from the hippocampus

and amygdala into the left neocortex (Solomon & Heide, 2005). Here particular experiences are integrated into the fabric of one's total life experience. The process of incorporating such an experience into one's life narrative is the process by which the "fight or flight" response, necessary for survival at the time of the original stressor, is recognized as no longer adaptive or appropriate as one recalls or is reminded of a fearful experience. The understanding of the meaning of the event as a past (but no longer imminent) threat such that "fight or flight" is no longer reactivated is the process of extinction learning.

The orbitofrontal cortex also plays a role in facilitating a response to the emotional meaning of events. Via its connections with the hypothalamus and limbic system, the orbitofrontal cortex regulates autonomic responses to social stimuli and thus mediates "emotionally attuned" interpersonal communication, by facilitating the understanding of others' emotional experience and enabling an empathic response. Studies of the orbitofrontal cortex and its limbic connections demonstrate that impaired development results in decreased capacity to regulate affect. Positron emission tomography

(PET) scans of individuals asked to write detailed narratives of their traumatic experience demonstrate increased right limbic (and visual cortex) activity. Cortical activity in the anterior cingulate region thought to modulate the limbic system is diminished (Rauch *et al.*, 1996). Hence, pathological responses to trauma may be conceptualized as a failure of higher cortical structures, via noradrenergic communication through the anterior cingulate, to inhibit limbic brainstem structures and responses.

Traumatic events may overwhelm the brain's capacity to process information. Episodic memory may persist within the limbic system indefinitely, generating vivid images of traumatic events, terrifying thoughts, and physical manifestations of the "fight or flight" response associated with the initial stressor. Such unprocessed (or not yet integrated) memories may result in loop re-activation of the "fight or flight" response, excessive arousal and vigilance, and the psychological and behavioral manifestations of post-traumatic distress. Moreover, since these unprocessed memories remain terrifying, the individual avoids thinking about or talking about the experience, and learns to avoid other reminders of his or her experience. This avoidance continues to prevent adaptive processing of the information or extinction of the immediate traumatic stress response (Solomon & Heide, 2005).

The neural circuitry model outlined above emphasizes the central role of noradrenergic hyperactivity on arousal, memory, fear response, fear conditioning, and therefore post-traumatic symptom development. The noradrenergic system, however, does not operate in isolation. Serotonergic projections from the raphe nuclei, in addition to having a modulatory influence on the LC, communicate directly with limbic and cortical structures important to the "fight or flight" response and may therefore have both a direct and an indirect role in the development of symptoms related to heightened arousal, irritability, and aggression (Nisenbaum & Abercrombie, 1993) – see Figure 7.2. Finally, the

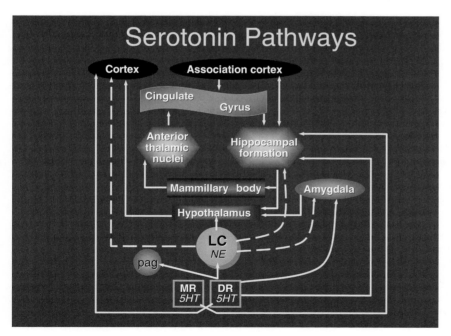

Figure 7.2 Serotonergic pathways in the traumatic stress response. Acute response: "fight or flight," rage, attenuation of fear, ASD/PTSD; associated symptoms: aggression/violence, anger, impulsivity, anxiety, depression

inhibitory and excitatory influences of γ-aminobutyric acid (GABA) and glutamate on these systems (or the regulatory role of neuropeptide Y on GABA/glutamate) are also the focus of current investigation and present potential targets for pharmacological intervention (Pitman & Delahanty, 2005). As the mechanisms underlying their influence on aspects of the traumatic response are elucidated, additional biologic therapies targeting these neuropeptides and their receptor sites may be identified.

Management in the disaster setting

In the disaster or postdisaster setting the management of ASD – and eventually PTSD – involves first the identification of affected individuals and then the initiation of treatment for those with significant symptoms. Given the magnitude of the population that may develop symptoms of ASD or PTSD in the event of a large-scale disaster, management must incorporate aspects of primary prevention to decrease the likelihood of persons developing significant illness, and a methodology for rapid triage and identification of vulnerable individuals within the larger population (secondary prevention) to inform targeted interventions and to enhance the possibility that screening efforts will identify persons in need of more individualized treatment.

Assessment and screening

The timing and nature of initial assessment in the aftermath of disaster will be influenced by the type of event, the scope of destruction caused by the event, and the resources available for assessment and management. In large-scale disasters (e.g., earthquakes) an initial triage may take place before any assessment for the presence of specific psychiatric disorders. For example, persons may be sorted and prioritized for further assessment by the presence of physical injury or obvious signs of psychological distress (e.g., agitation, disorientation), or by membership of groups at greatest risk

for psychiatric sequelae (e.g., children, the elderly, those with known medical or psychiatric illnesses) before any effort is made to further qualify diagnosis. In large-scale disasters (just as individual traumas) priority must be given to the provision of stabilizing medical care or first aid, rest, nutrition, and control if there is injury-related pain. Assuring physical health and enhancing the experience of safety to acutely traumatized populations facilitate the development of therapeutic relationships. To this end, assessment and care should be initiated within a safe environment whenever possible. In large-scale disasters this may not be feasible however, and reassurance that efforts are being made to make the environment safer (assuming that this is the case) may reduce anxiety that would otherwise cloud the diagnostic picture. During the first 48–72 h after a traumatic event some individuals may be very anxious, aroused or angry, while others may appear minimally affected, or "numb," as a result of injury, pain, or dissociative phenomena (Shalev, 2002). In the triage or emergency setting, a detailed history may be required for medical or safety reasons (or as part of a criminal investigation) but this may still increase distress. In circumstances involving the death or injury of family members a clinician may need to obtain or discuss upsetting information. In such instances evaluators must carefully gauge the individual's needs and capacities to respond to distressing questions. Care must be taken when group settings are used as a triage tool to identify those in need of intervention, as discussion of extremely stressful memories or events in heterogeneously exposed groups may adversely affect those with little or no exposure as they hear of the terrifying experiences of others.

At a minimum, the assessment of ASD or PTSD requires an elaboration of the individual's trauma history to include information on both the objective features (e.g., whether the person was exposed to an event involving actual or threatened injury, death or loss of physical integrity to self or others) and the person's subjective reaction (e.g., whether the person responded with intense fear or horror). Because of the presumed etiologic link between

Table 7.5 Domains of assessment in comprehensive post-trauma evaluation

Clinical domain	Component
Trauma history	Type, age, and duration
Safety	Threat of harm from others and dangerousness to self or others
Dissociative symptoms	Necessary for diagnosis of ASD: numbing, detachment, derealization/depersonalization, dissociative amnesia in acute response to trauma
ASD/PTSD symptoms	Re-experiencing, avoidance and numbing, hyperarousal as a consequence of trauma (PTSD is diagnosed if symptom onset is >30 days after the traumatic event; if <30 days, and if dissociative symptoms are present, ASD is diagnosed)
Military history	Prior exposure(s), training and preparedness for exposure
Behavioral and health risks	Substance use/abuse, sexually transmitted diseases, pre-existing mental illness, non adherence to treatment, impulsivity, and potential for further exposure to violence
Personal characteristics	Coping skills, resilience, interpersonal relatedness/attachment, history of developmental trauma or psychodynamic conflict(s), motivation for treatment
Psychosocial situation	Home environment, social support, employment status, ongoing violence (e.g., interpersonal, disaster, war), parenting/caregiver skills or burdens
Stressors	Acute and/or chronic trauma, poverty, loss, bereavement
Legal system involvement	Meaning of symptoms, compensation based on disability determination or degree of distress

traumatic exposure and ASD or PTSD the temporal relationship between trauma and symptoms must be established. The nature and duration of symptoms and the resulting functional impairment should be clarified to determine whether or not individuals meet threshold diagnostic criteria for ASD or PTSD. Finally as these disorders are highly co-morbid with other psychiatric disorders (especially other anxiety disorders, mood disorders, and substance-misuse disorders), assessment should include inquiry into possible co-occurrences of other psychiatric illness. Table 7.5 summarizes clinical domains that should be assessed in a comprehensive evaluation of ASD or PTSD.

The clinical interview remains the "gold standard" for the assessment of ASD or PTSD for several reasons. An interview allows for a detailed explanation of the nature of the traumatic stressor, and for the patient's initial emotional response. It permits the clearest understanding of the development of potentially confusing symptoms (e.g., a patient may not be able to distinguish or articulate the difference between intrusive recollections and flashbacks without an interactive explanation from an interviewer). Finally, the clinical interview allows for the progressive elaboration of symptoms in a manner sensitive to the emotional needs of the patient at the time of assessment. However, in a disaster setting resources will not be available to permit in-depth interview of all affected persons requesting or requiring mental health assistance or potentially meeting diagnostic criteria for these disorders. In disaster situations, several clinician-administered and self-report instruments can be used to obtain diagnostic information (and in some cases indications of the degree of severity or response) in the aftermath of traumatic exposure. The most widely used instruments are listed in Table 7.6.

Because ASD has only become recognized as a specific diagnostic entity relatively recently, there are few measures of acute stress validated against DSM-IV criteria. The Acute Stress Disorder Interview (ASDI) is a clinician-administered interview that covers all diagnostic criteria in a yes/no format. It can quickly yield diagnostic information, but does not provide any measure of syndrome severity. The Acute Stress Disorder Scale (ASDS) is

Table 7.6 Instruments used in the assessment and diagnosis of ASD and PTSD

- The Structured Clinical Interview for DSM IV (SCID-IV)[a]
- The Clinician-Administered PTSD Scale (CAPS)[a]
- The Davidson Trauma Scale (DTS)
- The PTSD Symptom Scale Interview (PSSI)[a]
- The PTSD Symptom Scale Self-Report (PSS-SR)
- The Impact of Event Scale (IES)
- Acute Stress Disorder Interview (ASDI)[a]
- Acute Stress Disorder Scale (ASDS)

[a] Clinician administered.

a self-report measure of the ASD in which the patient classifies the severity of each symptom "since the event" on a 5-point scale. The scale yields a severity index ranging from 19 to 95 (Bryant & Harvey, 2000). A cut-off score of >156 has been found to correctly classify 91% subsequently diagnosed with PTSD and 93% of those who did not develop PTSD (Bryant *et al.*, 2000). The scale does not assess the nature of the traumatic exposure, the duration of disturbance, or the degree of social, occupational or other functional impairment, so it must be augmented by clinical interview or other measure to confirm a diagnosis of ASD.

There are several reliable and valid instruments used to obtain diagnostic information (and in some cases index of severity) for PTSD. The PTSD module of the Structured Clinical Interview for DSM-IV (SCID-IV) uses open-ended questions about traumatic exposure (supplemented with examples) as well as questions about each of the 17 symptoms of PTSD, duration of disturbance, and functional impairment. The evaluator must judge whether each symptom and its functional criteria are either absent, subthreshold, or at/above threshold. The result leads to a determination of the presence or absence of disorder as well as a severity index of mild, moderate, or severe (First *et al.*, 1995). The most commonly used PTSD measure in research, the Clinician-Administered PTSD scale (CAPS), asks the patient about the frequency and severity of each symptom rating each on a scale of 1 to 4 yielding a

total score of between 0 and 136. A minimum score of 50 is often used as an entry criterion for PTSD research (Blake *et al.*, 1990). The Davidson Trauma Scale (DTS) is a similarly designed self-report scale asking patients (rather than clinicians) to score frequency and severity for each of the 17 PTSD symptoms on a 0–4 point scale (Davidson *et al.*, 1997). The PTSD Symptom Scale (PSS-I) and the PTSD Symptom Scale Self-Report (PSSI-SR) combine information on frequency and severity for each symptom on a point scale of 0–3 and yield total scores between 0 and 51 (Foa *et al.*, 1993). These instruments are briefer than the CAPS, which takes an average of 90 min to administer. The PSS-I and PSS-SR are highly correlated with one another, and the PSS-I correlates highly with the CAPS (Foa & Tolin, 2000). However, neither the PSS nor the CAPS has been validated against clinical interview in a postdisaster setting to a sufficient degree. Finally, the Impact of Events Scale (IES) is a 15-item scale developed prior to the introduction of PTSD into the DSM-III yielding separate scores on seven-item intrusion and eight-item avoidance subscales. Although it does not correspond with current DSM symptom criteria for either ASD or PTSD, it has been found to be sensitive to treatment-related changes in post-trauma symptomatology in both psychotherapy and psychopharmacology studies (Horowitz, 1976).

The instruments described above may each serve unique purposes in terms of characterizing post-traumatic symptomatology and all have been utilized in treatment studies. None has been extensively validated against clinical interview in the mass trauma environment. Since clinical resources may be dramatically overwhelmed by needs during initial assessment, and postdisaster triage, the availability of preprinted self-report forms or focused clinical interview guides should augment traditional clinical assessment. Modifications of recognized assessment instruments may also allow for the classification of persons requiring additional interview or short-term follow-up. Although no combination of symptom checklist and abbreviated interview allows for the sensitivity of a thorough and detailed individual

Table 7.7 Limitations of ASD and PTSD practice guidelines

Emphasis on published randomized controlled trials (RCT) limits the contributions of clinical experience

Restrictive eligibility, short treatment duration, and high drop-out rates of RCT diminish generalizability of findings to clinical populations

Medication adherence in RCT protocol may not reflect medication adherence in clinical populations

Negative trials often unpublished therefore results are not synthesized into guideline recommendations

Different criteria used for evaluating quality of evidence leads to disparate recommendations

Guidelines rarely assess population-based approaches

Limited evidence basis to support current early intervention strategies

Interest group representation on guideline committees may affect recommendations

Clinical advances occurring during guideline development may not be included

assessment, the administration of abbreviated interviews and checklists in group format may be necessitated by disaster and may prove critical in targeting therapeutic intervention.

Treatment and prevention

Professional organizations and institutions, including the U.S. Departments of Defense and Veterans Affairs and the American Psychiatric Association, have developed and published practice guidelines for the treatment of ASD and PTSD. Practice Guidelines do not define the standard of care (see Table 7.7). However, their synthesis of research and expert consensus augments clinical experience in treating patients, educating the public, guiding research, and establishing credibility for medical care delivery. In the final section of this chapter, essential recommendations of these practice guidelines are summarized. The developments in

treatment and prevention that have subsequently emerged are outlined, and areas for future research are noted.

Psychopharmacology

Although it is hypothesized that pharmacological treatment soon after trauma exposure may prevent the development of ASD or PTSD, existing evidence may be considered only as preliminary. Given the significance of noradrenergic mechanisms within the amygdala in the consolidation of memory and learning of fear in response to stressful events it is not surprising that disruption of this process with postsynaptic beta-blocking agents has been proposed as a preventive intervention. Preliminary studies of beta-blockers administered acutely after trauma exposure have demonstrated reductions in physiological correlates of PTSD and trends in the reduction of PTSD symptoms but have not yet demonstrated efficacy in preventing the development of the syndrome (Pitman & Delahunty, 2005). Thus, existing practice guidelines make no specific recommendations regarding pharmacologic intervention for the prevention of ASD or PTSD. For persons with ASD, the uses of SSRIs and other antidepressants is supported by limited research in ASD and by findings of considerable clinical benefit in persons with PTSD.

SSRIs are considered the first-line medication treatment for PTSD. In both male and female patients, treatment with SSRIs has been associated with reductions of core PTSD symptoms in all three symptom clusters. Other antidepressants, including tricyclic antidepressants (TCAs) and monoamine oxidase inhibitors (MAOIs), have demonstrated efficacy in earlier – and in some cases less rigorous – studies (American Psychiatric Association, 2004). More recently, prazocin, a centrally active alpha-1 receptor antagonist, has been shown to reduce trauma-related nightmares and overall levels of PTSD in a series of combat veterans and other trauma victims (Raskind *et al.*, 2003).

Benzodiazepines appear to reduce anxiety and improve sleep. They also oppose norepinephrine's memory-potentiating activity in the amygdala (although to a lesser degree than beta-blockers). They are often used in trauma-exposed individuals including those with PTSD. Their efficacy in treating the core symptoms of PTSD has not been established. Because of observations including increased incidence of PTSD after early treatment, worsening symptoms upon withdrawal, and the possibility of dependence, benzodiazepines are not recommended as monotherapy for PTSD (American Psychiatric Association, 2004).

Limited studies suggest that second-generation antipsychotic medications (e.g., olanzapine, quetiapine, and resperidone) may be helpful in some patients with PTSD. Although flashbacks and intrusive symptoms are considered to be distinct from psychotic phenomena the similarity between particularly intense flashbacks and other impairments in reality testing may provide a partial explanation for these observations. The neurophysiological kindling model suggests a theoretical basis for the anticonvulsant medications (e.g., divalproate, carbamazepine, topiramate, and lamotrigine) in terms of preventive as well as therapeutic efficacy. While preventive effects have not been quantified, limited studies suggest therapeutic benefit particularly in the re-experiencing symptom cluster with these agents (Connor & Butterfield, 2003).

Psychosocial interventions

Some evidence exists to support the effectiveness of psychotherapeutic approaches immediately after trauma in preventing the development of ASD or PTSD. Cognitive-behavioral therapy (CBT) attempts to correct cognitive distortions (e.g., overgeneralization of threat levels) and reduce the frequency and symptomatology associated with traumatic memories by re-exposure (imagined or in vivo) in a controlled setting. Studies of CBT in rape and sexual assault victims as well as motor vehicle and industrial accident survivors suggest that CBT delivered over a few sessions on the weeks following trauma may speed recovery and prevent

the development of PTSD (American Psychiatric Association, 2004).

Imagery rehearsal, prolonged exposure, cognitive processing (CPT), and virtual reality (VRT) therapies share with traditional CBT the incorporation of an element of progressive and guided re-exposure to traumatic recollections as part of the therapeutic process. The other exposure-based psychotherapies have received less attention in clinical trials. CPT has demonstrated good outcomes in a group setting with sexual assault victims; however, the degree to which this would translate to success in a postdisaster setting has not been examined (Resick *et al.*, 2002). Eye movement desensitization and reprocessing (EMDR) combines a re-exposure element with eye movement, memory recall, and verbalization. Numerous studies have demonstrated the efficacy of CBT in reducing symptoms of PTSD. EMDR has also been widely studied and appears effective – although the eye movement component of the treatment may be unnecessary (Davidson & Parker, 2001).

The idea that trauma exposure and the development of ASD or PTSD occurred simultaneously in large groups or communities was recognized long before it was confirmed in epidemiologic studies of combat veterans or survivors of the September 11 terrorist attacks. Military commanders have long used after-action reviews in an effort to evaluate the effectiveness of, and damage resulting from, combat operations. More recently this process has evolved into a number of techniques applied to groups of law-enforcement personnel, emergency service providers, and civilians, collectively referred to as psychological debriefing. Critical Incident Stress Debriefing (CISD) is a popular form of a semi-structured, staged, group psychological debriefing. While there are reports that many who receive debriefing experience the process as beneficial there is no evidence to suggest that debriefings prevent PTSD and some studies suggest that the process may be harmful (Bryant, 2005). The current American Psychiatric Association practice guidelines do not recommend CISD or other forms of psychological debriefing for the prevention or treatment of ASD or PTSD. The guidelines do call for the development of population-based approaches to exposure to mass violence aimed at the reduction of distress and maladaptive distress behavior in communities and populations as well the prevention of acute ASD and PTSD (American Psychiatric Association, 2004).

Future directions

Early interventions

In the hours or days after a disaster or even as a prolonged event is unfolding, the aim of early intervention must be to reduce immediate distress. Ideally, interventions targeted at reducing acute distress and dysfunctional behavior might also prevent the development of ASD or PTSD. One model of early intervention after disaster recommended by expert panelists is Psychological First Aid (PFA). One component of PFA is the establishment of a sense of safety (e.g., through evacuation or protection from re-traumatization). Other components include facilitation of social connectedness, fostering optimism, decreasing arousal, and restoring a sense of self-efficacy (e.g., through psychoeducation, basic relaxation training, and cognitive reframing). These interventions have not been tested empirically. Moreover, the process does not include individual assessment or monitoring for follow-up or response, so the extent to which PFA or its components prevents or reduces the development of ASD or PTSD will require further research. Targeting PFA (or other preventive strategies) to specific subsegments of the population will require a greater understanding of the extent to which ASD or other factors are associated with the subsequent development of PTSD. The characterization of biological or genetic markers, psychological traits, life experiences, or ethnocultural variables that relate to the development or severity of ASD or PTSD after initial or subsequent exposures could

inform such targeting strategies (Charney, 2004; Hembree & Foa, 2000).

Subthreshold and complex PTSD

The variability of human response to traumatic events has been noted above. Persons may develop significant symptoms in one or more of the three ASD or PTSD symptom clusters but not meet full diagnostic criteria for either illness (Stein *et al.*, 1997; Zlotnick *et al.*, 2002). That such persons may be significantly impaired raises questions about the current symptom threshold criteria for PTSD. Randomized controlled trials of medication and therapy have focused on reducing readily identifiable core symptoms (since these symptoms most readily lend themselves to quantification with severity scales). The changes in belief systems, view of self, ability to trust others, and related changes in social occupational functioning may affect patients' lives to a far greater extent than easily recognized and reportable symptoms. The extent to which these symptoms represent disabling aspects of the disorders, and the extent to which they are targeted by available treatments are questions to be answered by further research. So too are questions about whether changes in the view of self, society, or the ability to trust should be incorporated into refinements in diagnostic criteria, or into the development of further diagnostic subcategories.

Response to loss and loss-related intrusive symptoms are often a focus of treatment in persons who have confronted the traumatic death of loved ones. Therefore, another question for research is whether the presence of complicated or traumatic grief represents further diagnostic classifications (Shear *et al.*, 2001). Prigerson and others have called for the addition of Complicated Grief to the fifth edition of *Diagnostic and Statistical Manual*. In their proposed diagnostic criteria, the diagnosis of Complicated Grief would require the bereaved person to have persistent and disruptive yearning, pining, and longing for the deceased. Additionally, four of the following eight symptoms would be experienced at least several times a day and/or to a severely distressing and disruptive degree: trouble accepting the death; inability to trust others since the loss; excessive bitterness related to the death; feeling uneasy about moving on; detachment from formerly close others; feeling life is meaningless without the deceased; feeling that the future holds no prospect for fulfillment without the deceased; feeling agitated since the death. The symptomatic distress must continue for at least 6 months and be associated with significant impairment in social, occupational, or other important domains of functioning (Prigerson, 2004; Prigerson *et al.*, 1996).

In their conceptualization Complicated Grief would be distinguished from PTSD in that avoidance of fear-inducing stimuli associated with psychic trauma need not necessarily occur with Complicated Grief. It is the excessive and disruptive focus on the loss and reminders of the deceased and a desire for reconnection with the deceased rather than aversive physiological reactivity when exposed to cues or reminders of the deceased that characterize the proposed criteria. Additionally, the unique separation distress symptoms of Complicated Grief such as longing and pining for the deceased, and interpersonal attachment issues of mistrust of others and difficulty forming new relationships are not included among criteria for PTSD. Complicated Grief may affect survivors of naturally occurring deaths (e.g., deaths not occurring in the context of disaster). However, traumatic losses of very close others as might occur in disaster would be circumstances in which symptoms of both Complicated Grief and PTSD may co-occur. Since co-morbid PTSD and Complicated Grief have been noted in studies of widows and widowers (Barry *et al.*, 2001), efforts to develop effective treatments for the symptoms of Complicated Grief when these occur in addition to PTSD must also be initiated.

Generalizing research to postdisaster populations

As with most disorders, the generalizability of medication or therapy trials for the treatment of

ASD or PTSD is limited by the stringent subject exclusion criteria, relatively short duration of follow-up, and high drop-out rates in research trials. Robust treatment responses observed in the research setting may not be seen in clinical settings where access to care, co-morbidity, and not fully understood ethnocultural considerations may reduce the applicability of tested approaches. Effectiveness trials may clarify the potentially adverse effects of treatment and/or patient factors that may reduce adherence in the clinical setting. Given the high degree of co-morbidity with mood disorders and substance abuse, and observed co-morbidity in persons with schizophrenia or bipolar disorder the effectiveness of known or proposed interventions must also be studied in these vulnerable populations (Zatzick, 2003).

Conclusion

Social scientists, historians, and psychiatrists concerned themselves with the consequences of traumatic experiences on individuals and populations for decades before the diagnoses of ASD and PTSD were specifically identified. Descriptive literature, clinical experience, and case study guided the characterization and treatment of persons suffering from the aftermath of trauma before epidemiologic studies and randomized controlled trials became the standards for disease classification and treatment evaluation. History and scientific investigation have refined our understanding of the mechanisms underlying the highly variable range of human response to traumatic events. Such study has led to the characterization and refinement of the diagnosis of PTSD and more recently ASD as distinct but related entities along the continuum of neuropsychological response to the terror, loss, and disruption created by events such as natural or manmade disasters. Research and clinical experience to date have led to the development of effective evidence-based pharmacological and psychosocial treatments for ASD and PTSD, and others that have demonstrated promise in terms of preventing these disorders. While the assessment and treatment strategies identified thus far have not been systematically applied to populations in the aftermath of disaster, these strategies inform current thinking regarding population-based approaches. Future research should help to identify individual and group-specific risk factors or vulnerabilities. Identification of at-risk groups as well as factors impacting on treatment response or adherence will advance the application of population-based approaches to the recognition and management of ASD and PTSD during and after future disasters.

REFERENCES

American Psychiatric Association (1987). *Diagnostic and Statistical Manual of Mental Disorders*, 3rd edn., revision. Arlington, Va.: American Psychiatric Press

American Psychiatric Association (2000). *Diagnostic and Statistical Manual of Mental Disorders*, 4th edn., text revision. Arlington, Va.: American Psychiatric Press.

American Psychiatric Association (2004). Practice guidelines for the treatment of patients with acute stress disorder and post traumatic stress disorder. *American Journal of Psychiatry, Suppl,* **161**(11).

Barry, L. C., Kasl, S. V. & Prigerson, H. G. (2001). Psychiatric disorders among bereaved persons: the role of perceived circumstances of death and preparedness for death. *American Journal of Geriatric Psychiatry,* **10**, 447–457.

Benedikt, R. A. & Kolb, L. C. (1986). Preliminary findings on chronic pain and posttraumatic stress disorder. *American Journal of Psychiatry,* **143**, 908–910.

Blake, D. D., Weathers, F. W., Nagy, L. M. *et al.* (1990). A clinician rating scale for current and lifetime PTSD: the CAPS-1. *Behavior Therapist,* **18**, 187–188.

Breslau, N. (2002). Gender differences in trauma and post traumatic stress disorder. *Journal of Gender Specific Medicine,* **5**, 34–40.

Breslau, N., Davis, G. C., Andreski, P. & Peterson, E. (1991). Traumatic events and posttraumatic stress disorder in an urban population of young adults. *Archives of General Psychiatry,* **48**, 216–222.

Breslau, N., Kessler, R. C., Chilcoat, H. D. *et al.* (1998). Trauma and posttraumatic stress disorder in the community: the 1996 Detroit area survey of trauma. *Archives of General Psychiatry,* **55**, 626–632.

Brewin, C. R., Andrews, B. & Valentine, J. D. (2000). Meta-analysis of risk factors for post-traumatic stress disorder in trauma-exposed adults. *Journal of Consulting and Clinical Psychology,* **68**, 748–766.

Bromet, E., Sonnega, A. & Kessler, R. C. (1998). Risk factors for DSM-III-R posttraumatic stress disorder: findings from the national comorbidity survey. *American Journal of Epidemiology,* **147**, 353–361.

Bryant, R. A. (2005). Psychosocial approaches to acute stress reactions. *CNS Spectrums,* **10**, 116–122.

Bryant, R. A. & Harvey, A. G. (2000). *Acute Stress Disorder: A Handbook of Theory, Assessment and Treatment.* Washington, D.C.: American Psychological Association.

Bryant, R. A., Moulds, M. L. & Guthrie, R. M. (2000). Acute stress disorder scale: a self-report measure of acute stress disorder. *Psychologic Assessment,* **12**, 61–68.

Charney, D. S. (2002). Update on treatment of anxiety disorders. *Journal of Clinical Psychiatry CNS Discourses,* **2**, 1–4.

Charney, D. S. (2004). Psychobiological mechanisms or resilience and vulnerability: implications for successful adaptation to extreme stress. *American Journal of Psychiatry,* **161**, 194–216.

Connor, K. M. & Butterfield, M. I. (2003). Posttraumatic stress disorder. *FOCUS,* **I**, 247–262.

Davidson, J. R., Hughes, D., Blazer, D. G. & George, L. K. (1991). Post-traumatic stress disorder in the community: an epidemiological study. *Psychological Medicine,* **21**, 713–721.

Davidson, J. R. T., Book, S. W., Colket, J. T. *et al.* (1997). Assessment of a new self-rating scale of post-traumatic stress disorder. *Psychological Medicine,* **27**, 153–160.

Davidson, P. R. & Parker, K. C. (2001). Eye movement desensitization and reprocessing (EMDR): a meta-analysis. *Journal of Consulting and Clinical Psychology,* **69**, 305–316.

Delahanty, D. L., Raimonde, J. & Spoonster, E. (2000). Initial post-traumatic urinary cortisol levels predict subsequent symptoms in motor vehicle accident victims. *Biological Psychiatry,* **48**, 940–947.

Drossman, D. A. (1995). Sexual and physical abuse and gastrointestinal illness. *Scandinavian Journal of Gastroenterology,* **30** (Suppl 208), 90–96.

First, M. B., Spitzer, R. L., Gibbon, M. & Williams, J. B. (1995). *Structured Clinical Interview for DSM–IV Axis I Disorders-Patient Edition (SCID I/P Version 2).* New York: Biometrics Research Department, New York State Psychiatric Institute.

Foa, E. B. & Tolin, D. F. (2000). A comparison of the PTSD symptom scale interview and the clinician-administered PTSD scale. *Journal of Traumatic Stress*, **13**, 181–191.

Foa, E. B., Riggs, D. S., Dancu, C. B. & Rothbaum, B. O. (1993). Reliability and validity of a brief instrument for assessing post-traumatic stress disorder. *Journal of Traumatic Stress*, **6**, 459–473.

Galea, S., Ahern, J., Resnick, H. *et al.* (2002). Psychological sequelae of the September 11th terrorist attacks in New York City. *New England Journal of Medicine*, **346**, 982–987.

Galea, S., Boscarino, J., Resick, H. & Vlahov, D. (2003a). Mental Health in New York City after the September 11th terrorist attacks: results from two populations surveys. In *Mental Health, United States, 2002*, eds. R.W. Mandersheid, & M.J. Henderson. Washington, D.C.: US Government Printing Office.

Galea, S., Vlahov, D., Resick, H. *et al.* (2003b). Trends of probable post-traumatic stress disorder in New York City after the September 11th terrorist attacks. *American Journal of Epidemiology*, **158**, 514–524.

Grieger, A., Cozza, S. J., Ursano, R. J. *et al.* (2006). Post-traumatic stress disorder and depression in battle-injured soldiers. *American Journal of Psychiatry*, **163**, 1777–1783.

Harvey, A. G. & Bryant, R. A. (1998). The relationship between acute stress disorder and posttraumatic stress disorder: a prospective evaluation of motor vehicle accident survivors. *Journal of Consulting and Clinical Psychology*, **66**, 507–512.

Helzer, J. E., Robins, L. N. & McEvoy, L. (1987). Posttraumatic stress disorder in the general population: findings of the Epidemiological Catchment Survey. *New England Journal of Medicine*, **317**, 1630–1634.

Hembree, E. A. & Foa, E. B. (2000). Posttraumatic stress disorder: psychological factors and psychosocial interventions. *Journal of Clinical Psychiatry*, **61** (Suppl 7), 33–39.

Horowitz, M. J. (1976). *Stress Response Syndromes*. New York: Jason Aronson.

Horowitz, M. J., Siegel, B., Holen, A. *et al.* (1997). Diagnostic criteria for complicated grief disorder. *American Journal of Psychiatry*, **154**, 904–910.

Jordan, B. K., Schlenger, W. E., Hough, R. *et al.* (1991). Lifetime and current prevalence of specific psychiatric disorders among Vietnam veterans and controls. *Archives of General Psychiatry*, **48**, 207–215.

Keane, T. M. & Wolf, J. (1990). Comorbidity in posttraumatic stress disorder: an analysis of community and clinical studies. *Journal of Applied Social Psychology*, **20**, 1776–1778.

Kessler, R. C., Sonnega, A., Bromet, E., Hughes, M. & Nelson, C. B. (1995). Posttraumatic stress disorder in the National Comorbidity Survey. *Archives of General Psychiatry*, **52**, 1048–1060.

Kulka, R. A., Schlenger, W. E., Fairbank, J. A. *et al.* (1990). *Trauma and the Vietnam War Generation: Report of Findings from the National Vietnam Veterans Readjustment Study*. New York: Brunner/Mazel.

McFarlane, A. C. (1998). Epidemiological evidence about the relationship between PTSD and alcohol abuse: the nature of the association. *Addictive Behaviors*, **23**, 813–825.

McFarlane, A. C., Yehuda, R. & Clark, C. R. (2002). Biologic models of traumatic memories and post-traumatic stress disorder: the role of neural networks. *Psychiatric Clinics of North America*, **25**, 253–270.

Mellman, L. (1998). Consequences of violence against women. In: *Women's Health: A Lifelong Guide*. New York: Scientific American Digital.

Nisenbaum, L. K. & Abercrombie, E. D. (1993). Presynaptic alterations associated with enhancement of evoked release and synthesis of norepinephrine in hippocampus of chronically cold-stressed rats. *Brain Research*, **608**, 280–287.

Norris, F. H. (1992). Epidemiology of trauma: frequency and impact of different potentially traumatic events on different demographic groups. *Journal of Consulting and Clinical Psychology*, **60**, 409–418.

North, C. S., Nixon, S. J., Shariat, S. *et al.* (1999). Psychiatric disorders among survivors of the Oklahoma City Bombing. *Journal of the American Medical Association*, **282**, 755–762.

Pitman, R. K. & Delahanty, D. L. (2005). Conceptually driven pharmacologic approaches to acute trauma. *CNS Spectrums*, **10**, 99–106.

Pitman, R. K., Shalev, A. Y. & Orr, S. P. (2000). Posttraumatic stress disorder: emotion, conditioning and memory. In *The New Cognitive Neuroscience, 2nd edn.*, eds. M.D. Corbetta & M. Gazzaniga, pp. 1133–1147. New York: Plenum Press.

Prigerson, H. G. (2004). Complicated grief: when the path of adjustment leads to a dead-end. *Bereavement Care*, **23**, 38–40.

Prigerson, H. G., Bierhals, A. J., Kasl, S. V. *et al.* (1996). Complicated grief as a disorder distinct from bereavement-related depression and anxiety: a replication study. *American Journal of Psychiatry*, **153**, 1484–1486.

Prigerson, H. G., Shear, M. K., Jacobs, S. C. *et al.* (1999). Consensus criteria for traumatic grief: a preliminary empirical test. *British Journal of Psychiatry*, **174**, 67–73.

Raskind, M. A., Peskind, E. R., Kanter, E. D. *et al.* (2003). Reduction of nightmares and other PTSD symptoms in combat veterans by prazosin: a placebo-controlled study. *American Journal of Psychiatry*, **160**, 371–373.

Rauch, S. L., van der Kolk, B. A., Fisler, R. E. *et al.* (1996). A symptom provocation study of posttraumatic stress disorder using positron emission tomography and script-driven imagery. *Archives of General Psychiatry*, **53**, 380–387.

Resick, P. A., Nishith, P., Weaver, T. L., Astin, M. C. & Feuer, C. A. (2002). A comparison of cognitive processing therapy with prolonged exposure and a waiting condition for the treatment of chronic posttraumatic stress disorder in female rape victims. *Journal of Consulting and Clinical Psychology*, **70**, 867–879.

Resnick, H. S., Kilpatrick, D. G., Dansky, B. S., Saunders, B. E. & Best, C. L. (1993). Prevalence of civilian trauma and posttraumatic stress disorder in a representative national sample of women. *Journal of Consulting and Clinical Psychology*, **61**, 984–991.

Rothbaum, B. O., Foa, E. B., Murdock, T. & Walsh, W. (1992). A prospective examination of post-traumatic stress disorder in rape victims. *Journal of Traumatic Stress*, **5**, 455–475.

Salmon, P. & Calderbank, S. (1996). The relationship of childhood physical and sexual abuse to adult illness behavior. *Journal of Psychosomatic Research*, **40**, 329–336.

Shalev, A. Y. (2002). Acute stress reactions in adults. *Biological Psychiatry*, **181**, 158–162.

Shalev, A. Y., Sahar, T., Freedman, S. *et al.* (1998). A prospective study of heart rate response following trauma and the subsequent development of posttraumatic stress disorder. *Archives of General Psychiatry*, **55**, 553–559.

Shear, M. K., Zuckoff, A. & Frank, E. (2001). The syndrome of traumatic grief. *CNS Spectrums*, **6**, 336–346.

Solomon, E. P. & Heide, K. M. (2005). The biology of trauma: implications for treatment. *Journal of Interpersonal Violence*, **20**, 51–60.

Southwick, S. M., Bremner, J. D., Rasmusson, A. *et al.* (1999). Role of norepinephrine in the pathophysiology and treatment of posttraumatic stress disorder. *Biological Psychiatry*, **46**, 1192–1204.

Stein, M. B., Walker, J. R., Hazen, A. L. & Forde, D. R. (1997). Full and partial posttraumatic stress disorder: findings from a community survey. *American Journal of Psychiatry*, **154**, 1114–1119.

Ursano, R. J., Fullerton, C. S., Epstein, R. S. *et al.* (1999). Acute and chronic posttraumatic stress disorder in motor vehicle accidents. *American Journal of Psychiatry*, **156**, 589–595.

van der Kolk, B. A. (1997). The psychobiology of posttraumatic stress disorder. *Journal of Clinical Psychiatry*, **58** (Suppl 9), 16–24.

Vlahov, D., Galea, S., Resnick, H. *et al.* (2002). Increased use of cigarettes, alcohol, and marijuana among Manhattan, New York residents after the September 11th terrorist attacks. *American Journal of Epidemiology*, **155**, 988–996.

Watson, P. & Shalev, A. (2005). Assessment and treatment of adualt acute response to traumatic stress. *CNS Spectrums*, **10 (2)**, 96–98.

Zatzick, D. (2003). Posttraumatic stress, functional impairment and service utilization after injury: a public health approach. *Seminars in Clinical Neuropsychiatry*, **8**, 149–157.

Zlotnick, C., Franklin, C. L. & Zimmerman, M. (2002). Does "subthreshold" posttraumatic stress disorder have any clinical relevance? *Comprehensive Psychiatry*, **43**, 413–419.

8

Assessment and management of medical-surgical disaster casualties

James R. Rundell

Introduction

Having medical or surgical injuries or conditions following a disaster or terrorist attack increases the likelihood a psychiatric condition is also present. Fear of exposure to toxic agents can drive many times more patients to medical facilities than actual terrorism-related toxic exposures. Existing post-disaster and post-terrorism algorithms consider predominantly medical and surgical triage and patient management. There are few specific empirical data about the potential effectiveness of neuropsychiatric triage and treatment integrated into the medical-surgical triage and management processes (Burkle, 1991). This is unfortunate, since there are lines of evidence to suggest that early identification of psychiatric casualties can help decrease medical-surgical treatment burden, decrease inappropriate treatments of patients, and possibly decrease long-term psychological sequelae in some patients (Rundell, 2000). Physicians and mental health professionals involved in disaster/terrorism response planning should understand the importance of considering behavioral symptoms within the context of concurrent medical-surgical assessment and treatment (Rundell, 2003). Effective medical-psychiatric differential diagnosis and adequate attention to public risk communication lessen the risk of medical or psychiatric misdiagnoses, and decrease the odds that healthcare systems may be overwhelmed (Rundell & Christopher, 2004). This chapter will identify how postdisaster patient triage and management can incorporate behavioral/psychiatric assessment and treatment, merging behavioral and medical approaches in the differential diagnosis and early management of common psychiatric syndromes among medical-surgical disaster or terrorism casualties.

Phases of individual and community responses to terrorism and disasters: integrating psychiatric management into disaster victim medical-surgical triage and treatment

Disasters include natural disasters as well as human-made disasters such as terrorist attacks with explosives, chemicals, and biological agents. In cases of disaster or terrorism, particularly when the scope of potential casualties could overwhelm local response capabilities, the ability to separate medical-surgical casualties, psychiatric casualties, mixed casualties, and the worried well becomes crucial to targeting aid to the correct patients. The principles of differential diagnosis discussed in this chapter are aimed to be clinically useful across the range of disaster etiologies.

Following a potential terrorism or disaster-related toxic (biological, chemical or nuclear) exposure, or a possible toxic exposure, three types of patients present themselves for medical evaluation, (1) people with disease or injuries due to the toxic agent,

(2) people who have organic disease plus a concurrent psychiatric condition that may confuse the clinical picture, and (3) people who have not been exposed but fear they have. Anxiety and fear provoked by concerns about having been potentially exposed can complicate the medical picture; physiological signs of autonomic nervous system arousal, along with normal somatizing behaviors and dysphoria, can mimic symptoms and signs of diseases due to biological and chemical agents.

The numbers of people who present for healthcare in each of the three categories above are neither proportional nor linear across the life of a bioterrorism epidemic. When there is an explosive event, such as a suicide bombing or a building bombing, physical injuries are often clear, definable, and obvious. If exposure is covert, as in potential release of a chemical or biological agent, patients with organic disease will present before any wave of patients who present with fear, anxiety, or psychiatric illness. If a biological or chemical attack is announced by the perpetrators, the first wave of people presenting for health evaluation is more likely to feature behavioral manifestations, given the incubation periods of potential biological agents. Figure 8.1 summarizes the differences between these two types of individual and community responses to toxic agent exposure.

Covert exposure

If a terrorist group unleashes a biological agent covertly, organic disease will emerge before the general public is aware of the terrorist event. The duration of the period when illnesses attributable to the agent comprise all of the patients presenting or referred for medical evaluation depends on three variables: (1) the incubation period, the duration of the prodrome, and the time to definitive diagnosis, (2) the length of time it takes public health authorities to identify a bioterrorist event, and (3) the length of time it takes the public to be informed about the event. Once there is general public awareness there has been a terrorist event or disaster-related release of toxic substances, people who fear they may have been exposed will

begin to present to medical facilities for evaluation – some will contract illness and some won't. The experience in the United States following the anthrax terrorism of October 2001 was that the number of people who feared exposure, or were exposed but never developed disease, was over a thousand times greater than the number of people who actually developed anthrax (CDC, 2001a). The ratio will depend on the virulence of the agent, the mode of delivery, and the effectiveness of risk communication to the general public. After the clinical illnesses have run their courses, there will continue to be patients presenting for health evaluations who fear they have been exposed and displaying anxiety, fear, or idiosyncratic manifestations of psychiatric illnesses. The principles presented in this discussion and in Figure 8.1 may occur serially or continuously if there is an ongoing bioterrorism event (e.g., anthrax-tainted letters mailed over several months), producing waves of exposures and fear.

Announced exposure

Some terrorists may estimate that the greatest impact on a population will occur if they announce they have perpetrated a bioterrorist act. An actual attack may or may not follow. If an attack does not follow, all presentations will represent behavioral and physical manifestations of fear, anxiety, and idiosyncratic presentations of psychiatric illness. If an actual exposure occurs in the context of an announcement, the length of time for actual clinical prodromes or illnesses to appear that are attributable to the agent will depend on the incubation period of the disease produced by the agent. Prior to the onset of the organic infectious disease, all patients presenting to medical facilities will be people who fear exposure and might be misinterpreting signs and symptoms of other physical illnesses, psychiatric illnesses, or autonomic hyperactivity. After patients stop presenting with clinical illnesses attributable to the biological agent there will be a period during which the worried well or the medically ill who fear their symptoms may be due to the biological agent continue to present, often with symptoms of fear,

COVERT EXPOSURE

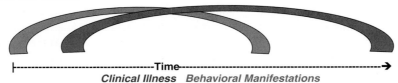

├----------------------------------Time--------------------------------------→

Clinical Illness   Behavioral Manifestations

▓ Clinical illness: first wave of people who present with clinical symptoms and signs of agent before the general public becomes aware of the bioterrorism event

▓ Behavioral symptoms and signs: as the outbreak becomes defined and publicized, patients present with a mixture of clinical illness attributable to the agent, behavioral manifestations attributable to fears of having been exposed, and psychiatric disorders. After the exposures attributable to the biological agent illnesses have run their course, fears of having been exposed remain and result in continued presentations to medical facilities

ANNOUNCED EXPOSURE

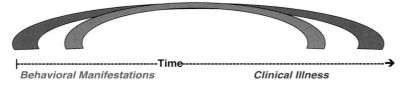

├----------------------------------Time--------------------------------------→

Behavioral Manifestations   Clinical Illness

▓ Behavioral manifestations: initially, the latency period and clinical course of the biological agent dictate that there has not been time yet for actual illnesses attributable to the biological agent to have occurred. Behavioral manifestations will remain after clinical cases have run their course among those worried they may have been exposed

▓ Clinical illness: it is important to address anxiety and concurrent psychiatric disorders in the overall medical management of patients with confirmed illness due to biological agents

Figure 8.1 Phases of individual and community responses to chemical or biological agent exposure. Adapted with permission from Rundell & Christopher (2004)

anxiety, or psychiatric illness. If there are ongoing or serial bioterrorism events, the simple curves and phases presented in Figure 8.1 may become complicated, serial, and merge together into an ongoing need to attend to medical-behavioral differential diagnosis issues.

Factors determining presentations to healthcare providers and facilities

The number and types of patient presentations to healthcare providers following a bioterrorism event will be determined by a number of factors, listed in Table 8.1. These are a combination of individual medical factors (risk factors and nature of the illnesses produced by the agent as delivered) and public health/education factors. Explosive events will produce initial injuries, and then those casualties due to secondary or delayed effects of the initial injuries, such as those related to infection, blood loss, head injury, etc. The nature of various biological and chemical agents likely to be used in terrorist activities is presented later in this chapter. It is important, however, to emphasize how crucial it is

Table 8.1 Factors that determine the timing, number and types of presentations to healthcare providers following a biological or chemical terrorism event

1. Whether the event is covert or announced
2. The toxicity of the agent employed
3. The duration and magnitude of the exposure
4. The effectiveness of the delivery mechanism
5. The incubation period and duration of prodromal syndromes and illnesses caused by the agent
6. The duration of time it takes public health authorities to identify and characterize the threat
7. Effectiveness of public education and risk communication efforts
8. Individual behavioral and medical risk factors of those potentially exposed
   a. General health
   b. Concurrent medical illnesses
   c. Concurrent psychiatric illnesses
   d. Psychiatric predispositions
   e. Underlying degree of anxiety regarding terrorism threat
   f. Individual social supports and overall sense of community
   g. General sense of efficacy of and confidence in governmental and public health officials

Adapted with permission: Rundell & Christopher (2004).

for competent, credible public health authorities to provide the general public with timely, truthful, and accurate information. The degree of behavioral contagion possible in the context of a bioterrorism event is inversely associated with the efficacy of the public information campaign. Bioterrorism is a particularly challenging public health problem because of the different agents' latency periods and the large number of variables that can affect the number, nature, and severity of casualties. Figure 8.2 summarizes the phases of public understanding following a bioterrorism event that will drive the nature of presentations to healthcare providers and medical facilities.

Following a bioterrorism event, there will be an initial period during which patients present with prodromes and clinical illnesses that eventually become part of a pattern recognized and defined by public health officials. The duration of time before the epidemic is defined depends on the complexity of the presentations and how much warning there was, either through intelligence or announcement of the event by the perpetrators. For obvious reasons, there will be very little specific public fear or anxiety driving referrals to healthcare providers or facilities during the initial phases of a covert bioterrorism event. However, as the nature of the threat becomes defined and publicized, there will be a period of uncertainty that will increase public anxiety and fear, lowering individuals' thresholds for seeking medical attention for unexplained physical symptoms or physiological sensations. Fear and anxiety itself leads to autonomic arousal, which may cause people to experience signs and symptoms leading to medical referrals. This intermediate phase of uncertainty (Figure 8.2) is associated with the highest degree of public fear and anxiety. The risk of behavioral contagion overwhelming a healthcare system is greatest during this phase, and can be minimized by truthful, thoughtful, and reassuring information from governmental and public health authorities. As the illnesses attributable to the biological agent become defined, and risk communication to the general public has occurred, there is a third (consolidation) phase. As the illnesses caused by the agent decrease in frequency, and public knowledge about risks increases, public fear and anxiety decrease to more moderate and realistic levels. Multiple, serial, or ongoing bioterrorism events will result in overlapping curves of the graphs in Figures 8.1 and 8.2, which translate into the need for healthcare providers and systems to be as effective as possible with differential diagnosis and patient education.

The ATLS® primary and secondary surveys

Since 1980 the American College of Surgeons has taught Advanced Trauma Life Support®, an approach for providing care to people suffering major, life-threatening physical injury. The underlying concept of ATLS® is simple: the greatest threats to life are treated first – loss of airway, loss of breathing ability, loss of circulating blood volume,

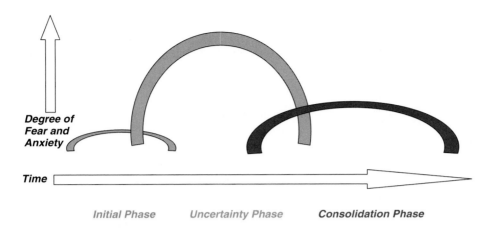

Degree of Fear and Anxiety

Time

Initial Phase   *Uncertainty Phase*   **Consolidation Phase**

Initial phase: initial presentations of cases as they develop prodromes and illnesses prior to general public awareness – little if any public fear or anxiety

Uncertainty phase: "There's something going on but we're not sure what" period of general public knowledge and perception – highest amount of public fear and anxiety. Requires thoughtful public education and risk communication

Consolidation phase: the outbreak and risks to individuals and the community become defined and publicized – moderate and manageable public fear and anxiety

Figure 8.2 Phases of public understanding following a disaster or terrorism event that will drive nature of presentations to medical facilities. Adapted with permission from Rundell & Christopher (2004).

and effects of an expanding intracerebral mass (American College of Surgeons, 2004). ATLS® principles are sure to be applied when there are explosive injuries to large numbers of patients. The rapid, targeted examination of the patient necessary to identify these life-threatening injuries is called the "primary survey." The victim's airway is checked for obstruction, while taking care to protect the spine and spinal cord. Next, adequate air flow to the lungs is ensured, and provided to the patient by artificial means if needed. Next, blood circulation is assessed, points of hemorrhage addressed, fluids replaced, and cardiac compressions administered if indicated. A brief alertness assessment is made; the patient is described as alert/responsive to verbal stimuli, responsive to painful stimuli, or unresponsive. The

more alert the patient, the more reassured the triager is that the individual is stable for the moment. The final step of the primary survey is to completely undress a patient and observe for obvious injury, taking care to prevent hypothermia.

Once the primary survey of a trauma victim is completed, resuscitative efforts are well established, and the patient has stable vital signs, the "secondary survey" is initiated. The secondary survey (American College of Surgeons, 2004) is a "head to toe" evaluation of the trauma patient – each region of the body is systematically examined. Available and relevant aspects of medical history are reviewed at this juncture as well: especially allergies, current medications, significant past illnesses, and events related to the injury.

The "tertiary" psychiatric survey: early identification of psychiatric casualties

There are many advantages if psychiatrists likely to participate in disaster or terrorism response have training, and ideally current certification, in ATLS® and Advanced Cardiac Life Support (ACLS) (American Heart Association, 2002). The history and physical examination findings collected during the primary and secondary surveys are the very data needed for the differential diagnosis of psychiatric symptoms in the medical-surgical and trauma settings. Psychiatrists who are skilled in or at least understand ATLS® and ACLS principles can be highly effective in the disaster or emergency room setting when the time comes to evaluate potential victims. First, they have credibility with medical-surgical colleagues because they speak the language inherent in ACLS and ATLS® algorithms and understand the concepts of clinical management defined by those two approaches. Credibility with disaster leaders is key to influencing their leadership behaviors (Bartone et al., 1994). Second, they can apply the triage philosophies behind ATLS® and ACLS to the differential diagnosis of neuropsychiatric symptoms and to early identification of psychiatric disaster casualties.

A postdisaster or post-terrorism psychiatric screening examination to triage and identify early psychiatric casualties can be thought of as a "tertiary" survey that focuses on the most common psychiatric sequelae (Holloway et al., 1997; Rundell & Ursano, 1996; Ursano & Rundell, 1994) and those most likely to adversely affect medical-surgical outcomes. There will be time for a more comprehensive mental health evaluation later, along with psychotherapy, medication evaluations, and debriefings when indicated. The screening psychiatric examination of the disaster, terrorism, or trauma victim is easy if the primary and secondary surveys are unremarkable. Psychiatric examination findings in that instance are likely to represent the warning signs of primary psychiatric disorders. However, when there are behavioral signs as well as significant primary and secondary survey findings, differential diagnosis can

be difficult, and multiple disorders may be present. Table 8.2 summarizes key principles of psychiatric screening of medical-surgical disaster victims following primary and secondary surveys and medical stabilization.

The mental status examination in critically injured patients

Conducting a good mental status examination in a critically injured patient is a challenge, but it is indispensable for differential diagnosis. Following explosive and exposure events, many patients will have altered mental status examinations. First, note the patient's level of consciousness. Next, establish a method of communication. If the patient cannot communicate verbally, have him or her write answers on a tablet. Writing may show spatial disorientation, misspellings, inappropriate repetition of letters (perseveration), and linguistic errors. If a patient is unable to speak or write, use either an eye blink method of communication (one blink for yes, two blinks for no), or have the patient squeeze your finger with his or her hand (one squeeze for yes, two squeezes for no). Phrase questions to allow for a yes or no response (e.g., "are you feeling frightened?"). To determine whether a patient is confused, insert nonsense questions such as "Do catfish fly" or "Do beagles yodel?" (Wise & Rundell, 2005). If the patient looks surprised or amused and properly answers the question, a secondary psychiatric disorder (medical or toxic etiology) is less likely.

Medical-psychiatric differential diagnosis

Unique attributes of biological and chemical terrorist attacks

While there is ample recent evidence that natural disasters and explosive devices can cause considerable death and destruction, an incident of chemical or biological terrorism has the potential to generate tens of thousands of casualties requiring prompt medical attention. Chemical and biological terrorism

Table 8.2 Screening psychiatric examination of medical-surgical disaster casualties: the "tertiary" survey

Examination parameter	Finding increases likelihood of:
History	
Physical injuries during traumatic event	Secondary psychiatric disorder,[a] ASD,[b] PTSD, dissociation
Past history of psychiatric disorder	That psychiatric disorder
Patient is on routine, ongoing medication	Substance intoxication, substance withdrawal, secondary psychiatric disorder
Received ATLS® or ACLS medications	Secondary psychiatric disorder[a]
Physical findings	
Elevated heart rate, blood pressure	Substance withdrawal, generalized anxiety disorder, panic disorder ASD,[b] PTSD,[c] secondary psychiatric disorder[a]
Easy startle	ASD,[b] PTSD,[c] generalized anxiety disorder
Lateralizing neurological signs	Head or vertebral column injury, secondary psychiatric disorder[a]
Physical complaints out of proportion to objective findings	Conversion disorder, hypochondriasis, factitious disorder, malingering,[d] undiagnosed physical condition
Mental status examination	
Disoriented	Delirium, secondary psychiatric disorder[a]
Clouded consciousness	Delirium, secondary psychiatric disorder,[a] dissociation
Dysarthria	Substance intoxication, head injury
Dysgraphia, dyscalculia	Head injury, delirium
Impaired short-term memory	Head injury, substance intoxication, delirium, generalized anxiety disorder, panic attack
Hallucinations or delusions	Substance intoxication, secondary psychiatric disorder,[a] substance withdrawal, primary psychotic disorder

[a] Psychiatric disorders due to general medical conditions or due to toxins/psychoactive substances.
[b] Acute stress disorder.
[c] Post-traumatic stress disorder.
[d] Malingering is not a psychiatric disorder; it is a legal accusation.
Adapted with permission from Rundell (2003).

is of particular interest to mental health professionals because the news or rumor of a chemical or biological attack could also cause tens of thousands of people to fear they have been exposed who could rapidly overwhelm local medical resources. Biological and chemical warfare are not new. Since antiquity biological and chemical agents have been used to contaminate sources of water and food, or to cause uncontrollable diseases among populations (Christoper *et al.*, 1997). In recent years, the technical capabilities of those who would use biological or chemical agents of terror have surged (Franz *et al.*, 1997). Because of the potential impacts of large-scale exposure and psychological contagion, local- and

national-level response effectiveness to chemical and biological potential threats depends as much or more on effective public education and public health efforts as on individual medical treatments. Because the signs and symptoms of chemical and biological attacks can be nonspecific and mimic neuropsychiatric syndromes, differential diagnosis by skilled clinicians is crucial to effectively triage large populations. In many cases the presence or absence of fever may be the only reliable early differentiator between those exposed to a biological agent and those not exposed but fearful they may have been.

When a patient presents to a health provider with signs or symptoms suggesting disease caused by a chemical or biological agent, or fears he or she may have been exposed, a number of infectious diseases, psychiatric syndromes, or behavioral contagion issues may account for the presentation. There may be multiple simultaneous presentations; having an illness due to a biological agent does not exclude psychiatric disorders or fear/anxiety, it makes these behavioral manifestations more likely. In addition, patients with pre-existing medical or psychiatric illnesses are at risk for exaggerated responses to potential exposure, including idiosyncratic or unusual presentations. This is particularly true of the chronically and persistently mentally ill with severe psychiatric disorders, such as schizophrenia and bipolar disorder. Other predictors of having a maladaptive psychological response to the chemical and biological warfare or terrorist event environment include anticipatory anxiety, low perceived social support (especially when stress is high), lack of effective preparatory training, and fatigue (Fullerton *et al.*, 1996).

Table 8.3 summarizes the medical, psychiatric, and behavioral conditions important in the aftermath of a terrorist event related to possible biological or chemical agents. These will be discussed individually in the remainder of this section of the chapter.

Nerve agents

The nerve agents are derived from organophosphorus compounds related to insecticides such as diazinon and parathion. They can be very toxic; for example, 0.4 mg of agent VX or 0.8 mg of Soman can be lethal to humans (Jones, 1995). Other nerve agents, such as Sarin, can penetrate ordinary clothes with ease. Nerve agents in the liquid state can penetrate unbroken skin. Nerve agents are irreversible inhibitors of acetylcholinesterase, an enzyme present in the central nervous system, skeletal muscle, several endocrine glands, and other cholinergically innervated organs. Poisoning with these agents results in an inability to break down acetycholine, leading to a functional denervation state or subsensitivity of the postsynaptic receptor in response to overwhelm-

ing stimulation (Heath, 1961). Resulting symptoms include cholinergic signs such as lacrimation, salivation, nausea, hyperpnea, rhinorrhea, bronchoconstriction, vomiting, muscle twitching, progressive respiratory paralysis, and death. The usual cause of death is respiratory paralysis.

Nerve agents have the greatest potential among toxic agents for causing diagnostic confusion. Psychological findings may be more prevalent than physical findings, especially in early stages of exposure (DiGiovanni, 1999). Persistent long-term neuropsychiatric effects can be seen as well, including drowsiness, memory impairment, depression, fatigue, and increased irritability. These effects can last weeks to years after the exposure.

Acute treatment is atropine. As much as 10–40 mg of atropine may be necessary within 24 h, and atropinization is usually maintained for at least 24–48 h (Grob & Harvey, 1953). Treatment protocols also include pralidoxime (2-PAM chloride), which acts by removing bound agent from the enzyme, reactivating the enzyme. Atropine causes neuropsychiatric effects which may be worse than the nerve agent itself in some cases. Doses necessary for treatment may cause significant drowsiness, concentration disturbance, hyperactivity, hallucinations, and stupor or coma (DiGiovanni, 1999).

Time is of the essence in treating nerve agent poisoning, and symptoms should not be mistaken for anxiety or panic attacks. Key in the differential diagnosis is history of nerve agent use and presence of early cholinergic symptoms, such as lacrimation, salivation, and rhinorrhea. Poisoning with nerve agents at a sublethal level may cause or mimic psychiatric disturbances such as anxiety disorders, mood disorders, and delirium (Jones, 1995). Atropine itself can cause psychosis. These should not be treated with highly anticholinergic antipsychotic agents, as they may worsen the syndrome.

Cyanide

Cyanide is a nonpersistent gas, especially dangerous because it may saturate the active material in gas masks, rendering them useless (Jones, 1995).

Table 8.3 Medical-psychiatric differential diagnosis of patients in the aftermath of a chemical or biological terrorism event

	Latency to initial prodrome	Time to onset of full illness	Time for lab to identify specimen or agent	Key elements of prodrome or mild exposure	Key elements of illness	Treatment	Comments
Nerve agents	Minutes to hours	Minutes to hours	Rapid presumptive ID can be made in field	Lacrimation, salivation, nausea, hyperpnea, rhinorrhea, broncho-constriction, vomiting	Progressive respiratory paralysis, muscle twitching, and death	Atropine, pralidoxime	Avoid anticholinergic antipsychotics if treating anticholinergic psychosis due to atropine
Cyanide	Minutes to hours	Minutes to hours	No rapid lab diagnosis	Anxiety, confusion, giddiness, and hyperventilation	Anxiety, confusion, giddiness, and hyperventilation	Symptomatic	Exposure symptoms are difficult to distinguish from situational anxiety
Incapacitating agents	Instant	Instant	No lab diagnosis	Lacrimation, pain	Lacrimation, pain	Symptomatic	May be confused with nerve agent exposure; avoid premature atropine use
Mustard	Several hours	Several hours	Rapid presumptive ID can be made in field	Conjunctivitis	Higher doses burn the eyes and cause blindness, pulmonary injury if inhaled, and disfiguring facial and other skin	Symptomatic and supportive	Conjunctivitis and blindness can be permanent or last for several days or weeks
Cutaneous anthrax	2–5 days	2–5 days	1–2 days	Pruritic macules or papules	Ulcerated lesions turning into eschars	Doxycycline Penicillin Ciprofloxacin	
Inhalation anthrax	1–5 days	2–60 days	1–2 days	Malaise, fatigue, cough, headache, vomiting, fever	Hemorrhage, edema, dyspnea, stridor,	Ciprofloxacin or Doxycycline plus one or	Key differentiating feature between prodrome and depressive disorders or

					diaphoresis, cyanosis.	two additional agents	hypochondriacal concern is presence or absence of fever
Smallpox	12–14 days	13–15 days	Days–weeks	Fever, malaise, prostration, headache, backache	Maculopapular rash in mouth, pharynx, face, and forearms – spreads to trunk and legs, progresses through vesicles, pustules, and scabs	Postexposure vaccination; supportive care (cidofovir, effective in vitro)	Key differentiating feature between prodrome and depressive disorders or hypochondriacal concern is presence or absence of fever. Vaccine as postexposure prophylaxis
Tularemia	3–5 days	Days–weeks	2–10 days	Fever, chills, headache, bodyache	Pneumonitis, pharyngitis, bronchiolitis, lymphadenopathy	Streptomycin, gentamicin, doxycycline, ciprofloxacin	Key differentiating feature between prodrome and depressive disorders or hypochondriacal concern is presence or absence of fever and chills
Plague	×1–6 days	3–10 days	1–2 days	Fever, cough, chest pain, hemoptysis	Pneumonia, progressing to septic shock	Streptomycin, gentamicin, tetracycline	Droplet isolation pending negative cultures, postexposure prophylaxis
Botulism	1–3 days	1–3 days	3–5 days	Diplopia, dysphonia, dysarthria	Descending flaccid paralysis with bulbar signs and autonomic dysfunction	Antitoxin, supportive care	Key differentiating feature between prodrome and anxiety disorders or hypochondriacal concerns is presence or absence of viscous secretions, especially in throat
Delirium	Variable	Variable	No lab diagnosis	Confusion, insomnia, restlessness, irritability	Short-term memory deficit, disorientation, disorganized thinking, sleep-wake cycle disturbance, visual hallucinations, hypoactivity or hyperactivity	Symptomatic management with sedating or antipsychotic medication; remove etiology	Medications used in resuscitation or life support may cause delirium

Table 8.3 (cont.)

	Latency to initial prodrome	Time to onset of full illness	Time for lab to identify specimen or agent	Key elements of prodrome or mild exposure	Key elements of illness	Treatment	Comments
Depression and mood disorders	Variable	Variable	No lab diagnosis	Malaise, lassitude, dysphoria, low energy	Two or more weeks: sleep disturbance, loss of interest and pleasure, depressed mood, low energy, low concentration, appetite disturbance, psychomotor disturbance, guilt, suicidality	Antidepressant medications Cognitive-behavioral psychotherapy	Depressed mood or resignation in the aftermath of bioterrorism or other traumatic event may be difficult to distinguish from the malaise and lassitude common among the prodromes of infectious diseases. Look for presence of fever as a discriminator
Acute stress disorder (ASD)	1–2 days	2–28 days	No lab diagnosis	Sleep disturbance, arousal, anxiety, dissociation	Dissociation, re-experiencing phenomena, avoidance of associated stimuli, increased arousal, disrupted social/ occupational functioning	Antidepressant medication Psychotherapy	Not everyone who has re-experiencing and arousal goes on to develop ASD – focus on social and occupational functioning to guide diagnosis
Post-traumatic stress disorder (PTSD)	2–28 days	>30 days	No lab diagnosis	ASD or arousal, anxiety, or dissociation	Dissociation, re-experiencing phenomena, avoidance of associated stimuli, increased arousal, disrupted social/ occupational functioning	Antidepressant medication Psychotherapy	Half of patients with ASD go on to develop PTSD

Generalized anxiety disorder (GAD)	Variable	Variable	No lab diagnosis	Worry, restlessness, fatigue, irritability	Incessant worry, restlessness, fatigue, autonomic arousal, irritability, muscle tension, sleep disturbance	Benzodiazepine or antidepressant medication Cognitive psychotherapy	Look for mucous secretions to help differentiate botulism prodrome from GAD. Situational anxiety is differentiated from GAD by degree of worry and impact on social and occupational functioning
Panic disorder	Variable	Variable	No lab diagnosis	No prodrome	Recurrent attacks characterized by massive autonomic discharge for several minutes, followed by worry and behavior changes related to attack	Antidepressant or benzodiazepine medication Cognitive and behavioral psychotherapy techniques	
Hypochondriasis	Variable	Chronic disorder	No lab diagnosis	No prodrome	Fear and belief that one has a disease, based on misinterpretation of body symptoms. Reassurance exceedingly difficult	Reassurance, high tolerance for patients' requests for appointments and examinations	Six full months of symptoms necessary to make diagnosis. Mild hypochondriacal concerns may be common among general population following disasters or terrorist events
Conversion symptoms	Variable	Variable	No lab diagnosis	Variable	Physical symptoms without medical basis or etiology	Sometimes suggestive; reassurance, education	Prevention enhanced by effective training in prevention of exposure to chemical/biological agent
Dissociative disorder	Variable	Variable	No lab diagnosis	No prodrome	Depersonalization or environmental perception disturbance that is persistent or recurrent, and results in a feeling of detachment or unreality. Must cause social/occupational dysfunction	Psychotherapy	Dissociative disorder can resemble organic or traumatic central nervous system disorders (e.g., consequences of head trauma)

Table 8.3 (cont.)

	Latency to initial prodrome	Time to onset of full illness	Time for lab to identify specimen or agent	Key elements of prodrome or mild exposure	Key elements of illness	Treatment	Comments
Situational dissociation	Variable	Variable	No lab diagnosis	No prodrome	Depersonalization or derealization in the context of a traumatic event not rising to threshold of dissociative disorder	Do not overstimulate. May be a normal, expectable response	Can be confused with neuropsychiatric disorder secondary to disaster or terrorist event, especially head trauma or smoke inhalation. Important to recognize, and manage conservatively
Situational anxiety	Variable	Variable	No lab diagnosis	No prodrome	Worry, insomnia, restlessness, fatigue, irritability, autonomic signs	Benzodiazepine medication (short-term) Behavioral and cognitive therapies	Unrecognized anxiety symptoms can resemble prodrome of botulism and be an adverse effect of medications used in disaster/mass violence settings
Substance-related disorders	Variable	Variable	Alcohol and drug screens can take minutes to hours	Intoxication seconds to minutes. Withdrawal hours to days	Toxicity state depends on substance. Withdrawal/ abstinence states characterized by autonomic hyperactivity	Supportive management for toxicity states; standard algorithms exist for managing withdrawal states	Toxicity and withdrawal states can mimic effects of chemical/ biological agents, metabolic derangements, and medications used to treat medical-surgical conditions in the disaster/ terrorism setting

Early symptoms of cyanide exposure are anxiety, confusion, giddiness, and hyperventilation. These symptoms are difficult to distinguish from situational anxiety, sure to be common in the disaster or terror setting.

Incapacitating agents

Tear gas has long been used as a harassing agent, as it is rarely lethal. It is intended to cause temporary unconsciousness or immobilization. Tear gas may produce inappropriate responses by mimicking the early symptoms of more lethal agents. For example, tear gas effects may be confused with lacrimation produced by nerve gases and lead to inappropriate treatment with anticholinergic medication.

Blister agents

Mustard gas is insidious and several hours may pass before characteristic burns and blisters appear. Low doses of mustard produce painful conjunctivitis, and are disabling and anxiety-producing. Higher doses burn the eyes and cause blindness, pulmonary injury if inhaled, and disfiguring facial and other skin burns (Jones, 1995). Blister agents such as mustard and Lewisite have been reported to produce long-term psychological symptoms such as apathy and depression (Grinstad, 1964). Acutely, blister agents can also cause delirium, and psychological distress resulting from the disfiguring lesions, most commonly in the face and genitalia (DiGiovanni, 1999).

Cutaneous anthrax

Cutaneous anthrax occurs when spores of *Bacillus anthracis* are introduced into superficial, and often unapparent cuts or abrasions. After a brief incubation period of a few days, a small pruritic macule will develop. This lesion will evolve into a round ulcer, with a black, depressed, painless eschar that will dry and fall off within 2 weeks. Cutaneous anthrax carries a very narrow differential diagnosis, possibly including spider bites (Franz *et al.*, 1997; Inglesby *et al.*, 2000).

Inhalation anthrax

Inhalation anthrax results when aerosolized spore-bearing particles of 1–5 µm are deposited into the alveoli. Macrophages phagocytize the spores, which resist intracellular lysis due to the presence of a protective capsule. Surviving spores are transported to mediastinal lymph nodes, where germination occurs 2–60 days later. Once germination occurs, disease follows rapidly. Replicating bacteria release toxins leading to mediastinal hemorrhage, edema and necrosis, followed by bacteremia and sepsis. Inhalation anthrax features a nonspecific prodrome of malaise, fatigue, myalgia, headache, abdominal pain, nausea, vomiting, dry cough, chest tightness, and fever (Franz *et al.*, 1997; Henderson *et al.*, 1999). There may be a brief 2- to 3-day period of improvement, followed by an abrupt onset of severe respiratory distress with dyspnea, stridor, diaphoresis, and cyanosis (Franz *et al.*, 1997). Septic shock portends death within 24–36 h. During the 1979 Sverdlovsk anthrax epidemic, there were reportedly only 2 patients with cutaneous lesions among 77 cases of inhalation anthrax (Meselson *et al.*, 1994), and no cutaneous lesions reported among the 42 patients who underwent autopsy (Abramova *et al.*, 1993). Preliminary diagnosis may be made via culture within 6–24 h. Laboratory confirmation requires an additional 1–2 days of testing in laboratories with additional technical capability (Papaparaskevas *et al.*, 2004). Recommended therapy for inhalation anthrax utilizes combinations of two or three parenteral antibiotics, to include either ciprofloxacin or doxycycline (CDC, 2001b). Early treatment is important to prevent progression to septic shock, meningitis, and death.

Smallpox

A global campaign, begun in 1967 under the auspices of the World Health Organization, succeeded in eradicating smallpox in 1977. In 1980, vaccination of the general population ceased worldwide. The terrorist reintroduction of smallpox would be an unprecedented public health catastrophe, due to the lack of herd immunity, the virulence and contagiousness of the organism, and a relatively long incubation period of 7–17 days. Each index case may produce as many as 10–20 second-generation cases, raising human rights and public panic issues associated with the inevitable need for isolation or quarantine of potentially exposed populations. Postexposure vaccination within 4 days of exposure has been shown to reduce morbidity and mortality, and to potentially prevent disease (Fenner, 1988). Postexposure vaccination would be indicated for those potentially exposed during the initial release, healthcare providers treating cases, and other contacts of cases (CDC, 2001c). At this time, the mainstay of therapy of cases would be supportive care by vaccinated caregivers. Patients must be isolated, and contacts must be placed under epidemiologic surveillance (Franz et al., 1997; Henderson et al., 1999). In some cases quarantine will be necessary, for example when there is uncontrolled contagion or where individuals are uncooperative with isolation and surveillance procedures.

Tularemia

Francisella tularensis has long been considered a potential biological weapon. In 1969, a World Health Organization committee estimated that an aerosol dispersal of 50 kg of virulent *F. tularensis* over a metropolitan area with 500 000 people would result in 125 000 cases, including 30 000 deaths (World Health Organization, 1970). Within 3–5 days of exposure, pneumonic tularemia will begin with an acute and nonspecific febrile prodrome with chills, headache, and bodyache. Within days to weeks, a pneumonitis, pharyngitis, or bronchiolitis, possibly with hilar or mediastinal lymphadenopathy, or a prolonged typhoidal illness would follow (Dennis et al., 2001; Franz et al., 1997). The presence of the febrile prodrome is key to differentiating tularemia from any psychiatric conditions.

Plague

Plague, caused by *Yersinia pestis*, occurs naturally in bubonic and pneumonic forms. An aerosolized plague weapon could cause pneumonic plague, with fever, cough, chest pain, and hemoptysis due to severe pneumonia 1–6 days after exposure. Rapid evolution of disease would occur during the first 2–4 days of illness, with septic shock with high mortality without early treatment (Butler, 1995; Perry & Fetherston, 1997). There are no widely available rapid diagnostic tests for plague. Since the diagnosis may be missed with laboratory methods, case reports will be a primary source of information for public health authorities and clinicians. Prompt treatment is essential. Plague is an internationally quarantinable disease (Franz et al., 1997; Inglesby et al., 2000).

Botulism

Clostridium botulinum is a spore-forming, obligate anaerobe that produces botulinum toxin. Botulinum toxin binds to the neuronal cell membrane at the nerve terminus and enters the neuron by endocytosis. The toxin cleaves specific sites on neuronal proteins, preventing complete assembly of synaptic fusion complexes and thereby blocking acetylcholine release. The absence of acetylcholine results in neuromuscular paralysis and autonomic dysfunction, producing the signs of botulism. An aerosolized or foodborne botulinum weapon would cause acute, symmetric, descending flaccid paralysis with prominent bulbar palsies, manifested 12–72 h after exposure as diplopia, dysarthria, dysphonia, and dysphagia (Arnon et al., 2001). Autonomic complications may include dry mouth, ileus, and urinary retention. Patients who may fear they have been exposed, but haven't, could report similar symptoms due to anxiety and worry. By the second day of clinical illness, however, difficulty moving eyes, indistinct speech, unsteady gait, and extreme weakness will leave little doubt as to the presence of a severe neurological disturbance.

Delirium

In the disaster or terrorism victim with major illness or injuries due to explosive devices, volume depletion and metabolic derangements can cause delirium: clouded consciousness, agitation or diminished responsiveness, and disorientation (American Psychiatric Association, 2000). A prodrome of confusion, restlessness, irritability and insomnia may portend a full syndrome which includes short-term memory deficit, distractibility, difficulty abstracting, disorganized thinking, dysarthria, reduced comprehension, illusions, visual hallucinations, sleep-wake cycle disturbance ("sundowning"), and either hypoactivity or hyperactivity. While medication treatment of the delirious patient can help decrease agitation and mitigate a safety problem, this is not the ideal management. The medications used to manage agitation can further complicate both medical assessment and an already difficult clinical course. Onset of signs and symptoms can occur within hours of exposure to the offending agent. Symptomatic management of the patient's behavioral problems with sedating medication should be initially reserved to protect the life or safety of the patient and other patients or staff. Resolution of the delirium itself should be the primary goal, and requires resolving the metabolic sequelae of the injury. Common causes of delirium in disaster settings include hypovolemia, hypoxemia, central nervous system mass effect, infection, and adverse effects of ATLS® and ACLS medications.

Depression

Depressed mood or resignation in the aftermath of a disaster or terrorist event may be difficult to distinguish from the malaise and lassitude common among the prodromes of many chemical and bioterrorism exposures (Table 8.3). When depressed mood and associated depressive symptoms disrupt social and occupational functioning, major depressive disorder is diagnosed. Antidepressant medications and cognitive-behavioral psychotherapy are the mainstays of treatment for major depressive disorder, and may assist with managing subsyndromal depression.

Acute stress disorder and post-traumatic stress disorder

There can be a substantial burden of acute stress disorder (ASD), acute post-traumatic stress disorder (PTSD) and depression following a major terrorist event. Among 1008 adults interviewed in New York City between 1 and 2 months after the attacks on the World Trade Center, 7.5% reported symptoms consistent with a diagnosis of current PTSD and 9.7% reported symptoms consistent with current depression (Galea et al., 2002). ASD and PTSD do not occur in vacuums. When one of these disorders exists, it is highly probable that other psychiatric conditions exist as well, especially major depressive disorder, panic disorder, substance use disorder, and generalized anxiety disorder (Ursano et al., 1995). Having a physical injury increases the risk of ASD and PTSD. Treatment involves antidepressant medication and psychotherapy.

Generalized anxiety disorder

Excessive anxiety plus apprehensive expectations about events or activities (American Psychiatric Association, 2000) characterize generalized anxiety disorder (GAD). A patient's incessant worry is difficult to control and commonly evokes restlessness, fatigue, irritability, muscle tension, and sleep disturbance. Motor tension is prominent, and may include trembling and twitching. Treatment is with benzodiazepine medications, antidepressant medications, beta-blockers, and/or cognitive psychotherapy.

Panic disorder

Panic disorder (American Psychiatric Association, 2000) entails recurrent, unexpected panic attacks followed by worry, concern, and behavior changes related to the attacks. The attacks are not due to a general medical condition or the direct effects of a substance. Panic attacks are characterized by massive autonomic discharge for several minutes. Treatment is with antidepressant medication, benzodiazepines, and/or psychotherapy (behavioral, relaxation, and cognitive).

Hypochondriasis

Hypochondriasis is the fear or belief that one has a serious disease based on the misinterpretation of bodily symptoms. Anxiety and fear about the disease persist despite normal medical evaluations and reassurance (American Psychiatric Association, 2000). In the generally anxious atmosphere and uncertainty following disasters and terrorist events, patients with hypochondriasis may have particular problems managing their anxiety and beliefs, and people without a history of hypochondriasis may present with it for the first time. There is bodily pre-occupation and vigilance regarding body sensations. Concern about the feared illness is a central feature of the individual's self-image, and a topic of social discourses. Because of the generally increased anxiety following a stressful event, six full months of symptoms are required before making this diagnosis. Hypochondriasis is a chronic condition with a poor prognosis. Subsyndromal hypochondriacal fears, on the other hand, may be widespread among the general population following a bioterrorist event, and should be managed with reassurance and a degree of tolerance for patients' requests for appointments and examinations by their primary care providers.

Unexplained physical symptoms and conversion symptoms

Unexplained physical symptoms are common after terrorism and war. Not all unexplained physical symptoms are conversion symptoms, though conversion is well documented anecdotally after terrorist and combat events. Unfortunately, there is at present little scientific basis for future prevention and care of unexplained physical symptoms (Clauw *et al.*, 2003). However, it is important that persons with unexplained symptoms be identified in the triage process so that inappropriate and potentially harmful treatments are not conducted that could also draw resources away from victims needing them.

Use of biological or chemical agents presents a challenging differential diagnosis and contagion problem. People may not be easily talked out of the notion they have been exposed, even in the face of information certifying their risk to be nonexistent or exceedingly low (Stuart *et al.*, 2003). During World War I "gas hysteria" was common and threatened the integrity of entire military units (Miller, 1944). Psychological casualties in chemical and biological threat scenarios may outnumber and prove more costly in personnel losses than physical casualties, as occurred in World War I (Cadigan, 1982). Acute symptoms of gas hysteria often mimicked some of the symptoms of gas poisoning (dyspnea, coughing, aphonia, burning of the skin). The degree of exact exposure was unrelated to the symptoms presented. Patients frequently presented with air hunger and other symptoms consistent with anxiety and panic. Factors that predispose to psychiatric casualties related to psychological contagion include rates of wounding/exposure in the unit, lack of sleep, and lack of prior experience with these phenomena/attacks (Jones, 1995).

Dissociative disorders

The essential feature of dissociative disorders is a disruption in the usually integrated functions of consciousness, memory, identity, or perception of the environment. The onset may be sudden, gradual, transient, or chronic (American Psychiatric Association, 2000). There are several subtypes of dissociative disorder, including amnesia, fugue, depersonalization, and derealization. The centerpiece of the diagnosis, to discriminate it from situational dissociation, is the presence of significant distress, or significant disruption in social or occupational functioning. People who have been exposed to traumatic events are at increased risk for developing dissociative disorder. Differential diagnosis of head injury and dissociation is one of the most important roles of psychiatrists participating in large-scale triage operations following explosive terrorist events.

Situational dissociation

Dissociation which falls short of diagnostic criteria for dissociative disorder is common in the context of any traumatic or terrorist event. Dissociation is generally under-recognized in the immediate aftermath of a traumatic event or terrorist event. Among the USS Cole casualties evacuated to Landstuhl Regional Medical Center in October 2000, dissociation was the most common behavioral response observed (author, personal communication). There was a fatal train crash in Silver Spring, Maryland, in February 1996, and the author lived nearby and was a first responder. At least 4 of the first 12 initial casualties brought to a hastily arranged medical triage area initially labeled as "urgent" casualties because of apparent unresponsiveness were later found to simply be dissociating. Their misidentification as potential head injury patients resulted in misdirected rescue resources early in a mass casualty situation with heavy demands on local rescue resources.

Dissociation may be adaptive in the immediate aftermath of a trauma – dissociating may prevent the eruption of intolerable affects or the unleashing of potentially dangerous impulses or behaviors (e.g., to flee the scene). It is easy to confuse dissociation and diminished neurological responsiveness. A key role of a psychiatrist in the immediate aftermath of a disaster, while primary and secondary surveys are occurring, can be to help identify dissociation. Gently tap the patient on the shoulder and ask if there is anything they need and do they know where they are/what day it is. Watch for a muted but appropriate response in a dissociating person; this indicates his or her level of consciousness and orientation is grossly intact. Identifying otherwise uninjured disaster victims who are simply dissociating frees up scarce evaluation and treatment resources for other emergency patients. If dissociation subsequently becomes frequent, ongoing, and disabling, it may then be formally diagnosed as a psychiatric disorder – dissociative disorder. Serial examinations of the patient can help differentiate adaptive dissociation from dissociative disorder.

Situational anxiety and worry

Sometimes anxiety associated with potential exposure to bioterrorism agents and worry that one might have been exposed can cause troublesome anxiety symptoms that cause disruption of normal func-tioning and can complicate the overall differential diagnosis. While not rising to the threshold for diagnosis of an anxiety disorder per se, the anxiety signs and symptoms can be managed to the benefit of the patient. A number of techniques and interventions are employed, including relaxation techniques, systematic desensitization, biofeedback, meditation, and short-term use of anti-anxiety or antidepressant medications. Behavior and cognitive psychotherapies provide an opportunity for reduction of acute anxiety, enhancement of the patient's sense of mastery, and clarification of measurable goals. Israeli studies on how terrorist victims and their families cope in the early post-terrorism period is instructive; the most prevalent coping mechanisms are active information search about loved ones and seeking out social support (Bleich et al., 2003).

Substance use disorders

Following a disaster or terrorism event, people may increase their use of alcohol or drugs as a way to decrease the acute despair or anxiety associated with the event. The substance use can then evolve into a problematic condition in its own right and should be screened for. Rescue and healthcare workers are at risk because of the types of scenes they may be participating in and exposed to. Disaster response leaders must educate and model for their workers the avoidance of alcohol and drugs during the disaster management period and its aftermath. Patients who have substance-related disorders may present at a triage or patient management area intoxicated or in withdrawal. Either can be confused with toxicities associated with chemical agents, biological agents, metabolic derangements, or medications used to treat patients' medical-surgical conditions.

Effects of disaster medications

A mainstay of managing patients under ATLS® and ACLS paradigms is medication, many of which can cause neuropsychiatric or autonomic symptoms. It is important to find out what medications an injured patient has received, in what amounts, and over what time period. Agents such as intravenous fluids (water), epinephrine, lidocaine, atropine, sedatives, nitroglycerin, and morphine are commonly used and have significant psychiatric or autonomic effects. These can resemble primary psychiatric disorders. For example, atropine causes significant anxiety and anticholinergic effects. Epinephrine causes blood pressure and heart rate elevations, and causes patients to feel anxious or panicky. Morphine causes sedation and impairs orientation and responsiveness.

It is also important to know what substances a patient has *not* been exposed to. Following a faked chemical or biological agent threat, there may be a large number of individuals who fear they have been exposed and will present with realistic symptoms based on their knowledge of the alleged agent and vital sign abnormalities produced by anxiety/fear (Fullerton *et al.*, 1996). To minimize the effects of mass hysteria, disaster leaders need accurate information from investigating authorities, as soon as it can be provided, along with a preplanned public information campaign.

Effective medical-psychiatric differential diagnosis

Initial presentation of patients in the emergency department or triage setting

A terrorist attack is psychological warfare, intended to disrupt normal societal and individual functioning. Following a terrorist attack, whether explosive, chemical, or biological, there will be patients, exposed and not exposed, who will have anxiety, tachycardia, tachypnea, shakiness, and other autonomic signs and symptoms that could be due to a toxic agent or to anxiety or fear associated with the incident. When there are not pathognomonic signs of a toxic agent, or when differential assessment is not conducted, patients may receive inappropriate treatments that could worsen their condition, or have a delay in appropriate treatment. Psychiatrists assisting with a focused mental status examination and a brief history can help identify patients who do

not need medical-surgical treatments (e.g., atropine), help differentiate dissociation from delirium, and help identify patients who have mental status findings consistent with delirium instead of anxiety. Psychiatrists can also conduct brief interventions with individuals convinced they have been exposed to a toxic or biological agent but who are judged by disaster managers to be at no or extremely low risk (Stuart *et al.*, 2003; Ursano *et al.*, 2003, 2004).

Key elements in the differential diagnosis

When triage and evaluation occur for people who have potentially been exposed to a chemical or bioterrorism agent, including behavioral and psychiatric considerations in the medical differential diagnosis increases the efficacy of overall management. This is particularly important because behavioral responses to bioterrorism may exceed in number and magnitude the medical and surgical consequences. In addition, the signs of psychiatric illness and behavioral contagion can overlap with medical signs of injury, toxicity or infection. Table 8.3 summarizes the medical-psychiatric differential diagnosis of history and examination findings that may present in patients coming in for healthcare in the aftermath of a bioterrorism event. There are three critically important elements that point the examiner in the direction of a higher likelihood of underlying psychiatric disorder: past history of similar psychiatric symptoms/diagnosis, family history of similar psychiatric symptoms/diagnosis, and having a clinical presentation which is more consistent with a psychiatric disorder than with the feared injury, chemical exposure, or infectious disease.

There is a need for research on gender- and age-related differences in the aftermath of terrorist, combat, or disaster events. Data from Operation Enduring Freedom and Operation Iraqi Freedom patients seen at Landstuhl Regional Medical Center, where women are serving in danger settings in unprecedented numbers, suggest that there are gender differences in types of injuries and return to duty rates (Rundell & Baine, 2002). For children, there is a need for appropriate management protocols unique to different age groups of children, tailored to their specific needs and abilities (Committee on Environmental Health and Committee on Infectious Diseases, 2000).

Effective community prevention and response to disasters and terrorist attacks as tools to mitigate psychiatric casualties

Government and organizational responses may play an important role in limiting psychological contagion and may help to lessen overburdening of the healthcare system after a terrorist event or disaster. A well-designed, well-coordinated and rehearsed community management strategy based on empirical evidence will do much to reduce public anxiety and increase the confidence of healthcare workers (Alexander & Klein, 2003; CDC, 2000; Everly & Mitchell, 2001; Stern, 1999; Tucker, 1997). There are mass trauma casualty predictors which can help leaders in planning community responses (CDC, 2003b). Communities must work together to coordinate the disaster response so that triage systems are consistent, clear, simple, and implementable in a short period of time (Ihlenfeld, 2003; Nocera & Garner, 1999). After a terrorist attack or disaster, communicating health information to an alarmed public is crucial to limiting psychological contagion; effective use of the internet for risk communication will be increasingly important (Hobbs *et al.*, 2004).

Training and confidence in containment procedures may be important factors in limiting psychological contagion and unexplained physical symptoms. Military experience is that the risk of psychiatric casualties such as conversion disorder is lessened when potentially exposed personnel receive good training to allow them to feel confident in their odds of survival in the chemical or biological threat scenario (Marshall, 1979). In addition to training, there is focus on vaccinating groups at highest risk of coming into contact with biological agents or with persons exposed to them, including healthcare workers (CDC, 2002, 2003a; Wharton *et al.*, 2003). Hospitals are being urged to update their infection control procedures to increase responders' confidence that the level of risk can be managed for aerosolized biological threat agents (Keim & Kaufmann, 1999).

Clinical issues in medical-surgical disaster/terrorism casualties

Clinical treatments that aim to prevent psychiatric sequelae

It is natural and proper that mental health professionals strive to prevent long-term psychiatric sequelae of exposure to traumatic events by intervening early. Unfortunately, some well-intentioned attempts prove in the end to be either not beneficial or even potentially harmful for some people (Wessely *et al.*, 1999). There are, however, anecdotal and case series that describe potentially effective interventions for well-defined groups of people (Benedek *et al.*, 2002; Bryant *et al.*, 1999; Cloak & Edwards, 2004; Holloway *et al.*, 1997; Yori, 2002). Evidence-based approaches exist to treat patients with identified psychiatric disorders. This makes psychiatric triage and case identification important in the early post-terrorism management scenario. The efficacy of group interventions aimed at preventing later sequelae needs further research.

Burns patients

During the first 24–72 h after a severe burn, there is typically a brief period of initial lucidity, during which patients usually are told their prognosis. After that, between 30% and 70% of hospitalized severe burns patients develop delirium, presumably caused by biologic stress and burn-induced metabolic disturbances (Rundell & Wise, 2000). Watch closely for substance withdrawal syndromes; unfortunately, the time courses for most withdrawal syndromes coincide with the critical periods of burns patients' medical courses. Substance withdrawal can greatly complicate medical care if not managed early and aggressively.

Strongly consider the possibility of a medically induced secondary mood syndrome when burns patients appear depressed (Raison *et al.*, 2002). Burns patients lose water at a rate several times faster than normal; hypovolemic shock is common. Following the shock phase is a period of intense catabolism and negative nitrogen balance. The usual anorexia, weight loss, exhaustion, and lassitude of this period may lead unsuspecting clinicians to diagnose primary depression.

Pain is a continuing and critical issue for burns patients; it becomes especially important during dressing changes and debridement. Narcotics are the drugs of choice for treating acute burn pains – this is not the time to worry about addiction. Dressing changes often require pre-emptive analgesia.

Agitated patients

Patients who are agitated in the emergency or triage setting can present the potential for considerable harm to self, to others, and to the effectiveness of the medical management scenario. Clinicians must balance patients' rights, rights of others to be treated or work safely, the potential for complicating an already uncertain diagnostic situation by adding another medication, the patient's degree of suffering, and the potential for drug/drug or chemical agent/drug interactions when deciding whether to control a patient's agitation with medication in the disaster or terrorism setting.

A recently developed algorithm for treating patients who present to the Emergency Department with acute psychotic agitation and require control for safety is potentially helpful in the postdisaster or post-terrorism setting since it focuses on medications less likely than in previous years to worsen or complicate the mental status examination. The algorithm was developed by experts in Emergency Medicine and Psychiatry from a number of academic centers (Currier *et al.*, 2004). An agitated patient must first of all be assessed for potentially reversible causes of agitation, using vital signs, physical examination, finger-stick glucose, history, and if indicated drug and alcohol screens, and a screen for suspected agents of exposure. If patients cannot be reassured and remain uncooperative and a risk to self or others, chemical restraint is appropriate. If the patient can take oral medication, oral risperidone (2 mg), oral lorazepam (2 mg), or orally disintegrating olanzapine (5–10 mg) are first line. Often risperidone and lorazepam are given together. If oral medications are not appropriate because the patient is uncooperative or not fully alert, the first-line parenteral medication is ziprasidone 20 mg intramuscularly, supplemented as needed with lorazepam 20 mg intramuscularly. Intramuscular or intravenous haloperidol is considered second line in these scenarios because of the higher risk for extrapyramidal symptoms, potentially disabling and confusing in the bioterrorism or chemical terrorism settings.

Losses of body parts and functions

The larger the disaster or terrorist event, the higher the probability that medical-surgical needs will outstrip available resources, particularly in the crucial "golden hour" following an event. This means that there will be a number of victims who have lost body parts and functions that might have been salvaged if the disaster had been on a smaller scale. For example, victims who might have received early comprehensive intervention at a trauma center following a car accident might be triaged into a less emergent category and attended to much later following a large train accident. This can become an important psychotherapy issue after the original survival crisis, when inevitable "what if" and "if only" thoughts emerge. When there is acute vision loss, there is a high risk for delirium, psychosis, and dissociation.

Disfigurement and body image

Facial disfigurement and facial burns usually cause more psychological difficulty than injuries and burns to other body areas. Give patients honest explanations and prognoses, but do not force a patient to view a deformity until ready; he or she may choose to wait several days or even weeks before looking in a mirror. Longer-term individual or group psychotherapy is sometimes required to help severely injured or burned patients adjust to permanent disfigurement and changes in body image. In one study, 35.3% of burns patients met criteria for PTSD at 2 months, 40% met the criteria at 6 months, and 45.2% met the criteria at 12 months (Perry *et al.*, 1992).

Guilt and grief

It is a rare disaster or terrorist event where bereaved families are not offered grief counseling or therapy. However, survivors and their families will also have to face important grief and guilt issues – particularly over losses of body parts and functions. Having a serious injury does not make a survivor immune from the survivor guilt experienced by those disaster victims who walk away uninjured. Unassuaged survivor guilt may complicate and slow psychotherapy aimed at body image and disfigurement issues. There also may be secondary effects among surviving children of victims of terrorist events or other disasters.

The dead and dying

It is often easy in a busy postdisaster setting to ignore those individuals who are "expectant." It is a fact that people die in disasters, and sometimes not instantly – avoid avoiding them. The dead deserve a respectful transition from disaster scene to family funeral director. When resources are available, a great deal can be done to ease the suffering of disaster victims who are dying (Breitbart & Lintz 2002; Shuster *et al.*, 1999). The dying patient is generally comfortable talking about death. It is usually the family, and sometimes the disaster management team, who are reluctant to engage in such conversations. Don't underestimate the importance of religious belief and the belief in an afterlife in dying patients. Discuss "do not resuscitate" orders, wills, and comfort measures early.

In a postdisaster hospital or hospice setting, depression is common. The utility of antidepressant medications is limited by the several weeks needed for the agents to be effective. The threat of impending death can also obviously cause a great deal of anxiety. If an individual does not mention fears of dying, inquire either indirectly (e.g., "You look scared; how are you doing?") or inquire directly (e.g., "Are you worried you may die?"). If death is imminent and the patient is lucid, ask "What frightens you most about dying?" Three common fears are abandonment, uncontrollable pain, and shortness of breath (Cassem, 2004). Therapists should not be afraid to speak the unspeakable or confirm reality (Blacher, 1987). Anti-anxiety medications are very effective for dying patients if symptomatic or disabling anxiety persists after psychological support and the opportunity for abreaction is provided (Rundell & Wise, 2000).

Heroes in hospitals

Being a hero presents unique psychological challenges. Released prisoners of war, disaster victims who saved others' lives, and rescue personnel who went beyond the efforts of their peers frequently become public heroes. The hero must meet expectations of adoring audiences and communities. They must grin when they might want to cry. They must avoid or be extremely cautious in how they publicly discuss their own survivor guilt and grief. Heroes' families may insist on special treatment for themselves and their hero relatives. Medical personnel, with the best of intentions, may set up scenarios which make heroes' own postdisaster recoveries more problematic, particularly when the expressions of community support and adoration fade away. For example, heroes with relatively minor physical injuries may be offered ongoing narcotic analgesic "prn" medication even in the absence of nocioceptive pain. The hero may accept these medications because it may help temporarily relieve psychological pain, guilt, and anxiety.

Hospitalized heroes become the centers of politician, press, and community attention. Then when the public's short attention span wanders to other topics, heroes have to become regular people again.

This dizzying rise and steep fall need to be addressed in psychotherapy. Preventing post-traumatic psychiatric syndromes in these unique individuals requires that they be protected from overstimulation during the immediate postdisaster period. Jealously protect the individual's "quiet time." Hospitalized heroes' real achievements should be acknowledged and rewarded, but pampering and overinflating achievements increase the chances there will be a psychological "crash and burn."

Conclusion

Healthcare professionals should consider behavioral and psychiatric issues in the context of an overall differential diagnosis in the aftermath of a terrorism event, especially following chemical and biological attacks. When psychiatric signs and symptoms confuse or coexist with medical-surgical injuries and conditions, psychiatric consultation early in the triage and management process can ensure more timely, accurate, efficacious, and cost-effective management of disaster or terrorism victims. Psychiatrists can increase their potential effectiveness in the disaster arena by taking ACLS and ATLS® courses, and using the programs' algorithm-based concepts to guide their own assessment and management of disaster victims.

In the instance of chemical and biological terrorism, the symptoms and signs of psychiatric conditions and effects of exposure and its treatment overlap. Knowledge of the way infectious diseases, chemical agent exposures, psychiatric disorders, and behavioral contagion present can help to ensure that patients receive the right treatments for the right disorders. When there is a surgical or medical condition that presents following physical trauma or exposure to a chemical or biological agent, the risk for the psychiatric disorders described in this chapter increase and should be managed along with the effects of the chemical or primary infectious disease in order to decrease morbidity and mortality. Careful management of the public education and risk communication aspects of disaster and terrorism has multiplier effects in terms of preventing inappropriate and costly utilization of healthcare resources.

REFERENCES

Abramova, F. A., Grinberg, L. M., Yampolskaya, O. V. & Walker, D. H. (1993). Pathology of inhalational anthrax in 42 cases from the Sverdlovsk outbreak of 1979. *Proceedings of the National Academy of Sciences of the United States of America*, **90**, 2291–2294.

Alexander, D. A. & Klein, S. (2003). Biochemical terrorism: too awful to contemplate, too serious to ignore: subjective literature review. *British Journal of Psychiatry*, **183**, 491–497.

American College of Surgeons (2004). *Advanced Trauma Life Support® for Doctors – Student Course Manual*, 7th edn. Chicago, IU.: American College of Surgeons.

American Heart Association. (2002). *Advanced Cardiac Life Support*. Dallas, Tex.: American Heart Association.

American Psychiatric Association. (2000). *Diagnostic and Statistical Manual of Mental Disorders*, 4th edn., Text revision. Washington, D.C.: American Psychiatric Publishing.

Arnon, S. S., Schecter, R. & Inglesby, T. V. (2001). Botulinum toxin as a biological weapon: medical and public health management. *Journal of the American Medical Association*, **285**, 1059–1070.

Bartone, P. T., Wright, K. M. & Radke, A. (1994). Psychiatric effects of disaster in the military community. In *Military Psychiatry: Preparing in Peace for War*, eds. F. D. Jones, L. R. Sparacino, V. L. Wilcox & J. M. Rothberg. Washington, D.C.: TMM Publications.

Benedek, D. M., Holloway, H. C. & Becker, S. M. (2002). Emergency mental health management in bioterrorism events. *Emergency Medicine Clinics of North America*, **20**, 393–407.

Blacher, R. (1987). Brief psychotherapeutic interventions for the surgical patient. In *The Psychological Experience of Surgery*, ed. R. S. Blacher. New York: John Wiley and Sons.

Bleich, A., Gelkopf, M. & Solomon, Z. (2003). Exposure to terrorism, stress-related mental health symptoms, and coping behaviors among a nationally representative sample in Israel. *The Journal of the American Medical Association*, **290**, 612–620.

Breitbart, W. & Lintz, K. (2002). Psychiatric issues in the care of dying patients. In *The American Psychiatric*

Publishing Textbook of Consultation-Liaison Psychiatry, 2nd edn., eds. M. G. Wise & J. R. Rundell. Washington, D.C.: American Psychiatric Publishing.

Bryant, R. A., Sackville, T., Dang, S. T., Moulds, M. & Guthrie, R. (1999). Treating acute stress disorder: an evaluation of cognitive behavior therapy and supportive counseling techniques. *The American Journal of Psychiatry,* **156,** 1780–1786.

Burkle, F. M. (1991). Triage of disaster-related neuropsychiatric casualties. *Emergency Medicine Clinics of North America,* **9,** 87–105.

Butler, T. (1995). *Yersinia* species. In *Principles and Practice of Infectious Diseases,* eds. G. L. Mandell, J. E. Bennett & R. Dolin. New York: Churchill Livingstone.

Cadigan, F. D. (1982). Battleshock, the chemical dimension. *Journal of the Army Medical Corps,* **128,** 89–92.

Cassem, N. H. (2004). End of life issues: principles of care and ethics. In *Massachusetts General Hospital Handbook of General Psychiatry,* 5th edn., ed. T. A. Stern. Philadelphia, Pa.: Elsevier.

CDC. (2000). Biological and chemical terrorism: strategic plan for preparedness and response. Recommendations of the CDC Strategic Planning Workgroup. *Morbidity and Mortality Weekly Report,* **49** (Suppl), RR–4.

CDC. (2001a). Update: investigation of bioterrorism-related anthrax and adverse effects from antimicrobial prophylaxis. *Morbidity and Mortality Weekly Report,* **50,** 973.

CDC. (2001b). Update: investigation of bioterrorism-related anthrax and interim guidelines for exposure management and antimicrobial therapy. *Morbidity and Mortality Weekly Report,* **50,** 909–919.

CDC. (2001c). Vaccinia (Smallpox) vaccine. Recommendations of the Advisory Committee on Immunization Practices (ACIP). *Morbidity and Mortality Weekly Report,* **50** (Suppl), RR–10.

CDC. (2002). Use of anthrax vaccine in response to terrorism: supplemental recommendations of the advisory committee on immunization practices. *Morbidity and Mortality Weekly Report,* **51,** 1024–1025.

CDC. (2003a). Recommendations for using smallpox vaccine in a pre-event vaccination program. *Morbidity and Mortality Weekly Report,* **52,** 1–16.

CDC. (2003b). Mass trauma casualty predictor. *Centers for Disease Control Emergency Preparedness and Response Website,* updated March 17, 2003. http://www.bt.cdc.gov/masscasualties/predictor.asp.

Christopher, G. W., Cieslak, T. J., Pavlin, J. A. & Eitzen, E. M. (1997). Biological warfare: a historical perspective.

Journal of the American Medical Association, **278,** 412–417.

Clauw, D. J., Engel, C. C., Aronowitz, R. *et al.* (2003). Unexplained symptoms after terrorism and war: an expert consensus statement. *The Journal of Occupational and Environmental Medicine,* **45,** 1040–1048.

Cloak, N. L. & Edwards, P. (2004). Psychological first aid: emergency care for terrorism and disaster survivors. *Current Psychiatry Online,* **3,** 1–8.

Committee on Environmental Health and Committee on Infectious Diseases. (2000). Chemical-biological terrorism and its impact on children: a subject review. *Pediatrics,* **105,** 662–670.

Currier, G. W., Allen, M. H., Bunney, E. B. *et al.* (2004). Updated treatment algorithm. *The Journal of Emergency Medicine, Supplemental Issue,* **27,** S25–S26.

Dennis, D. T., Inglesby, T. V., Henderson, D. A. *et al.* (2001). Tularemia as a biological weapon: medical and public health management. *Journal of the American Medical Association,* **285,** 2763–2773.

DiGiovanni, C. (1999). Domestic terrorism with chemical or biological agents: psychiatric aspects. *The American Journal of Psychiatry,* **156,** 1500–1505.

Everly, G. S. & Mitchell, J. T. (2001). America under attack: the "10 Commandments" of responding to mass terror attacks. *International Journal of Emergency Mental Health,* **3,** 133–135.

Fenner, F. (1988). *Smallpox and its Eradication.* Geneva: World Health Organization.

Franz, D. R., Jahrling, P. B., Friedlander, A. M. *et al.* (1997). Clinical recognition and management of patients exposed to biological warfare agents. *Journal of the American Medical Association,* **278,** 399–411.

Fullerton, C. S., Brandt, G. T. & Ursano, R. J. (1996). Chemical and biological weapons: silent agents of terror. In *Emotional Aftermath of the Persian Gulf War: Veterans, Families, Communities, and Nations,* eds. R. J. Ursano & A. E. Norwood. Washington, D.C.: American Psychiatric Press.

Galea, S., Ahern, J., Resnick, H. *et al.* (2002). Psychological sequelae of the September 11 terrorist attacks in New York City. *The New England Journal of Medicine,* **346,** 982–987.

Grinstad, B. (1964). *BC Warfare Agents.* Stockholm: Forsvarets Forskningsanstalt.

Grob, D. & Harvey, A. M. (1953). The effects and treatment of nerve gas poisoning. *American Journal of Medicine,* **14,** 52–63.

Heath, D. F. (1961). *Organophosphorus Poisons.* New York: Paragon Press.

Henderson, D. A., Inglesby, T. V., Bartlett, J. G. *et al.* (1999). Smallpox as a biological weapon: medical and public health management. *Journal of the American Medical Association*, **281**, 2127–2137.

Hobbs, J., Kittler, A., Fox, S., Middleton, B. & Bates, D. W. (2004). Communicating health information to an alarmed public facing a threat such as a bioterrorist attack. *Journal of Health Communication*, **9**, 67–75.

Holloway, H. C., Norwood, A. E., Fullerton, C. S., Engel, C. C. & Ursano, R. J. (1997). The threat of biological weapons: prophylaxis and mitigation of psychological and social consequences. *The Journal of the American Medical Association*, **278**, 425–427.

Ihlenfeld, J. T. (2003). Precepting student nurses in the intensive care unit. *Dimensions of Critical Care Nursing*, **22**, 204–207.

Inglesby, T. V., Dennis, D. T., Henderson, D. A. *et al.* (2000). Plague as a biological weapon: medical and public health management. *Journal of the American Medical Association*, **283**, 2281–2290.

Jones, F. D. (1995). Neuropsychiatric casualties of nuclear, biological, and chemical warfare. In *War Psychiatry*, eds. F. D. Jones, L. R. Sparacino, V. L. Wilcox, J. M. Rothberg & J. W. Stokes. Washington, D.C.: TMM Publications.

Keim, M. & Kaufmann, F. (1999). Principles for emergency response to bioterrorism. *Annals of Emergency Medicine*, **34**, 177–182.

Marshall, S. L. A. (1979). *Bringing Up the Rear: A Memoir.* San Rafal, Calif.: Presidio Press.

Meselson, M., Guillemin, J. G., Hugh-Jones, M. *et al.* (1994). The Sverdlovsk anthrax outbreak of 1979. *Science*, **226**, 1202–1207.

Miller, E. (1944). *Neurosis in War.* New York: Macmillan.

Nocera, A. & Garner, A. (1999). Australian disaster triage: a colour maze in the Tower of Babel. *Australia and New Zealand Journal of Surgery*, **69**, 598–602.

Papaparaskevas, J., Houhoula, D. P., Papadimitrious, M. *et al.* (2004). Ruling out *Bacillus anthracis*. *Emerging Infectious Diseases*, **10**, 1–6.

Perry, R. D. & Fetherston, J. D. (1997). *Yersinia pestis –* etiologic agent of plague. *Clinical Microbiology Review*, **10**, 35–66.

Perry, S. W., Difede, J., Musngi, G., Frances, A. J. & Jocobsberg, L. (1992). Predictors of posttraumatic stress disorder after burn injury. *American Journal of Psychiatry*, **149**, 931–935.

Raison, C. L., Pasnau, R. O., Fawzy, F. I. *et al.* (2002). Surgery and surgical subspecialties. In *The American Psychiatric Publishing Textbook of Consultation – Liaison Psychiatry*, 2nd edn., eds. M. G. Wise & J. R. Rundell. Washington, D.C.: American Psychiatric Publishing.

Rundell, J. R. (2000). Psychiatric issues in medical-surgical disaster casualties: a consultation-liaison approach. *Psychiatric Quarterly*, **71**, 245–258.

Rundell, J. R. (2003). A consultation-liaison psychiatry approach to disaster/terrorism victim assessment and management. In *Terrorism and Disaster: Individual and Community Mental Health Interventions*, eds. R. J. Ursano, C. S. Fullerton & A. E. Norwood. New York: Cambridge University Press.

Rundell, J. R. & Baine, D. (2002). The first OEF patients evacuated to Landstuhl Regional Medical Center. *Journal of the U.S. Army Medical Department*, **8–02–10**, 6–13.

Rundell, J. R. & Christopher, G. W. (2004). Differentiating manifestations of infection from psychiatric disorders and fears of having been exposed to bioterrorism. In *Bioterrorism*, eds. R. J. Ursano & A. E. Norwood. New York: Cambridge University Press.

Rundell, J. R. & Ursano, R. J. (1996). Psychiatric responses to war trauma. In *Emotional Aftermath of the Persian Gulf War*, eds. R. J. Ursano & A. E. Norwood, Washington, D.C.: American Psychiatric Press.

Rundell, J. & Wise, M. G. (2000) Medical conditions associated with psychiatric disorder. In *New Oxford Textbook of Psychiatry*, eds. M. G. Gelder, J. J. Lopez-lbor & N. C. Andreasen, pp. 1157–1168. New York: Oxford University Press.

Shuster, J. L., Breitbart, W. & Chochinov, H. M. (1999). Psychiatric aspects of excellent end-of-life care. *Psychosomatics*, **40**, 1–4.

Stern, J. (1999). The prospect of domestic bioterrorism. *Emerging Infectious Diseases*, **5**, 517–522.

Stuart, J., Ursano, R. J., Fullerton, C. S., Norwood, A. E. & Murray, K. (2003). Belief in exposure to terrorist agents: reported exposure to nerve/mustard gas by Gulf War Veterans. *Journal of Nervous and Mental Disease*, **191**, 431–436.

Tucker, J. B. (1997). National health and medical services response to incidents of chemical and biological terrorism. *Journal of the American Medical Association*, **278**, 362–368.

Ursano, R. J. & Rundell, J. R. (1994). The prisoner of war. In *Military Psychiatry: Preparing in Peace for War*, eds. F. D. Jones, L. R. Sparacino, V. L. Wilcox & J. M. Rothberg, Washington, D. C.: TMM Publications.

Ursano, R. J., Fullerton, C. S. & Norwood, A. E. (1995). Psychiatric dimensions of disaster: patient care, community consultation, and preventive medicine. *Harvard Review of Psychiatry*, **3**, 196–200.

Ursano, R. J., Fullerton, C. S. & Norwood, A. E. (2003). *Terrorism and Disaster: Individual and Community Mental Health Interventions*. Cambridge: Cambridge University Press.

Ursano, R. J., Norwood, A. E. & Fullerton, C. S. (2004). *Bioterrorism: Psychological and Public Health Interventions*. Cambridge: Cambridge University Press.

Wessely, S., Rose, S. & Bisson, J. (1999). Brief psychological interventions ("debriefing") for treating immediate trauma-related symptoms and the prevention of post-traumatic stress disorder (Cochrane Review). In *The Cochrane Library*. Oxford: Update Software Ltd.

Wharton, M., Strikas, R. A., Harpaz, R. *et al.* (2003). Recommendations for using smallpox vaccine in a pre-event vaccination program. MMWR Recommendations and Reports, **52 (RR07)**, 1–16.

Wise, M. G. & Rundell, J. R. (2005). Special consultation-liaison settings and situations. In *Concise Guide to Consultation-Liaison Psychiatry*, 5th edn., eds. M. G. Wise & J. R. Rundell. Washington, D.C.: American Psychiatric Press.

World Health Organization. (1970). *Health Aspects of Chemical and Biological Weapons*. Geneva: World Health Organization.

Yori, G. (2002). Posttraumatic stress disorder after terrorist attacks: a review. *The Journal of Nervous and Mental Disease*, **190**, 118–121.

9

Interventions for acutely injured survivors of individual and mass trauma

Douglas Zatzick

Introduction

Natural and human-made disasters entail the threat of physical injury. Injured trauma survivors initially receive care in the acute care medical setting. For example, the Centers for Disease Control report that within 48 h after the September 11, 2001 attack on the World Trade Center, 1 103 physically injured survivors were triaged through five acute care facilities in New York (Centers for Disease Control and Prevention, 2002). Injured survivors of mass disasters have been identified as a high-risk group that may require specialized early screening and evaluation procedures (United States Department of Defense et al., 2001; United States Department of Health and Human Services, 2003).

Trauma exposure when coupled with physical injury confers a higher risk for the development of post-traumatic stress disorder (PTSD) (Abenhaim et al., 1992; Green, 1993; Helzer et al., 1987; Hoge et al., 2004; Koren et al., 2005). Between 10% and 40% of hospitalized adolescent and adult injury survivors in the United States may go on to develop symptoms consistent with a diagnosis of PTSD (Holbrook et al., 2001; Marshall & Schell, 2002; Michaels et al., 1999b; Ursano et al., 1999; Zatzick et al., 2002a, 2002b, 2004c, 2006). Among injury survivors, PTSD is often complicated by comorbid, depressive symptoms (O'Donnell et al., 2004; Shalev et al., 1998b; Zatzick et al., 2004c, 2006) and medically unexplained somatic complaints (Engel et al., 2000; Katon et al., 2001b; Zatzick et al., 2003).

In trauma-exposed populations in general, and injured trauma survivors in particular, multiple demographic, clinical, and injury-related risk factors for the development of PTSD have been identified (Brewin et al., 2000; Green, 1993; Holbrook et al., 1999; Kessler et al., 1999; March, 2003; Marshall & Schell, 2002; Mayou et al., 1993, 1997; Mellman et al., 2001; Michaels et al., 1999a; O'Donnell et al., 2003, 2004; Pynoos et al., 1999; Shalev et al., 1998a; Winston et al., 2003; Yehuda, 1999; Zatzick et al., 2002b, 2005b). In acutely injured patients, higher initial post-traumatic distress, higher initial emergency department heart rate, female gender, and greater preinjury trauma are among the most consistently identified predictors of persistent PTSD symptoms (Bryant et al., 2000; Holbrook et al., 2001; Marshall & Schell, 2002; Michaels et al., 1999a, 1999b O'Donnell et al., 2003; Winston et al., 2003; Zatzick et al., 2002b, Zatzick et al., 2005a).

Post-traumatic high-risk behaviors and functional impairment

A body of investigation substantiates an association between mass trauma exposure and the development of high-risk health behaviors such as substance abuse (Boscarino et al., 2006; Galea et al., 2002; Reijneveld et al., 2003, 2005; Vlahov et al., 2004a, 2004b). One controlled prospective study of disaster-exposed adolescents found that while emotional distress diminished over time, problems related to alcohol misuse endured chronically (Reijneveld *et al.*, 2005). In civilian and veteran trauma-exposed populations these high-risk behaviors appear to be linked to recurrent traumatic life events including an increased risk of recurrent physical injury and mortality (Hearst *et al.*, 1986; Ramstad *et al.*, 2004; Rivara *et al.*, 1993).

In physically injured civilians (Holbrook *et al.*, 1999; Michaels *et al.*, 1999b; Zatzick *et al.*, 1997a, 1997b, 2002a), refugees (Mollica *et al.*, 1999), and veterans (Zatzick *et al.*, 1997a, 1997b), PTSD makes an independent contribution to post-trauma functional limitations and diminished quality of life above and beyond the impact of injury severity and comorbid medical conditions. In a randomly selected cohort of survivors of intentional and unintentional injury, PTSD was the strongest independent predictor of a broad profile of functional impairment 1 year after inpatient surgical hospitalization (Zatzick et al., 2002a). PTSD is associated with increased costs to society; these costs appear to be in part secondary to increased healthcare costs (Greenberg *et al.*, 1999; Kessler, 2000; Walker *et al.*, 1999, 2003). Thus, early interventions for injured survivors of individual and mass traumatic life events that reduce the likelihood of developing enduring post-trauma disturbances may be essential components of public health efforts targeting injury control (Zatzick, 2003b).

Trauma centers provide care for injured civilians after individual and mass traumatic life events

Acute care centers in the United States provide health services after mass trauma (Herman *et al.*, 2002; MacKenzie *et al.*, 2003; Ursano, 2002). Recent consensus guidelines recommend early mental health screening and evaluation procedures for injured trauma survivors who require medical/surgical attention, as this high-priority subgroup of patients is at risk for the development of PTSD (National Institute of Mental Health, 2002; United States Department of Health and Human Services, 2003).

The trauma care system is the service delivery sector in which injured patients receive treatment. A trauma care system is an organized and coordinated effort in a defined geographic area that is designated to deliver care to injured trauma victims (Bonnie *et al.*, 1999). This care begins immediately after the injury and includes paramedic and ambulance service, emergency department triage, and inpatient surgical hospitalization. Trauma centers are acute care hospitals that are designed to treat emergent medical complications related to physical injury. Level I trauma centers are designated and equipped to care for the most severely injured patients, while levels II–IV centers are designed to treat less severely injured patients and to triage to level I facilities.

The major goals of trauma care systems have been to prevent fatalities, and to triage patients who are more severely injured to the most appropriate and cost-effective level of trauma care within a region (Bonnie *et al.*, 1999). Guidelines for the operation of trauma care systems are only beginning to include comprehensive or even cursory approaches to the evaluation, referral, and treatment of injured patients with mental health problems (Committee on Trauma American College of Surgeons, 2006). In the United States, the American College of Surgeons Committee oversees verification/accreditation requirements for most of the country's 1154 trauma centers (Committee on Trauma American College of Surgeons, 2006).

Refinements in routine acute care mental health evaluation procedures may serve Americans in the wake of mass trauma

Although PTSD screening measures exist, these instruments may be difficult to administer in mass casualty conditions (Zatzick *et al.*, 2005a, 2005b). Routine acute care investigations are developing emergency department vital sign assessments that have the potential to be feasibly implemented with abbreviated symptom screens to predict PTSD after mass trauma (Bryant *et al.*, 2000; Kassam-Adams *et al.*, 2005; Shalev *et al.*, 1998b; Winston *et al.*, 2003; Zatzick *et al.*, 2005a). Health services research in the acute care medical setting presents a unique opportunity to test and develop routine screening and intervention procedures that may also benefit injured survivors of mass trauma (Zatzick *et al.*, 2004a, 2005b). In the United States 37 million individuals visit emergency departments each year after sustaining traumatic injuries and approximately 2.5 million Americans incur injuries so severe that they require inpatient hospitalization (Bonnie *et al.*, 1999).

Efficacious interventions for PTSD

Efficacy research suggests that patients with PTSD symptoms may respond to psychotherapeutic and psychopharmacological treatments (Foa & Meadows, 1997; Shalev *et al.*, 1996; Solomon *et al.*, 1992). There is evidence that brief, early cognitive-behavioral therapy (CBT) interventions can help curb the development of PTSD in injured trauma survivors (Bisson *et al.*, 2004; Bryant, 2002; Bryant *et al.*, 1998, 2003; Ehlers *et al.*, 2003; Foa *et al.*, 1995). Both selective serotonin reuptake inhibitors (SSRI) and tricyclic antidepressants are efficacious treatments for PTSD (Brady *et al.*, 2000; Davidson *et al.*, 2001; Marshall *et al.*, 2001; Solomon *et al.*, 1992). Guidelines based on this body of efficacy research have been formulated (Foa et al., 2000; Journal of Clinical Psychiatry Guidelines, 1999; Ursano *et al.*, 2004). These clinical guidelines have yet to be translated to the real world treatment of physically injured trauma survivors within trauma care systems.

Challenges to acute care mental health service delivery

The acute care medical setting presents a series of challenges for the delivery of efficacious mental health interventions (Litz *et al.*, 2002). Few investigations have successfully delivered efficacious PTSD interventions in the acute care setting (Zatzick *et al.*, 2006). Single-session debriefing interventions can be robustly delivered to representative samples of acute care patients (Bisson *et al.*, 1997; Mayou *et al.*, 2000). Unfortunately, debriefing has not been shown to be efficacious in preventing PTSD (Rose & Bisson, 1998; Van Emmerik *et al.*, 2002) and may actually be associated with poorer outcome among injured trauma survivors (Bisson *et al.*, 1997; Mayou *et al.*, 2000). Efficacy studies of psychotherapeutic and psychopharmacological interventions conducted under best practice conditions assume that well-developed clinical infrastructures exist for the delivery of treatments (Wells, 1999b). The acute care setting, however, poses a series of challenges to the delivery of efficacy-proven mental health interventions.

Acutely injured trauma survivors receive fragmented care that is not linked across inpatient, outpatient, and community service sectors. Currently, few resources exist for bridging acute care hospitalization to primary care and community services (Chesnut *et al.*, 1999; Horowitz *et al.*, 2001; Sabin, *et al.*, 2006; Zatzick *et al.*, 2003). Thus, the standardized regular appointments that constitute an implicit foundation of treatment delivery in efficacy trials may be difficult to implement, as injured patients move rapidly across surgical inpatient, primary care outpatient, and community health service delivery sectors in the days and weeks immediately following an injury. Furthermore, a substantial proportion of acute care patients are not connected to primary care providers (PCPs) (Sabin *et al.*, 2006; Zatzick *et al.*, 2003).

Currently, few patients treated in acute care receive comprehensive evaluation or evidence-based mental health treatment. Although over 50% of trauma surgery inpatients suffer from high levels of post-traumatic distress, depression, and alcohol use disorders (Zatzick *et al.*, 2004c), few symptomatic inpatients are detected (Cerda *et al.*, 2000; Zatzick *et al.*, 2000) or receive in-depth evaluation or referral (Danielsson *et al.*, 1999; Gentilello *et al.*, 1999a; Silver & McDuff, 1990; Zatzick *et al.*, 2005b).

Symptomatic patients infrequently access mental health services after hospital discharge (Dunn *et al.*, 2003; Jaycox *et al.*, 2004; McCarthy *et al.*, 2003; Sabin *et al.*, 2006; Zatzick *et al.*, 2001b). Thus, although evidence-based treatments for PTSD and related disorders exist, they are not routinely delivered as early interventions to injured trauma survivors in acute care.

The PhD/MD practitioners that deliver mental health interventions in efficacy trials are not representative of front-line acute care providers. Manuals for the operation of trauma centers clearly articulate roles for registered nurses, those with a Masters of Social Work, and trauma surgical providers, yet rarely mention PhD/MD mental health specialists (Committee on Trauma American College of Surgeons, 2006). Within trauma care systems, early interventions for PTSD and related conditions may ultimately be implemented by front-line acute care providers (Gentilello *et al.*, 1995). Review of the relevant literature revealed no studies that have tested the effectiveness of early PTSD interventions delivered by front-line acute care providers.

Front-line acute care providers are receptive to implementing mental health interventions, yet perceived and structural barriers to implementation exist. Surveys/interviews with acute care providers suggest that mental health interventions are viewed as highly relevant to trauma center care (Danielsson *et al.*, 1999; Schermer *et al.*, 2003; Tellez & Mackersie, 1996). When surveyed, front-line acute care providers express openness to implementing mental health interventions; these providers also endorse a number of barriers to routine implementation including time pressures encountered in emergency settings and lack of training [e.g., "not knowing where to start" (Danielsson *et al.*, 1999)].

Finally, longitudinal clinical investigations have consistently reported difficulties in engaging and retaining acutely traumatized patients in intervention protocols (Jack & Glied, 2002; Pitman *et al.*, 2002; Roy-Byrne *et al.*, 2004; Schelling *et al.*, 2004; Schwarz & Kowalski, 1992; Weisaeth, 2001). Data on patients' post-trauma concerns provide further insight into the observed difficulties in engaging

trauma victims in early interventions. For acutely injured patients multiple physical, financial, social, medical, and legal post-trauma concerns exist that may limit the ability to focus exclusively on the psychological sequelae of the trauma (Zatzick *et al.*, 2001a). Care management procedures that elicit and address patients' most pressing post-trauma concerns have the potential to initially engage traumatized patients in shared patient–provider treatment planning (Zatzick *et al.*, 2001a, 2004a).

Health services approaches to the problem of the development of early acute care intervention

Injured patients treated within trauma care systems are at high risk for developing PTSD. As is true for many Americans with psychiatric disorders, it appears that many injured patients who suffer from PTSD receive fragmented care and are not engaged in mental health services at strategic postinjury points (New Freedom Commission on Mental Health, 2003; Satcher, 1999). A literature review identified few early intervention trials targeting PTSD that have assessed symptomatic, functional, and utilization/cost outcomes for trauma survivors initially treated in acute care and followed through outpatient primary care visits and community rehabilitation.

Combined interventions have been developed as treatment strategies for chronically mentally ill, treatment-resistant, low-income, and primary care patients (Allness & Knoedler, 1998; Burns & Santos, 1995; Craske *et al.*, 2002; Deci *et al.*, 1995; Hoagwood *et al.*, 2001; Katon & Gonzales, 1994; Katon *et al.*, 1994, 1995, 1997, 1999, 2001a, 2001c, 2004; Roy-Byrne *et al.*, 2001, 2003; Santos *et al.*, 1995; Schoenwald & Hoagwood, 2001; Simon *et al.*, 1995, 2002; Stein & Santos, 1998; Unutzer *et al.*, 2001, 2002; Wells, 1999a; Wells *et al.*, 2000). These treatments bring together efficacious psychotherapy and medication interventions with disease management strategies such as care management; the care management intervention component serves to bridge medical and mental health care (Von Korff *et al.*, 1997; Wagner *et al.*, 1996).

Just as combined interventions have incorporated PCP into the provision of mental health services, the introduction of early combined interventions within trauma care systems may serve to integrate acute care providers into post-traumatic mental healthcare delivery. Using randomized effectiveness designs rooted in the structure, process, and outcome model of intervention delivery (McGlynn *et al.*, 1988), mental health services researchers have demonstrated that combined interventions can improve symptomatic outcomes for patients with depressive and anxiety disorders who are treated in primary care (Katon *et al.*, 1995, 1997, 1999, 2001a, 2004; Roy-Byrne *et al.*, 2001; Unutzer *et al.*, 2002; Wells *et al.*, 2000). Combined interventions in primary care settings have sought to find the optimal roles for PCP, practice nurses, and mental health specialists in the delivery of care for patients with psychiatric disorders and chronic conditions (Katon *et al.*, 2001c). Combined interventions hold promise for the delivery of mental health interventions in acute care as they can incorporate front-line trauma center providers into early mental health services delivery and can link trauma center care to outpatient services.

Clinical epidemiology as a foundation for a health services research approach to intervention development

This section is based on work published elsewhere (Engel & Katon, 1999; Engel *et al.*, 2004). Clinical epidemiology is the science of making predictions about individual patients by describing events in populations (Fletcher *et al.*, 1996). The methods used by clinical epidemiologists frame the care of the individual patient in the context of the larger population of patients that present for care in a specified health service delivery setting (Feinstein, 1987; Fletcher *et al.*, 1996; Sackett *et al.*, 1991; Walker-Barnes, 2003).

Acute care mental health services research programs aim to address the mental health needs of populations of injured patients presenting for treatment in the acute care medical setting. One

manner in which the acute care research programs have operationalized a clinical epidemiological approach is through the use of population-based automated data systems. These provide clinical and demographic information on all patients treated within the health service delivery system so that characteristics of an individual patient or subgroup of patients included in an investigation can be compared to the population of patients presenting for care. For instance, preliminary investigations have used automated medical record data to gain insight into the processes of care underlying the detection of patients with mental health symptoms/diagnoses (Zatzick *et al.*, 2000) and used the automated data systems to identify clinical populations to be targeted in a clinical trial (Zatzick *et al.*, 2002b, 2006). Automated data systems also provide key data related to the policy-relevant outcome domains, such as emergency department and inpatient surgical utilization data documenting recurrent injury admissions (Gentilello *et al.*, 1999a; Zatzick *et al.*, 2004b).

Developing early combined interventions for injured trauma survivors treated in the acute care trauma center setting

The rationale and design of the pilot randomized effectiveness trial (Zatzick *et al.*, 2001c) were strongly influenced by the results of the Gentilello *et al.* (1999a) intervention at the University of Washington's Harborview level I trauma center (Harborview). Gentilello *et al.* (1999a) demonstrated that a PhD-level clinician based in a trauma center could deliver a brief motivational interviewing (MI) intervention from a surgical inpatient unit that reduced post-traumatic alcohol use and hospital admissions secondary to new injury (Gentilello *et al.*, 1999a).

The pilot investigation sought to establish the feasibility of having three seasoned trauma center providers deliver a brief early intervention that aimed to reduce PTSD symptoms after the injury (i.e., secondary PTSD prevention) and high-risk behaviors such as postinjury alcohol consumption that were linked to injury recurrence (i.e., primary prevention of trauma/PTSD). One interventionist was a trauma surgery nurse practitioner who had over a decade of experience as a front-line provider with the University of California at Davis trauma surgery service; two interventionists were MD consultation liaison psychiatrists. These providers were trained in a care management procedure that aimed to engage injured trauma survivors by providing readily accessible, continuous trauma support in the days and weeks following the injury. A key component of the trauma support intervention was eliciting and targeting for improvement each patient's unique constellation of post-trauma concerns (Zatzick *et al.*, 2001c). Interventionists also received training in brief interventions for PTSD and alcohol use (Gentilello *et al.*, 1995; Litz, 2004). In accordance with a population-based/clinical epidemiological approach, patients were randomly selected to participate from the population of patients admitted to the University of California at Davis trauma surgery service. Only severely brain-injured and monolingual non-English-speaking patients were excluded from the investigation. Patients randomly selected for participation in the study had moderate levels of PTSD symptoms as well as substance-related comorbidities (Zatzick *et al.*, 2001c).

The pilot investigation found that patients in the intervention group, when compared to controls, manifested significantly decreased PTSD symptom levels at 1 month ($p < 0.05$) but not at 4 months after the injury (Zatzick *et al.*, 2001c). The observed reduction and subsequent recurrence of trauma survivors' PTSD and depressive symptoms followed the temporal "dosing" of the collaborative intervention. Examination of the interventionist's logs revealed that patients were engaged in the early intervention and that 75% of patient–interventionist contact occurred between the hospital admission and the 1-month telephone follow-up interview. Interventionists successfully worked with other acute care providers to integrate the early intervention activities with other aspects of acute care treatment delivery (e.g., pain control, discharge planning).

However, the trauma-center-based interventionists frequently encountered difficulty transitioning the care of patients to the community.

A randomized effectiveness trial of the early combined intervention at Harborview

The Harborview randomized effectiveness trial of early combined intervention expanded on the pilot trial by developing an early combined intervention that included continuous masters-level case managers over the first 6 months postinjury, and evidence-based medication and psychotherapy for PTSD delivered by MD/PhD-level mental health specialists (Zatzick *et al.*, 2004a). As with the University of California at Davis pilot, inclusion criteria for the Harborview pilot remained extremely broad. Patients screened into the study if they exhibited moderate levels of psychological distress in the surgical ward; patients with active alcohol and/or drug abuse were included in the study. The combined intervention components included: (1) care management targeting patient engagement and trauma center-to-community linkage; (2) medication and psychotherapy targeting PTSD; and (3) motivational interviewing targeting alcohol consumption and injury recurrence.

Care management targeting patient engagement and trauma center-to-community linkage

The goal of the 6-month care management intervention was to engage injured trauma survivors in early intervention, and to link injured trauma survivors to appropriate primary care and community services. The care manager began treatment by meeting the injured patient at the bedside and by eliciting, tracking, and targeting for improvement each patient's unique constellation of post-trauma concerns. The patient and care manager worked to formulate a comprehensive postinjury care plan.

In order to enhance engagement by encouraging spontaneous patient-initiated contact with the intervention team, the care manager pager was covered by team members 24 h per day, 7 days a week.

The care manager aimed to ensure that injured patients were linked to appropriate outpatient primary care and community services. The procedures for collaboration with PCPs were informed by previous trials of consultation psychiatry interventions for depressive and anxiety disorders in primary care (Katon *et al.*, 1995, 1999, 2001a; Roy-Byrne *et al.*, 2001). First the care manager ascertained whether patients had a regular PCP with whom they could follow-up after discharge from the trauma center. Over the initial weeks postinjury the care manager worked to obtain primary care services for any injured patient who did not have a regular provider. When patients had regular providers these practitioners were contacted by telephone to discuss the postinjury care plan. If necessary the care manager helped patients schedule primary care visits and provided reminders of scheduled appointments in order to facilitate attendance at office visits.

For the purposes of the trial a trauma center-to-community linkage team was developed. The team included practitioners with expertise in the care of homeless patients, first generation Americans, pastoral care services, and gender-specific community PTSD services. Providers on the team assisted the care manager in obtaining community services for injured patients.

In the later months of the care management intervention (e.g., months 3–6), PCPs were again contacted by intervention team members in order to summarize postinjury care and ensure adequate care transfer. For patients started on psychotropic medication, in addition to phone conversations, a letter was sent to PCPs notifying them of the current doses and making recommendations for ongoing prescription and side-effect management. Patients with symptomatic recurrences received stepped-up, evidence-based care, and/or extension of case management through the 6–12 months period postinjury.

Medication and psychotherapy targeting PTSD

At 3 months after the injury the care manager evaluated each intervention patient for PTSD with the Structured Clinical Interview for DSM (SCID) (First *et al.*, 1997). Patients diagnosed with PTSD were referred to the team's MD/PhD-level providers for the initiation of evidence-based medication and psychotherapy treatment. Team members shared information and deliberated (Charles *et al.*, 1999; Emanuel & Emanuel, 1992; Zatzick *et al.*, 2001c) with patients the importance of receiving guideline-level treatments for PTSD symptoms. All patients were given their choice regarding treatment options and patients could receive medications, CBT, or both. The investigation's expert CBT therapist, Amy Wagner, PhD, delivered an evidence-based protocol that derived from prior PTSD efficacy studies (Bryant *et al.*, 1998, 2003; Foa *et al.*, 1995; Wagner, 2003). The investigation's psychiatrist performed an initial medication evaluation and initiated guideline-concordant pharmacological treatment (Zatzick & Roy-Byrne, 2003). Once the patient was stabilized on an initial course of pharmacotherapy, the psychiatrist would work with each patient's primary care and community mental health providers to ensure guideline-level treatment was continued beyond the active study intervention phase.

Motivational interviewing (MI) targeting alcohol consumption and injury recurrence

The masters-level case manager had received prior training in the delivery of MI interventions (Johnston *et al.*, 2002) by the investigation's expert MI Supervisor, Chris Dunn, PhD. As with the previous MI intervention (Gentilello *et al.*, 1999a), an initial 30-min MI intervention was delivered in the surgical ward to patients with current or past histories of alcohol abuse/dependence; MI booster sessions were delivered on an as-needed basis to patients with ongoing alcohol abuse and/or drinking behaviors that risked new injury. For receptive patients, the care manager linked patients to community alcohol services [e.g., Alcoholics Anonymous (AA)].

Results of the early combined intervention (Zatzick *et al.*, 2004a)

Review of intervention logs revealed that the Case Management procedure effectively engaged 90% of intervention patients (Ghesquiere *et al.*, 2004). Approximately 50% of intervention patients reported no regular source of primary care services at the time of the surgical ward interview; over 60% of these patients required that their care be coordinated for follow-up with a PCP or other community provider. Successful trauma center–PCP linkage by the care manager often required multiple attempts over the weeks and months postinjury.

Table 9.1 Random regression results: PTSD

Variable	Estimate	SE	*p*
Time	0.30	0.20	0.125
Injury severity score	−0.09	0.06	0.144
Age	−0.05	0.04	0.214
Female gender	1.63	0.91	0.074
Chronic illness	1.43	1.21	0.226
Baseline alcohol	*2.05*	*0.91*	*0.024*
Baseline PTSD	3.38	1.00	0.001
Treatment group	1.72	1.01	0.090
Treatment group × time	0.67	0.27	0.013

Regression analyses revealed a significant treatment group by time interaction effect for PTSD (Table 9.1). The intervention effect coincided with the initiation of evidence-based medication and psychotherapy interventions for PTSD at the 3-month time point (Figures 9.1, 9.2). Post-hoc analyses revealed that the significant treatment group by time interaction was due to treatment group differences in the adjusted rates of change in PTSD over the 12 months postinjury ($p = 0.02$).

We previously reported that to further examine change over time we performed subgroup analyses of intervention and control group patients with PTSD 3 months postinjury (Figure 9.3, $n = 29$) and without PTSD 3 months postinjury ($n = 74$) (Zatzick *et al.*, 2005c). At 6 months, 91% of control patients versus 69% of intervention patients in the subgroup with PTSD at 3 months still had PTSD (effect size = 0.6), and at 12 months 78% of controls versus 58% of intervention patients had PTSD (effect size = 0.4) (Figure 9.3). The trajectories of PTSD decline in intervention and control patients in the with-PTSD subgroup were nonconverging (Figure 9.3). In the subgroup without PTSD at 3 months, 14% of controls and 14% of the intervention group had PTSD at 6 months, and 9% of the intervention group and 12% of controls had PTSD at 12 months (effect size = 0.1).

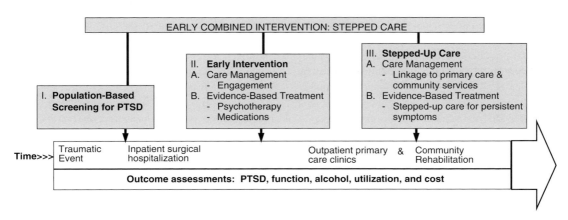

Figure 9.1 Implementing and assessing early combined intervention after traumatic injury

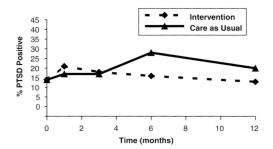

Figure 9.2 Percent of Patients who met DSM IV symptomatic criteria for PTSD (PCL: adjusted for injury severity, gender, age, chronic illness, and baseline alcohol and PTSD)

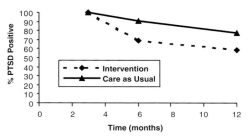

Figure 9.3 Course of symptoms in patients with PTSD 3 months postinjury

Regression analyses demonstrated a significant treatment group by time interaction effect for CIDI-diagnosed, where CIDI stands for composite international diagnostic interview (Kessler *et al.*, 1997) alcohol abuse/dependence (Zatzick *et al.*, 2004a). The intervention appears to have produced maintenance of drinking reductions beyond the 6 months post-injury time point. The significant treatment group by time interaction was due to treatment group differences in the adjusted rates of change in alcohol abuse/dependence for the two groups over the 12 months postinjury ($p < 0.001$) (Zatzick *et al.*, 2004a). Intervention patients demonstrated decreased new injury admissions (5%) relative to controls (10%). These differences did not, however, achieve statistical significance (adjusted odds ratio = 0.43, 95% CI = 0.10, 1.96) (Zatzick *et al.*, 2005c).

Looking to the future: how routine health services research in acute care medical settings may inform early intervention after mass trauma

Future investigations that refine routine acute care evaluation and treatment procedures have the potential to improve the quality of mental health care for Americans injured in the wake of mass trauma. For example, as discussed above, routine acute care prospective cohort studies have identified emergency department heart rate as a significant independent predictor of chronic PTSD symptoms. Brief PTSD screening instruments tailored for the acute care setting are now under development (Winston *et al.*, 2003). However, pragmatically oriented, time-efficient acute care providers have been slow to adopt mental health screening procedures that extend beyond established routine vital sign and physical exam assessments (Danielsson *et al.*, 1999; Gentilello *et al.*, 1999b; Zatzick *et al.*, 2005a). These tendencies can be expected to amplify under mass casualty conditions, leaving initial heart rate as potentially the most feasibly implemented acute care PTSD screen.

Recent investigation suggests that emergency department heart rate alone has only modest specificity (range 60%–65%) and sensitivity (range 49%–63%) for the prediction of chronic PTSD symptoms. The exclusive use of a heart rate screen, with sensitivities between 49% and 63%, risks screening out a substantial proportion of patients who will go on to develop PTSD. Previous acute care reports have enhanced the predictive value of initial emergency department heart rate by combining heart rate cut-offs with other clinical characteristics (Bryant *et al.*, 2000; Winston *et al.*, 2003). Future population-based investigations could test heart rate cutoffs as a screening tool alone and in combination with other demographic, injury, and clinical characteristics readily available among acutely injured patients.

Routine acute care studies of stepped care interventions, when combined with screening studies, could further inform care for injured patients after mass trauma. For example, postinjury care management interventions do not worsen PTSD symptoms and are an effective method of engaging injured trauma survivors in early intervention (Bordow & Porritt, 1979; Ursano *et al.*, 2004; Zatzick *et al.*, 2001a, 2004a).

Mental health professionals have been observed to converge on the scene of mass disasters. Rather than immediately preparing for early intervention targeting post-traumatic stress, newly arriving mental health professionals could be assigned as care managers to injured patients triaged through acute care settings. Reviews of initial emergency department heart rate data contained in acute care medical charts could inform triage efforts. Patients with higher heart rates and/or other demographic or clinical risk factors (e.g., multiple prior trauma exposures, female gender) could be identified for early care management contacts. Care manager problem solving around injured victims' most pressing post-traumatic concerns would be used to first engage injured patients in an initial postevent therapeutic alliance (Zatzick *et al.*, 2001a, 2004a). After initial engagement, patients with persistent symptoms could then be further evaluated and treated with evidence-based early interventions when indicated (Bryant *et al.*, 1998, 2003; Litz, 2004; Litz *et al.*, 2002; Ursano *et al.*, 2004). In this way evaluation and treatment procedures developed during routine acute care practice conditions can continue to inform the care of injured survivors of mass trauma.

ACKNOWLEDGEMENT

The author thanks Melissa Hanbey for her editorial assistance in preparing the manuscript.

REFERENCES

Abenhaim, L., Dab, W. & Salmi, L. R. (1992). Study of civilian victims of terrorist attacks (France 1982–1987). *Journal of Clinical Epidemiology*, **45**, 103–109.

Allness, D. J. & Knoedler, W. H. (1998). *The PACT Model of Community-Based Treatment for Persons with Severe and Persistent Mental Illnesses*. Arlington, Va.: NAMI.

Bisson, J. I., Jenkins, P. L., Alexander, J. & Bannister, C. (1997). Randomised controlled trial of psychological debriefing for victims of acute burn trauma. *British Journal of Psychiatry*, **171**, 78–81.

Bisson, J. I., Shepherd, J. P., Joy, D., Probert, R. & Newcombe, R. G. (2004). Early cognitive-behavioural therapy for post-traumatic stress symptoms after physical injury. Randomised controlled trial. *British Journal of Psychiatry*, **184**, 63–69.

Bonnie, R. J., Fulco, C. E. & Liverman, C. T. (1999). *Reducing the Burden of Injury: Advancing Prevention and Treatment*. Washington, D.C.: National Academy Press.

Bordow, S. & Porritt, D. (1979). An experimental evaluation of crisis intervention. *Social Science and Medicine*, **13A**, 251–256.

Boscarino, J. A., Adams, R. E. & Galea, S. (2006). Alcohol use in New York after the terrorist attacks: a study of the effects of psychological trauma on drinking behavior. *Addictive Behaviors*, **31**, 606–621.

Brady, K., Pearlstein, T., Asnis, G. M. *et al.* (2000). Efficacy and safety of sertraline treatment of posttraumatic stress disorder. *Journal of the American Medical Association*, **283**, 1837–1844.

Brewin, C. R., Andrews, B. & Valentine, J. D. (2000). Meta-analysis of risk factors for posttraumatic stress disorder in trauma-exposed adults. *Journal of Consulting and Clinical Psychology*, **68**, 748–766.

Bryant, R. A. (2002). Enhancing treatment effectiveness for acute stress disorder. Paper presented at the the 18th Annual Meeting of the International Society for Traumatic Stress Studies, Baltimore, Md.

Bryant, R. A., Harvey, A. G., Dang, S. T., Sackville, T. & Basten, C. (1998). Treatment of acute stress disorder: a comparison of cognitive-behavioral therapy and supportive counseling. *Journal of Consulting and Clinical Psychology*, **66**, 862–866.

Bryant, R. A., Harvey, A. G., Guthrie, R. M. & Moulds, M. L. (2000). A prospective study of psychophysiological arousal, acute stress disorder, and posttraumatic stress disorder. *Journal of Abnormal Psychology*, **109**, 341–344.

Bryant, R. A., Moulds, M. L., Guthrie, R. M., Dang, S. T. & Nixon, R. D. (2003). Imaginal exposure alone and imaginal exposure with cognitive restructuring in treatment of posttraumatic stress disorder. *Journal of Consulting and Clinical Psychology*, **71**, 706–712.

Burns, B. J. & Santos, A. B. (1995). Assertive community treatment; an update of randomized trials. *Psychiatric Services*, **46**, 669–675.

Centers for Disease Control and Prevention. (2002). Rapid assessment of injuries among survivors of the terrorist attack on the World Trade Center-New York City, September 2001. *Morbidity and Mortality Weekly Report*, **51**, 1–4.

Cerda, G., Zatzick, D., Wise, M. & Greenhalgh, D. (2000). Computerized registry recording of psychiatric disorders of pediatric patients with burns. *Journal of Burn Care and Rehabilitation*, **21**, 368–370.

Charles, C., Gafni, A. & Whelan, T. (1999). Decision-making in the physician-patient encounter: revisiting the shared treatment decision-making model. *Social Science and Medicine*, **49**, 651–661.

Chesnut, R. M., Carney, N., Maynard, H. *et al.* (1999). *Rehabilitation for Traumatic Brain Injury*. Rockville, Md.: Agency for Health Care Policy and Research.

Committee on Trauma American College of Surgeons. (2006). Performance improvement. In *Resources for the Optimal Care of the Injured Patient*. Chicago, Ill.: The American College of Surgeons.

Craske, M., Roy-Byrne, P., Stein, M. B. *et al.* (2002). Treating panic disorder in primary care: a collaborative care intervention. *General Hospital Psychiatry*, **24**, 148–155.

Danielsson, P. E., Rivara, F. P., Gentilello, L. M. & Maier, R. V. (1999). Reasons why trauma surgeons fail to screen for alcohol problems. *Archives of Surgery*, **134**, 564–568.

Davidson, J., Pearlstein, T., Londborg, P. *et al.* (2001). Efficacy of sertraline in preventing relapse of posttraumatic stress disorder: results of a 28-week double-blind, placebo-controlled study. *American Journal of Psychiatry*, **158**, 1974–1981.

Deci, P., Santos, A. B., Hiott, D. W., Schoenwald, S. & Dias, J. K. (1995). Dissemination of assertive community treatment programs. *Psychiatric Services*, **46**, 676–678.

Dunn, C., Zatzick, D., Russo, J. *et al.* (2003). Hazardous drinking by trauma patients during the year after injury. *Journal of Trauma Injury, Infection, and Critical Care*, **54**, 707–712.

Ehlers, A., Clark, D., Hackmann, A. *et al.* (2003). A randomized controlled trial of cognitive therapy, a self-help booklet, and repeated assessment as early interventions for posttraumatic stress disorder. *Archives of General Psychiatry*, **60**, 1024–1032.

Emanuel, E. J. & Emanuel, L. L. (1992). Four models of the patient-physician relationship. *The Journal of the American Medical Association*, **267**, 2221–2226.

Engel, C. C. & Katon, W. (1999). Population and need-based prevention of unexplained physical symptoms in the community. In *Institute of Medicine, Strategies to Protect the Health of U.S. Forces: Medical Surveillance, Record Taking and Risk Reduction*, pp. 173–212. Washington, D.C.: National Academy Press.

Engel, C. C., Liu, X., McCarthy, B. D., Miller, R. F. & Ursano, R. J. (2000). Relationship of physical symptoms to posttramatic stress disorder among veterans seeking care for gulf war-related health concerns. *Psychosomatic Medicine*, **62**, 739–745.

Engel, C. C., Hoge, C. W., Gonzalez, D., Bruner, V. & Zatzick, D. (2004). Improving access to quality military care for post-traumatic stress – stigma, barriers, and innovations. Paper presented at the 20th Annual Meeting of the International Society for Traumatic Stress Studies. New Orleans, LA.

Feinstein, A. R. (1987). *Clinimetrics*. New Haven, Conn.: Yale University Press.

First, M. B., Spitzer, R. L., Gibbon, M. & Williams, J. B.W. (1997). *Structured Clinical Interview for DSM-IV Axis I Disorders – Clinician Version (SCID-CV)*. Washington, D.C.: American Psychiatric Press.

Fletcher, R. H., Fletcher, S. W. & Wagner, E. H. (1996). *Clinical Epidemiology: The Essentials*, 3rd. edn. Baltimore, Md.: Williams & Wilkins.

Foa, E. B. & Meadows, E. A. (1997). Psychosocial treatments for posttraumatic stress disorder: a critical review. *Annual Review of Psychology*, **48**, 449–480.

Foa, E. B., Hearst-Ikeda, D. & Perry, K. J. (1995). Evaluation of a brief cognitive-behavioral program for the prevention of chronic PTSD in recent assault victims. *Journal of Consulting and Clinical Psychology*, **63**, 948–955.

Foa, E. B., Keane, T. M. & Friedman, M. J. (2000). *Effective Treatments for PTSD: Practice Guidelines from the International Society for Traumatic Stress Studies*. New York: Guilford Press.

Galea, S., Ahern, J., Resnick, H. *et al.* (2002). Psychological sequelae of the September 11 terrorist attacks in New York City. *New England Journal of Medicine*, **346**, 982–987.

Gentilello, L. M., Donovan, D. M., Dunn, C. W. & Rivara, F. P. (1995). Alcohol interventions in trauma centers: current practice and future directions. *Journal of the American Medical Association*, **274**, 1043–1048.

Gentilello, L. M., Rivara, F. P., Donovan, D. M. *et al.* (1999a). Alcohol interventions in a trauma center as a means of reducing the risk of injury recurrence. *Annals of Surgery*, **230**, 473–480.

Gentilello, L. M., Villaveces, A., Ries, R. R. *et al.* (1999b). Detection of acute alcohol intoxication and chronic alcohol dependence by trauma center staff. *Journal of Trauma*, **47**, 1131–1135.

Ghesquiere, A., Wagner, A., Russo, J. & Zatzick, D. (2004). Predicting injured trauma survivors' engagement in case management. Paper presented at the the the 20th Annual Meeting of the International Society for Traumatic Stress Studies, New Orleans, La.

Green, B. L. (1993). Identifying survivors at risk. In *International Handbook of Traumatic Stress Syndromes*, eds. J. P. Wilson & B. Raphael. New York: Plenum Press.

Greenberg, P. E., Sisitsky, T., Kessler, R. C. *et al.* (1999). The economic burden of anxiety disorders in the 1990's. *Journal of Clinical Psychiatry*, **60**, 427–435.

Hearst, N., Newman, T. B. & Hulley, S. B. (1986). Delayed effects of the military draft on mortality. A randomized natural experiment. *New England Journal of Medicine*, **314**, 620–624.

Helzer, J. E., Robins, L. N. & McEvoy, L. (1987). Posttraumatic stress disorder in the general population. Findings of the epidemiological catchment area survey. *New England Journal of Medicine*, **317**, 1630–1634.

Herman, D., Felton, C. & Susser, E. (2002). Mental health needs in New York state following the September 11th attacks. *Journal of Urban Health*, **79**, 322–331.

Hoagwood, K., Burns, B. J., Kiser, L., Ringeisen, H. & Schoenwald, S. K. (2001). Evidence-based practice in child and adolescent mental health services. *Psychiatric Services*, **52**, 1179–1189.

Hoge, C. W., Castro, C. A., Messer, S. C. *et al.* (2004). Combat duty in Iraq and Afghanistan, mental health problems, and barriers to care. *New England Journal of Medicine*, **351**, 13–22.

Holbrook, T. L., Anderson, J. P., Sieber, W. J., Browner, D. & Hoyt, D. B. (1999). Outcome after major trauma: 12-month and 18-month follow-up results from the trauma recovery project. *Journal of Trauma*, **46**, 765–773.

Holbrook, T. L., Hoyt, D. B., Stein, M. B. & Sieber, W. J. (2001). Perceived threat to life predicts posttraumatic stress disorder after major trauma: risk factors and functional outcome. *Journal of Trauma*, **51**, 287–293.

Horowitz, L., Kassam-Adams, N. & Bergstein, J. (2001). Mental health aspects of emergency medical services for children: summary of a consensus conference. *Academic Emergency Medicine*, **8**, 1187–1196.

Jack, K. & Glied, S. (2002). The public costs of mental health response: lessons from the New York City post-9/11 needs assessment. *Journal of Urban Health*, **79**, 332–339.

Jaycox, L. H., Marshall, G. N. & Schell, T. (2004). Use of mental health services by men injured through community violence. *Psychiatric Services*, **55**, 415–420.

Johnston, B. D., Rivara, F. P., Droesch, R. M., Dunn, C. & Copass, M. K. (2002). Behavior change counseling in the emergency department to reduce injury risk: a randomized, controlled trial. *Pediatrics*, **110**, 267–274.

Journal of Clinical Psychiatry Guidelines. (1999). Treatment of posttraumatic stress disorder. The expert consensus panels for PTSD. *Journal of Clinical Psychiatry*, **60**, 3–76.

Kassam-Adams, N., Garcia–Espana, J. F., Fein, J. A. & Winston, F. K. (2005). Heart rate and posttraumatic stress in injured children. *Archives of General Psychiatry*, **60**, 335–340.

Katon, W. & Gonzales, J. (1994). A review of randomized trials of psychiatric consultation-liaison studies in primary care. *Psychosomatics*, **35**, 268–278.

Katon, W., Von Korff, M., Lin, E. *et al.* (1994). Methodologic issues in randomized trials of liaison psychiatry in primary care. *Psychosomatic Medicine*, **56**, 97–103.

Katon, W., Von Korff, M., Lin, E. *et al.* (1995). Collaborative management to achieve treatment guidelines: impact on depression in primary care. *Journal of the American Medical Association*, **273**, 1026–1031.

Katon, W., Von Korff, M., Lin, E. *et al.* (1997). Population-based care of depression: effective disease management strategies to decrease prevalence. *General Hospital Psychiatry*, **19**, 169–178.

Katon, W., Von Korff, M., Lin, E. *et al.* (1999). Stepped collaborative care for primary care patients with persistent depression: a randomized trial. *Archives of General Psychiatry*, **56**, 1109–1115.

Katon, W., Rutter, C., Ludman, E. J. *et al.* (2001a). A randomized trial of relapse prevention of depression in primary care. *Archives of General Psychiatry*, **58**, 241–247.

Katon, W., Sullivan, M. & Walker, E. (2001b). Medical symptoms without identified pathology: relationship to psychiatric disorders, childhood and adult trauma, and personality traits. *Annals of Internal Medicine*, **134**, 917–925.

Katon, W., Von Korff, M., Lin, E. & Simon, G. (2001c). Rethinking practitioner roles in chronic illness: the specialist, primary care physician, and the practice nurse. *General Hospital Psychiatry*, **23**, 138–144.

Katon, W., Von Korff, M., Lin, E. H. *et al.* (2004). The pathways study: a randomized trial of collaborative care in patients with diabetes and depression. *Archives of General Psychiatry*, **61**, 1042–1049.

Kessler, R. C. (2000). Posttraumatic stress disorder: the burden to the individual and society. *Journal of Clinical Psychiatry*, **61**, 4–14.

Kessler, R. C., Crum, R. M., Warner, L. A. *et al.* (1997). Lifetime co-occurrence of DSM-III-R alcohol abuse and dependence with other psychiatric disorders in the National Comorbidity Survey. *Archives of General Psychiatry*, **54**, 313–321.

Kessler, R. C., Sonnega, A., Bromet, E. *et al.* (1999). Epidemiological risk factors for trauma and PTSD. In *Risk Factors for Posttraumatic Stress Disorder*, ed. R. Yehuda. Washington, D.C.: American Psychiatric Press.

Koren, D., Norman, D., Cohen, A., Berman, J. & Klein, E. M. (2005). Increased PTSD risk with combat-related injury: a matched comparison study of injured and uninjured soldiers experiencing the same combat events. *American Journal of Psychiatry*, **162**, 276–282.

Litz, B. T. (2004). *Early Intervention for Trauma and Traumatic Loss*. New York: Guilford Press.

Litz, B. T., Gray, M. J., Bryant, R. A. & Adler, A. B. (2002). Early interventions for trauma: current status and future directions. *Clinical Psychology: Science and Practice*, **9**, 112–134.

MacKenzie, E. J., Hoyt, D. B., Sacra, J. C. *et al.* (2003). National inventory of hospital trauma centers. *Journal of the American Medical Association*, **289**, 1515–1522.

March, J. S. (2003). Acute stress disorder in youth: a multivariate prediction model. *Society of Biological Psychiatry*, **53**, 809–816.

Marshall, G. N. & Schell, T. L. (2002). Reappraising the link between peritraumatic dissociation and PTSD symptom severity: evidence from a longitudinal study of community violence survivors. *Journal of Abnormal Psychology*, **111**, 626–636.

Marshall, R. D., Beebe, K. L., Oldham, M. & Zaninelli, R. (2001). Efficacy and safety of paroxetine treatment for chronic PTSD: a fixed-dose, placebo-controlled study. *American Journal of Psychiatry*, **158**, 1982–1988.

Mayou, R., Bryant, B. & Duthie, R. (1993). Psychiatric consequences of road traffic accidents. *British Medical Journal*, **307**, 647–651.

Mayou, R., Tyndel, S. & Bryant, B. (1997). Long-term outcome of motor vehicle accident injury. *Psychosomatic Medicine*, **59**, 578–584.

Mayou, R. A., Ehlers, A. & Hobbs, M. (2000). Psychological debriefing for road traffic accident victims. Three-year follow-up of a randomised controlled trial. *British Journal of Psychiatry*, **176**, 589–593.

McCarthy, M. L., MacKenzie, E. J., Edwin, D. *et al.* (2003). Psychological distress associated with severe lower-limb injury. *The Journal of Bone and Joint Surgery*, **85-A**, 1689–1697.

McGlynn, E. A., Norquist, G. S., Wells, K. B., Sullivan, G. & Liberman, R. P. (1988). Quality-of-care research in mental health: responding to the challenge. *Inquiry*, **25**, 157–170.

Mellman, T. A., David, D., Bustamante, V., Fins, A. I. & Esposito, K. (2001). Predictors of post-traumatic stress disorder following severe injury. *Depression and Anxiety*, **14**, 226–231.

Michaels, A. J., Michaels, C. E., Moon, C. H. *et al.* (1999a). Posttraumatic stress disorder after injury: impact on general health outcome and early risk assessment. *Journal of Trauma Injury, Infection, and Critical Care*, **47**, 460–467.

Michaels, A. J., Michaels, C. E., Zimmerman, M. A. *et al.* (1999b). Posttraumatic stress disorder in injured adults: etiology by path analysis. *Journal of Trauma*, **47**, 867–873.

Mollica, R. F., McInnes, K., Sarajlie, N. *et al.* (1999). Disability associated with psychiatric comorbidity and health status in Bosnian refugees living in Croatia. *Journal of the American Medical Association*, **282**, 433–439.

National Institute of Mental Health. (2002). *Mental Health and Mass Violence: Evidence-Based Early Psychological Intervention for Victims/Survivors of Mass Violence. A Workshop to Reach Consensus on Best Practices*. (NIH Publication No. 02-5138). Washington, D.C.: National Institute of Mental Health.

New Freedom Commission on Mental Health. (2003). *Achieving the Promise: Transforming Mental Health Care in America*. Rockville, Md.: DHHS.

O'Donnell, M. L., Creamer, M., Bryant, R. A., Schnyder, U. & Shalev, A. Y. (2003). Posttraumatic disorders following injury: an empirical and methodological review. *Clinical Psychology Review*, **23**, 587–603.

O'Donnell, M. L., Creamer, M. & Pattison, P. (2004). Posttraumatic stress disorder and depression following trauma: understanding comorbidity. *American Journal of Psychiatry*, **161**, 1390–1396.

Pitman, R. K., Sanders, K. M., Zusman, R. M. *et al.* (2002). Pilot study of secondary prevention of posttraumatic stress disorder with propranolol. *Biological Psychiatry*, **51**, 189–192.

Pynoos, R. S., Steinberg, A. M. & Piacentini, J. C. (1999). A development psychopathology model of childhood traumatic stress and intersection with anxiety disorders. *Society of Biological Psychiatry*, **46**, 1542–1554.

Ramstad, S. M., Russo, J. & Zatzick, D. F. (2004). Is it an accident? Recurrent traumatic life events in level I trauma center patients compared to the general population. *Journal of Traumatic Stress*, **17**, 529–534.

Reijneveld, S. A., Crone, M. R., Verhulst, F. C. & Verloove-Vanhorick, S. P. (2003). The effect of a severe disaster on the mental health of adolescents: a controlled study. *Lancet*, **362**, 691–696.

Reijneveld, S. A., Crone, M. R., Schuller, A. A., Verhulst, F. C. & Verloove-Vanhorick, S. P. (2005). The changing impact of a severe disaster on the mental health and substance misuse of adolescents: follow-up of a controlled study. *Psychological Medicine*, **35**, 367–376.

Rivara, F. P., Koepsell, T. D., Jurkovich, G. J., Gurney, J. G. & Soderberg, R. (1993). The effects of alcohol abuse on readmission for trauma. *Journal of the American Medical Association*, **270**, 1962–1964.

Rose, S. & Bisson, J. (1998). Brief early psychological interventions following trauma: a systematic review of the literature. *Journal of Traumatic Stress*, **11**, 697–710.

Roy-Byrne, P. P., Katon, W., Cowley, D. & Russo, J. (2001). A randomized effectiveness trial of collaborative care for patients with panic disorder in primary care. *Archives of General Psychiatry*, **58**, 869–876.

Roy-Byrne, P. P., Sherbourne, C., Craske, M. *et al.* (2003). Moving treatment research from clinical trials to the real world. *Psychiatric Services*, **53**, 327–332.

Roy-Byrne, P. P., Russo, J., Michelson, E. *et al.* (2004). Risk factors and outcome in ambulatory assault victims presenting to the acute emergency department setting: implications for secondary prevention studies in PTSD. *Depression and Anxiety*, **19**, 77–84.

Sabin, J., Zatzick, D., Jurkovich, G. & Rivara, F. (2006). Primary care utilization and detection of emotional distress after adolescent traumatic injury: identifying an unmet need. *Pediatrics*, **117**, 130–138.

Sackett, D. L., Haynes, R. B., Guyatt, G. H. & Tugwell, P. (1991). *Clinical Epidemiology: A Basic Science for Clinical Medicine*, 2nd edn. London.: Little, Brown and Co.

Santos, A. B., Henggeler, S. W., Burns, B. J., Arana, G. W. & Meisler, N. (1995). Research on field-based services: models for reform in the delivery of mental health care to populations with complex clinical problems. *American Journal of Psychiatry*, **152**, 1111–1123.

Satcher, D. (1999). *Mental health: A Report of the Surgeon General*. (Report). Rockville, Md.: US Department of Health and Human Services.

Schelling, G., Kilger, E., Roozendaal, B. *et al.* (2004). Stress doses of hydrocortisone, traumatic memories, and symptoms of posttraumatic stress disorder in patients after cardiac surgery: a randomized study. *Biological Psychiatry*, **55**, 627–633.

Schermer, C. R., Gentilello, L. M., Hoyt, D. B. *et al.* (2003). National survey of trauma surgeons' use of alcohol screening and brief intervention. *Journal of Trauma*, **55**, 849–856.

Schoenwald, S. K. & Hoagwood, K. (2001). Effectiveness, transportability, and dissemination of interventions: what matters when? *Psychiatric Services*, **52**, 1190–1197.

Schwarz, E. D. & Kowalski, J. M. (1992). Malignant memories: reluctance to utilize mental health services after a disaster. *The Journal of Nervous and Mental Disease*, **180**, 767–772.

Shalev, A. Y., Bonne, O. & Eth, S. (1996). Treatment of posttraumatic stress disorder: a review. *Psychosomatic Medicine*, **58**, 165–182.

Shalev, A. Y., Freedman, S., Peri, T. *et al.* (1998a). Prospective study of posttraumatic stress disorder and depression following trauma. *American Journal of Psychiatry*, **155**, 630–637.

Shalev, A. Y., Sahar, T., Freedman, S. *et al.* (1998b). A prospective study of heart rate response following trauma and the subsequent development of posttraumatic stress disorder. *Archives of General Psychiatry*, **55**, 553–559.

Silver, B. S. & McDuff, D. (1990). Behavioral correlates and staff recognition of alcohol use in a university hospital trauma service. *Psychosomatics*, **32**, 420–425.

Simon, G. E., Wagner, E. & Von Korff, M. (1995). Cost-effectiveness comparisons using "real world" randomized trials: the case of new antidepressant drugs. *Journal of Clinical Epidemiology*, **48**, 363–373.

Simon, G. E., Ludman, E., Unutzer, J. & Bauer, M. S. (2002). Design and implementation of a randomized trial evaluating systematic care for bipolar disorder. *Bipolar Disorders*, **4**, 226–236.

Solomon, S. D., Gerrity, E. T. & Muff, A. M. (1992). Efficacy of treatments for posttraumatic stress disorder. *Journal of the American Medical Association*, **268**, 633–638.

Stein, L. I. & Santos, A. B. (1998). *Assertive Community Treatment of Persons with Severe Mental Illness.* New York: W.W. Norton.

Tellez, M. & Mackersie, R. C. (1996). Violence prevention involvement among trauma surgeons: description and preliminary evaluation. *Journal of Trauma*, **40**, 602–606.

United States Department of Defense, U. S. Department of Health and Human Services, Health, N. I. O. M., Substance Abuse and Mental Health Services Administration, Services, C. f. M. H., U.S. Department of Justice, *et al.* (2001). Mental health and mass violence. Paper presented at the Evidence Based Early Psychological Intervention for Victims/Survivors of Mass Violence: A Workshop to Reach Consensus on Best Practices.

United States Department of Health and Human Services. (2003). *Mental Health All-Hazards Disaster Planning Guidance* (DHHS Publication No. SMA 3829). Rockville, Md.: Center for Mental Health Services, Substance Abuse and Mental Health Services Administration.

Unutzer, J., Katon, W., Williams, J. W. *et al.* (2001). Improving primary care for depression in late life: the design of a multicenter randomized trial. *Medical Care*, **39**, 785–799.

Unutzer, J., Katon, W., Callahan, C. M. *et al.* (2002). Collaborative care management of late-life depression in the primary care setting: a randomized controlled trial. *Journal of the American Medical Association*, **288**, 2836–2845.

Ursano, R. J. (2002). Post-traumatic stress disorder. *New England Journal of Medicine*, **346**, 130–132.

Ursano, R. J., Fullerton, C. S., Epstein, R. S. *et al.* (1999). Acute and chronic posttraumatic stress disorder in motor vehicle accident victims. *American Journal of Psychiatry*, **156**, 589–595.

Ursano, R. J., Bell, C., Eth, S. *et al.* (2004). Practice guideline for the treatment of patients with acute stress disorder and posttraumatic stress disorder. *American Journal of Psychiatry*, **161**, 3–31.

Van Emmerik, A., Kamphuis, J. H., Hulsbosch, A. M. & Emmelkamp, P. (2002). Single session debriefing after psychological trauma: a meta-analysis. *The Lancet*, **360**, 766–771.

Vlahov, D., Galea, S., Ahern, J. *et al.* (2004a). Consumption of cigarettes, alcohol, and marijuana among New York City residents six months after the September 11 terrorist attacks. *American Journal of Drug and Alcohol Abuse*, **30**, 385–407.

Vlahov, D., Galea, S., Ahern, J., Resnick, H. & Kilpatrick, D. (2004b). Sustained increased consumption of cigarettes, alcohol, and marijuana among Manhattan residents after September 11, 2001. *American Journal of Public Health*, **94**, 253–254.

Von Korff, M., Gruman, J., Schaefer, J., Curry, S. J. & Wagner, E. H. (1997). Collaborative management of chronic illness. *Annals of Internal Medicine*, **127**, 1097–1102.

Wagner, A. W. (2003). Cognitive-behavioral therapy for PTSD: applications to injured trauma survivors. *Seminars in Clinical Neuropsychiatry*, **8**, 175–187.

Wagner, E. H., Austin, B. T. & Von Korff, M. (1996). Organizing care for patients with chronic illness. *The Milbank Quarterly*, **74**, 511–543.

Walker, E., Unutzer, J., Rutter, C. *et al.* (1999). Costs of health care use by women HMO members with a history of childhood abuse and neglect. *Archives of General Psychiatry*, **56**, 609–613.

Walker, E. A., Katon, W., Russo, J. *et al.* (2003). Health care costs associated with posttraumatic stress disorder symptoms in women. *Archives of General Psychiatry*, **60**, 369–374.

Walker-Barnes, C. J. (2003). Developmental epidemiology: the perfect partner for clinical practice. *Journal of Clinical Child and Adolescent Psychology*, **32**, 181–186.

Weisaeth, L. (2001). Acute posttraumatic stress: non-acceptance of early intervention. *Journal of Psychiatry*, **62**, 35–40.

Wells, K. B. (1999a). The design of Partners in Care: evaluating the cost-effectiveness of improving care for depression in primary care. *Social Psychiatry and Psychiatric Epidemiology*, **34**, 20–43.

Wells, K. B. (1999b). Treatment research at the crossroads: the scientific interface of clinical trials and effectiveness research. *American Journal of Psychiatry*, **156**, 5–10.

Wells, K. B., Sherbourne, C., Schoenbaum, M. *et al.* (2000). Impact of disseminating quality improvement programs for depression in managed primary care: a randomized controlled trial. *Journal of the American Medical Association*, **283**, 212–220.

Winston, F. K., Kassam-Adams, N., Garcia-Espana, F., Ittenbach, R. & Cnaan, A. (2003). Screening for risk of persistent posttraumatic stress in injured children and their parents. *Journal of the American Medical Association*, **290**, 643–649.

Yehuda, R. (1999). *Risk Factors for Posttraumatic Stress Disorder*. Washington, D.C.: American Psychiatric Press.

Zatzick, D. F. (2003a). Collaborative care for injured victims of individual and mass trauma: a health services research approach to developing early interventions. In *Terrorism and Disaster: Individual and Community Mental Health Interventions*, eds. R. J. Ursano, C. S. Fullerton & A. E. Norwood. Cambridge: Cambridge University Press.

Zatzick, D. F. (2003b). Posttraumatic stress, functional impairment, and service utilization after injury: a public health approach. *Seminars in Clinical Neuropsychiatry*, **8**, 149–157.

Zatzick, D. F. & Roy-Byrne, P. (2003). Psychopharmacological approaches to the management of posttraumatic stress disorders in the acute care medical sector. *Seminars in Clinical Neuropsychiatry*, **8**, 168–174.

Zatzick, D. F., Marmar, C. R., Weiss, D. S. *et al.* (1997a). Posttraumatic stress disorder, and functioning and quality of life outcomes in a nationally representative sample of male Vietnam veterans. *American Journal of Psychiatry*, **154**, 1690–1695.

Zatzick, D. F., Weiss, D. S., Marmar, C. R. *et al.* (1997b). Post-traumatic stress disorder and functioning and quality of life outcomes in female Vietnam veterans. *Military Medicine*, **162**, 661–665.

Zatzick, D. F., Kang, S., Kim, S. *et al.* (2000). Patients with recognized psychiatric disorders in trauma surgery: incidence, inpatient length of stay, and cost. *Journal of Trauma Injury, Infection, and Critical Care*, **49**, 487–495.

Zatzick, D. F., Kang, S. M., Hinton, W. L. *et al.* (2001a). Posttraumatic concerns: a patient-centered approach to outcome assessment after traumatic physical injury. *Medical Care*, **39**, 327–339.

Zatzick, D. F., Roy-Byrne, P., Russo, J., Rivara, F. P. & Jurkovich, G. J. (2001b). Distress, functioning and service use in injured trauma survivors. Paper presented at the Reaching Undeserved Trauma Survivors Through Community-Based Programs: 17th Annual Meeting, New Orleans, Louisiana.

Zatzick, D. F., Roy-Byrne, P., Russo, J. *et al.* (2001c). Collaborative interventions for physically injured trauma survivors: a pilot randomized effectiveness trial. *General Hospital Psychiatry*, **23**, 114–123.

Zatzick, D. F., Jurkovich, G. J., Gentilello, L. M., Wisner, D. H. & Rivara, F. P. (2002a). Posttraumatic stress, problem drinking and functioning 1 year after injury. *Archives of Surgery*, **137**, 200–205.

Zatzick, D. F., Kang, S. M., Muller, H. G. *et al.* (2002b). Predicting posttraumatic distress in hospitalized trauma survivors with acute injuries. *American Journal of Psychiatry*, **159**, 941–946.

Zatzick, D. F., Russo, J. & Katon, W. (2003). Somatic, posttraumatic stress and depressive symptoms among injured patients treated in trauma surgery. *Psychosomatics*, **44**, 479–484.

Zatzick, D. F., Roy-Byrne, P., Russo, J. *et al.* (2004a). A randomized effectiveness trial of stepped collaborative care for acutely injured trauma survivors. *Archives of General Psychiatry*, **61**, 498–506.

Zatzick, D. F., Roy-Byrne, P., Russo, J. *et al.* (2004b). Effective early intervention for injury survivors: a randomized trial. Paper presented at the 20th Annual Meeting of the International Society for Traumatic Stress Studies, New Orleans, LA.

Zatzick, D. F., Jurkovich, G., Russo, J. *et al.* (2004c). Posttraumatic distress, alcohol disorders, and recurrent trauma across level 1 trauma centers. *Journal of Trauma: Injury, Infection, and Critical Care*, **57**, 360–366.

Zatzick, D. F., Russo, J., Pitman, R. K. *et al.* (2005a). Reevaluating the association between emergency department heart rate and the development of posttraumatic stress disorder: a public health approach. *Biological Psychiatry*, **57**, 91–95.

Zatzick, D. F., Russo, J., Rivara, F. *et al.* (2005b). The detection and treatment of posttraumatic distress and substance intoxication in the acute care inpatient setting. *General Hospital Psychiatry*, **27**, 57–62.

Zatzick, D. F., Roy-Byrne, P. P., Russo, J. *et al.* (2005c). Anxiety disorders and medical illness: risk factors, effectiveness trials, and quality of care. *CNS Spectrums*, **10**, 1.

Zatzick, D. F., Russo, J., Grossman, D. *et al.* (2006a). Posttraumatic stress and depressive symptoms, alcohol use, and recurrent traumatic life events in a representative sample of hospitalized injured adolescents and their parents. *Journal of Pediatric Psychology*, **31**, 377–387.

Zatzick, D., Simon, G. E. & Wagner, A. W. (2006b). Developing and implementing randomized effectiveness trails in general medical settings. *Clinical Psychology: Science and Practice*, **13** (1), 53–68.

10

Nongovernmental organizations and the role of the mental health professional

Joop de Jong

Introduction

A disaster is a serious event that causes an ecological breakdown in the relationship between humans and their environment on a scale that requires extraordinary efforts to allow the community to cope, and often requires outside help or international aid (Lechat, 1990; Noji, 1997). Berren *et al.* (1980) mention five factors that can be used conceptually to distinguish one disaster from another: (1) type of disaster: human-made or natural; (2) duration; (3) degree of personal impact; (4) potential of recurrence; and (5) control over future impact. In natural disasters, a natural hazard affects a population or area and may result in severe damage and destruction and increased morbidity and mortality that overwhelm local coping capacity. Similarly, in human-made disasters such as complex emergencies, wars or terrorist attacks, mortality among the civilian population substantially increases above the population baseline mortality, either as a result of the direct effects of war or conflict, or indirectly through the increased prevalence of malnutrition and/or transmission of communicable diseases, especially if the latter result from deliberate political and military policies and strategies (Salama *et al.*, 2004). In 2000, an estimated 1.6 million people worldwide died as a result of violence, and one-fifth were war related (World Health Organization, 2002b). As Chapter 2 shows, mental morbidity increases too, and varying risk groups need additional attention as well as preventative efforts to alleviate their plight.

This chapter highlights the role of (international) nongovernmental organizations [(I)NGOs]. NGOs are often a key player in both natural and "human-made" disasters. This chapter will focus on mental health professionals who plan to get involved in postdisaster or postconflict work. It addresses psychiatrists, psychologists, psychiatric nurses, social workers, and trainees who are, or who would like to get, involved in disaster work. The crux of this chapter may be well known to professionals from low- and middle-income (LIMA) countries. However, it illustrates various issues that colleagues from LIMA countries may not always be aware of, despite or because of these issues being part and parcel of their daily living environment. I will start with a brief outline of the world of (I)NGOs. Subsequently, the chapter addresses a series of challenges for mental health professionals and how they can prepare for a career in this field. Throughout the text I provide a series of caveats or recommendations for the professional who is preparing to work for an NGO. I asked several colleagues, i.e., Keven Bermudez, Mark Jordans, Wietse Tol, Marianne van der Veen, and Peter Ventevogel, to write some impressions of their work in Afghanistan, Nepal, Sri Lanka, Burundi, Indonesia, and Sudan. Their diaries or week diaries – inserted in boxes in the text – give the reader a sense of and some insight into what life is like "out there."

(International) nongovernmental organizations [(I)NGOs]

In the 1980s and 1990s, the Structural Adjustment Programmes of the International Monetary Fund (IMF) and the World Bank resulted in a reduction of government spending on health and education in a variety of countries. Neo-liberal economic policies further contributed to undermining the already weak governmental sector. To compensate for the decreased service delivery in sectors such as health and education, local and international NGOs tried to fill the gap and create a safety net with special attention paid to vulnerable, marginalized or minority populations. Although the interventions of the IMF often resulted in an overall economic growth, democratic changes and social mobility lagged behind causing increased economic disparities, regional and ethnic conflicts, human rights violations and ecological deterioration. These social changes are risk factors for breeding natural or human-made disasters – as several chapters of this book illustrate. Disasters overstretch existing service delivery capacities, even in high-income countries. Therefore, NGOs are extremely important for developing adequate services for survivors, especially in the emergency phase. The dynamics of the postdisaster context presents NGOs with choices in terms of service delivery models. Both curative and preventive health services can be provided using a horizontal or a vertical delivery mode. In a horizontal program services are delivered through public-financed health systems and are commonly referred to as comprehensive primary care as formulated by the World Health Organization (WHO) and UNICEF in Alma Ata in 1978 and later at the initiative of "Health for All by 2000" (World Health Organization, 1978). Vertical delivery of health services implies a selective targeting of specific interventions not fully integrated in health systems (Banerji, 1984; Rifkin & Walt, 1986).

The past few years have seen increased advocacy for vertical programming for a number of reasons. Vertical programs such as "National Immunization Days" to eradicate poliomyelitis attract donors and political establishments because they show quick results and they are easier to manage than horizontal programs. Vertical programs produce quick and visible results that fit media-hypes on themes such as child soldiers, woman and child trafficking or rape survivors. However, many policy-makers in developing countries see vertical programs diverting human and financial resources away from already resource-constrained health systems (Schreuder & Kostermans, 2001). Moreover, within the current context of health sector reform the tendency is towards health systems strengthening within horizontal programming. In addition, questions remain on the long-term sustainability of vertical programs in terms of outcomes and resources. This is especially important in the field of psychosocial and mental health care, which – despite its proven burden of disease – is less likely to receive the substantial funding that other public health priorities such as tuberculosis, acquired immunodeficiency syndrome (AIDS) or malaria attract (de Jong, 2002). The incentives driving donors and NGOs to provide services may be different (Msuya, 2003). Factors influencing the decisions made by donors on financing programs include the need for quick results to attract political or funding support from their constituents, as the examples of the Tsunami in 2004 and the floodings in the southern part of the United States in 2005 have shown. In making such choices, as a public official or as a donor, there are trade-offs in selecting horizontal or vertical programs. In postdisaster settings a transitional process of emergency through reconstruction to development paralleled by a transition from vertical to horizontal programming is likely to produce the highest level of sustainability. When we started our work it took us many years to develop a sustainable program that was completely implemented and managed by the local NGO to which we handed over all capacity, expertise, management responsibilities, and logistics including transport. For example, in Cambodia with a target population of about 2 million out of a total population of 13 million inhabitants, it took approximately 6 years; in northern Uganda among 170 000 Sudanese refugees, 8 years. After gaining more experience and being able to use expertise from the same region, we were able to shorten this period to 4–5 years, for example in Burundi where our program covers 4 million people, i.e., more than half of the population. Although we always tried to work toward horizontal integration with government public health services, this proved to be a difficult task because the government mostly did not have the capacity or the motivation to take over the services. This happened even when we offered to hand over the relatively easy task of integrating mental health into primary care including experienced trainers, supervisors, and supplies of drugs. Therefore, we sometimes continued to run the whole program under the aegis of the independent local NGO, or the local NGO continued to manage the psychosocial part while sharing (part of) the responsibility for mental disorders with government structures. In other words, although our final aim was to deliver an integrated horizontal public mental health program, we partially succeeded at the provincial or district level but not at a national level. This also happened in countries where we were the only service provider of community mental health and psychosocial care.

In addition to the government and the NGO sectors, a third, important and highly relevant player in the field, the United Nations (UN), further complicates the dynamic of positioning one's activities between the different actors. UN agencies are manifold, each with different though often overlapping mandates. UN agencies, like NGOs, may be challenged by competition. A mental health professional has to decide where she or he prefers to work. The worlds of the UN and of the NGO both have specific advantages and disadvantages. A mental health professional may be better off at the UN when status and income are important and when (s)he is able to deal with policy formulation, bureaucracy, hierarchy, distance to actual service delivery, and a system where diplomatic considerations may be more important than being qualified for a job. NGOs have their own peculiarities. On the one hand, the advantage is that NGOs are often more flexible, and that the professional has quick access to and stays in close contact with target groups. On the other hand,

one has to accept getting involved in many aspects of the work, varying from human resource capacity building to providing care to survivors, as well as management, research, funding, and accountability issues (as illustrated in the boxes in this chapter). In both worlds professional envy and fear of encroachment on one's turf go hand in hand with a compassionate humanitarian drive. A preference to coordinate over being coordinated is rampant, and loneliness may be an important personal aspect of life, whether working at the UN in New York or "en brousse." In the field professional isolation may be an additional challenge. In both worlds mental health professionals can play a supportive role in facilitating recovery of the core adaptive systems that hasten natural recovery from stress for the majority of the population. Where community mental health services are established, the emphasis should be on training local workers to train others and to assume leadership while designing and implementing interventions for families and individuals who are at greatest survival and adaptive risk.

Challenges for mental health professionals who plan to work in postdisaster and postconflict areas

In high-income countries the mental health profession of psychiatry, psychotherapy, psychology, nursing or social work is increasingly driven by evidence-based and manualized treatments, empirically supported treatments (EST), standardized guidelines, or diagnosis-related groupings. Messer (2002) mentions that there probably is no issue currently as contentious in the field of mental health treatment as that of the advocacy and use of manual-guided EST. Strupp (2001) also criticizes the EST development as being based "on a medical model that assumes that a psychotherapeutic treatment can be conceptualized independent of the human relationship in which it takes place. Psychotherapy and psychoanalysis are, however, treatments only in a metaphorical sense and are more akin to educational processes than medical treatments. Every therapeutic dyad is unique, and research that treats therapy as a standardized, disembodied entity will not contribute to our understanding." This has a particular bearing on postdisaster and postconflict settings that often have a disproportionally large impact in LIMA countries or among immigrant or minority groups in the "West" as the 2001 tragedies in New York and the 2005 tragedy in New Orleans have shown. In these (sub)cultures the collective, the group or the extended family are often more important than the individual, the ego, and the self (de Jong, 2004). The importance of human relationships in these collectivistic (sub)cultures underlines Strupp's criticism about therapy as a standardized disembodied entity. In theory, most scholars and practitioners agree that standardized treatment protocols and guidelines need thorough cultural adaptation, testing, and modification before they can be applied in a responsible way in low- and middle-income countries. Although much has been published on the use of allopathic, academic or "western" methods in culturally nondominant (or "nonwestern") settings, with a few exceptions little has been done to develop treatments based on local coping styles, culture-specific idioms of distress, and culturally appropriate helping methods. Examples of these exceptions are the use of healing, mourning, grief, reconciliation, and cleansing and purification rituals (de Jong, 2002, 2004; Van der Hart, 1983, 1988), the combination of cognitive-behavioral therapy with Taoist or Buddhist philosophy, or the influence of Buddhist approaches on western psychotherapeutic techniques (Bemak *et al.*, 1996; Boehnlein, 1987; Clifford, 1990; Epstein, 1995; Hinton *et al.*, 2004; Kabat-Zinn, 2003; Linehan, 1993; Otto *et al.*, 2003; Teasdale, 1997; Watts, 1969).

The existing evidence-based methods are thus of little avail to a mental health professional who plans to work in postdisaster and postconflict settings. More important even, one paradox of evidence-based medicine is that it may impede the development of creative skills that the mental health professional needs in LIMA countries. The following paragraphs describe several particular

Table 10.1 Challenges for mental health professionals

1. Addressing a multiplicity of causal factors
2. Addressing additional vulnerability factors within a contextual model
3. Addressing the scarcity of mental health professionals
4. Handling the complementarity between allopathic "western" and local healing methods
5. Taking specific characteristics of the survivors into account

challenges, obstacles, and pitfalls that warrant the attention of the future professional and that illustrate the high level of flexibility and creativity of the "disaster mental health professional" (see Table 10.1).

Addressing a multiplicity of causal factors

Most armed conflicts are the result of political, economic, and sociocultural processes. Known risk factors for major political conflicts are social and economic inequalities, rapidly changing demographics, lack of democracy, political instability, ethnic strife, deterioration of public services, and severe economic decline (Carnegie Commission on Preventing Deadly Conflict, 1997). Similarly to the development of individual psychopathology in adult or child psychiatry, an accumulation of risk factors or a critical mass of signs increases the likelihood of the occurrence of problems. The sequelae of conflicts are preferably resolved by multilevel, multisectoral public health approaches informed by social sciences (especially anthropology), behavioral sciences, and epidemiology (de Jong, 2002). (Multisectoral or intersectoral means via the sectors of health, education, social, and women's affairs, rural development and the like.)

Most protracted conflicts are related to competition for power and resources, and result in predatory social formations. They affect large, displaced and mostly poor populations, and they are often accompanied by cycles of violence (Hamburg *et al.*, 1999). Conflict-affected countries are among the most health deprived and access to health services is often extremely limited due to the combination of war superimposed on structural poverty (Lanjouw et al., 1999). This type of conflict requires flexible and sustainable solutions, both functionally and geographically, and may require that paraprofessionals from among the survivors move to other areas together with the refugees or displaced persons when the conflict dictates a continuation of their journey. A similar reasoning applies to natural disasters. Many natural disasters such as landslides, droughts, floodings, typhoons or volcano eruptions affect marginalized groups that often live in inhospitable or dangerous areas. Increasing industrialization, urbanization, decaying infrastructures, and deforestation are among the factors that place many of the world's countries at increasing risk (Quarantelli, 1994). As in human-made disaster, the public health infrastructure is often seriously affected and rebuilding it requires flexibility from the health workers. Consequences of chronic stress at the level of an individual [e.g., in diagnoses such as complex post-traumatic stress disorder (PTSD) or DESNOS] show conspicuous similarities to the prevailing political culture in countries where natural or human-made crises are highly prevalent. The "cultures of fear" in a number of these countries can be characterized by: (1) a sense of personal vulnerability and a feeling of powerlessness, (2) remaining in a state of alert, and (3) the impossibility of testing subjective experience against reality (Corradi et al., 1992; Salimovich et al., 1992). These "cultures of fear" interact with the individual consequences of traumatic stress and result in persistent fears among their populations. The prevailing fear and suspicion weave their way into society and affect support structures, commitments, belief in justice, democratization and human rights. In such a context, some agencies and NGOs work well with local governments. However, the government is often seen as the major cause of the crisis, especially when blamed for neglecting vital infrastructure or when known for its bad governance and human rights violations. In such contexts NGOs often retain critical positions. If the government did not prevent the crisis from happening, does not care about the survivors, or lacks the ability to provide support, the bulk of the relief work falls on the shoulders of the NGOs.

This sociopolitical context has important implications for a mental health professional getting involved in disaster work. A mental health professional designing interventions in crisis conditions should be able to reflect on the social, economic, political, biological, and cultural determinants of mental illness. He or she should be able to collaborate with public health specialists, anthropologists, economists, political scientists, historians, juridical experts, and epidemiologists. Ideally, the mental health professional should at least be acquainted with basic insights of public health and prevention, anthropology, political science, and epidemiology. He or she should be able to judge the (dis)advantages of working in an NGO setting while seeking more close or distant collaboration with the government structures that often contributed to the plight of the survivors. On a more personal level, the professional should also be aware of the impact of chronic sequential traumatization and its interaction with the "culture of fear" on one's own work. Over the past 30 years I have been involved in many post-disaster settings. At times I was seriously confronted with my naive fantasy that my local colleagues would not be affected by the suspicion, the mood swings, the ethnic strife or other sequelae that pervade our literature. And while being regarded as an expert in culture, and always paying attention to the cultural implications of our interventions, I was also confronted with my naiveté in the cultural realm. When we were requested to support an existing NGO (instead of developing our own NGO), I realized that those local NGOs that are able to smoothly interact with INGOs and donors have a large advantage in attracting professional expertise and funding. However, underneath we sometimes were confronted with a local management style that we regarded as feudal, dictatorial or nepotistic. While we always tried to stimulate good governance, democracy and ethnic collaboration by trying to realize these objectives at least in our own organization, we wondered whether we should emphasize our "universal" values or take a relativistic stance vis-à-vis these peculiarities that did not fit our management and human rights agenda.

Box 1: A day in Burundi

The green hills of Burundi are clouded in white morning haze when we leave Gitega, the ancient capital in the heart of the country. I am with Norbert who recently returned from Rwanda where HealthNet-TPO had him follow a 3-year course programme in psychiatric nursing. Now he is one of only two qualified psychiatric nurses in Burundi. We are accompanied by two general nurses who will be trained by Norbert and me. The road can hardly be called a road and the 90 km takes us three and a half hours. Upon our arrival dozens of patients have gathered for HealthNet-TPO's monthly mental health clinic. Before we start seeing patients we pass by the Provincial Director of Public Health. He is the only Governmental doctor in this province of 350 000 people. He is a young and energetic man, who welcomes us warmly. His desk is full with piles of health statistics that he has to compile for his monthly reports to the central Ministry of Health.

Many of the patients in the mobile clinic have walked for hours to come here and to receive their monthly medication. My task is to see some difficult diagnostic cases and to discuss treatment options with Norbert and the other nurses. The whole spectrum of severe psychiatry is demonstrated that morning: paranoid schizophrenia, severe depression, mania, autism, severe obsessive compulsive disorder and mental retardation. We also see dozens of cases of epilepsy, which in Africa belongs to the realm of psychiatry. Several of the epileptic patients bear visible signs of their illness, such as scars and burns. An old lady even has had her arm amputated after she fell in a fire during an attack. It is upsetting to see such severe disability that could have easily been prevented: since the mobile clinics started in Karuzi this patient has received monthly medication and is free of seizures.

At the end of the morning Daniel passes by. He is born in this area and is one of HealthNet-TPOs psychosocial assistants. During his field visits he encounters many severe psychiatric cases who he refers to the mobile clinic. People with milder psychopathology such as anxiety and depression, often related to psychosocial stress factors, are managed by Daniel himself. Some of them receive individual counseling, but others participate in psychosocial support groups. This afternoon Daniel facilitates a group of HIV-positive teenage mothers in a camp for internally displaced persons (IDPs). Since Norbert seems firmly in control of the mobile clinic I decide to join Daniel. The IDPs do not have refugee status since they remain within the borders of their own country. They are mainly ethnic Tutsis and some Twa (pygmees) who survived attacks by Hutu rebels in the previous decade. Their huts are small and crowded. I wonder how they have survived and lived here for 10 years. The support group takes place in an open field outside the camp. One by one the 15 participants gather, some of them accompanied by a baby or toddler. To my surprise they do not look demoralized and hopeless but rather strong and enthusiastic. Daniel tells me that when the group started, 6 months ago, most of them were too shy and embarrassed to share their stories. The stories are embarrassing indeed: young girls raped by neighbors or soldiers, or who sold their bodies in order to feed their siblings after the killing of their parents. The state of despair has clearly evaporated from this group. During the initial rounds of sharing experiences some of the women share their worries: Will they ever be strong again? What will happen to their child after they have died? The women console each other. In the last 40 min of the session the atmosphere becomes optimistic again after one of the participants proposes the plan to start an income-generating activity to create a mutual fund to help members who are in financial trouble. I am still thinking of this plan when we drive back to Gitega at the end of the day. I will discuss this in our management meeting, since I know that HealthNet-TPO Burundi has just received a small grant to initiate income-generating activities among vulnerable client groups. A small starting capital could really help this group of courageous women.

Peter Ventevogel, psychiatrist, Mental Health Advisor, HealthNet-TPO Burundi, Bujumbura.

Box 2: Jalalabad, Afghanistan

This region is currently recovering, as the rest of the country, from a quarter century of devastation brought on by multiple wars, amidst continuous threats to its stability posed by opponents to the reconstruction process. This makes it a "hardship context" in the (I)NGO lingo, and, as Psychosocial Advisor for Healthnet-TPO's Mental Health Program in this location, the following transcription of journal entries for three consecutive workdays may reflect some of the challenges an NGO worker dedicated to mental health concerns may be faced with.

August 28, 2005

I started the week with the typical question, "What will this week bring?" With all that is going on, I still can't consider this assignment anything else than a week-to-week, almost day-to-day affair. Things can shift at a moment's notice for any minor reason, as experience demonstrates. Now we're in the lead up to the Election Day, which at this late hour is still scheduled for September 18, 2005, and what that may bring is still uncertain to many. In terms of work activities, this will mean a slow down as international staff will be inevitably relocated to safer grounds prior to the date. At least this time the evacuation is a planned one, unlike the one which occurred last May, shortly after my arrival on site. Today was our weekly office-based training day, devoted to helping our local psychosocial staff members (two females and two males) build the necessary skills and confidence to run same-gender support groups in the targeted villages. They're entirely new at this but show high motivation to learn, although I also perceive their doubts that such a new way of approaching stress-related problems will take root in villages strongly anchored in traditional ways of addressing these kinds of problems. They are also conscious of the fact that, faced with extreme poverty, many villagers also turn to INGOs with the main expectation that they will provide needed material support, with little time left for those that don't. Fortunately, there also seems to be a wide recognition among the Afghan population that a quarter century of war has inevitably left scars in people's minds. Traditional healing approaches are, presently, not accessible to everyone in the rural areas where we operate or always effective to deal with such issues as arise from war-related experiences. There is, therefore, a chance that our support intervention will progress if adequately introduced.

August 29, 2005

Today we went to one of the three villages targeted in our psychosocial project. What is really tough about going out to the villages, which are no less than an hour away, is getting there given the current state of the roads. The pain has its rewards, however, once you reach the village, where you are invited to sit on a mat in the shade of a thick-trunk tree, remove your footwear, and are served *Chai* before anything else gets underway. This week only a few show up to the group, after a full and rather enthusiastic group last week. We obviously sought explanations, which came towards the end of our stay, when a few group members showed up. The reason: political rallies. Today, the village received a female candidate, and in a region where females are generally not supposed to be seen, this is a real public curiosity. This is not the only thing. The other is that food is served at these rallies. Villagers go to every possible political rally, even in villages different than their own and knowing they will never vote for such candidates, simply because they serve food. There's no way to beat that. One is left to wonder if the elected officials will be those that have served the best food.

August 30, 2005

Today we traveled to another target village, very low profile, as recommended by recent safety warnings due to the insurgent activity in this particular district. Shortly after taking our place in the shade of a tree, group participants started to arrive. The participants welcomed a discussion on the selected topic: the negative impact on general health and well-being of interpersonal conflicts among family and community members. Members of this ethnic group readily acknowledged the gravity of this problem among their own. However, they also expressed a sense of helplessness as these are, in many instances, situations that began generations ago. A participant managed to keep the group afloat by stating that if their ancestors had met in this way, perhaps those conflicts would have been resolved by now, so they better continue discussing this issue unless they wish to pass it down to their children as well. Everybody agreed. So far it follows the usual pattern. Community members turn out to see what is being offered, accept the need for such support, and then whether they continue to participate or not seems to depend on their real disposition to make room for such support in their lives. Many drop out alleging it's not doing enough for them quickly enough. Yet, since no one believes either that such problems can be solved as quickly as instant coffee, one is left with a sense that there's probably more to that demand than what appears on the surface ... A natural reservation to discuss a private issue surrounded with a certain degree of shame? A basic distrust in an alternative approach to their longstanding problems, especially if introduced by a foreign entity? A distrust in fellow-villagers, based on negative past experiences? The more than likely underlying reservations to engaging in such a process only underscore the importance of dedicating equal attention to basic aspects like these as to the identified major problem that brought the group together in the first place, by helping community members to feel comfortable in each others' presence, to form trusting relationships, to reconstruct their shared memories, and to provide them the chance to freely ask questions about their pressing concerns.

Keven E. Bermudez, MEd, LMHC, Psychosocial Advisor, Healthnet-TPO, Nangarhar Province, Eastern Afghanistan

Addressing additional vulnerability factors within a contextual model

Survivors of extreme stressors such as earthquakes, hurricanes, war, genocide, persecution, torture, ethnic cleansing or terrorism are prone to a range of additional vulnerability factors. Among these vulnerability or risk factors are increased economic hardship, poor physical conditions, a collapse of social networks, marginalization, discrimination, and a lack of acculturation and professional skills fitting the new environment (de Jong, 2002). Most mental health problems of survivors are not determined solely by traumatic events but also by the above-mentioned changes in the social context at the macro, the meso- and the micro-levels. Therefore, public mental health professionals should be able to handle a contextual approach, linking individuals, families, communities, and society-at-large. Trauma needs to be conceptualized in terms of an interaction between these different levels, and not merely as a reified psychological entity to be located and addressed within the individual or group psychology of those affected. Interventions that address one of these levels while taking account of the interaction with other levels are optimal. Interventions should straddle psychological and social domains.

Box 3: Life in a Nepali NGO

Introduction

Nepal has been submerged in a civil war, a conflict that has sharply escalated in the past years. Displacement, torture, unaccounted disappearances and vast losses of civilian lives have become rampant in this Himalayan Kingdom. Mark Jordans is a child psychologist who has

been working in Nepal for the past 6 years and is currently working for Transcultural Psychosocial Organization (TPO) with the Center for Victims of Torture, Nepal (CVICT). Together with CVICT he has been working on developing and conducting long-term training courses for psychosocial interventions and implementing psychosocial care programs for victims of child trafficking, for children in areas of armed conflict and victims of torture.

Monday

The day starts, be it the usual 30 min after the agreed upon time, with a team meeting in which resumption of the Post Graduate Diploma course in Psychosocial Interventions is discussed. TPO and CVICT jointly developed and conducted a one-year pilot course in 2004 for a group of students from Bangladesh, Pakistan, and Nepal. The course is the first postgraduate-level, skill-based course in this field of work in South Asia. The meeting focuses on the possibilities of future funding, either through structural support for the training institute as a whole or otherwise on student scholarship bases.

The afternoon is devoted to a national workshop, organized by Save the Children, on psychosocial and mental health issues for children in armed conflict. The meeting brings together some key organizations and touches on the impact of violence on children and the role of NGOs to counter such impact. I have been asked to give a presentation on screening for at-risk youth, which is seemingly well received, albeit by a group of participants that makes following workshops all but a profession.

Tuesday

In the morning a meeting of the Kathmandu Psychosocial Forum (KPF) is scheduled. KPF is an association, co-founded by TPO and CVICT, for organizations and individuals working in the field of psychosocial care and mental health in Kathmandu. It aims to encourage collaboration, technical exchange and professional sharing to increase the general awareness about and professionalism in mental health/ psychosocial care. The main agenda points are case sharing and a presentation on a mothers-to-mothers support program for underdeveloped urban populations.

The rest of the day is dedicated to a proposal for Healthnet-TPO International to conduct a five-country psychosocial care program in Sudan, Indonesia, Sri Lanka, Burundi, and Nepal. The project aims to develop a package of interventions, which includes a classroom-based psychosocial intervention (CBI) as well as youth groups, public awareness and family interventions for children affected by armed conflict. This process of writing has become increasingly frustrating as electricity supply is frequently interrupted (read: loss of unsaved data), which generally indicates heavy monsoon rains or governmental electricity supply control.

Wednesday

Today is the start of a new internship program; a 5-month training course in psychosocial counseling for a group of 12 participants, which is structured through interchanging cycles of classroom learning and supervised practical placements (Jordans *et al.*, 2002, 2003). This summarizes the core ideas of this training program; namely, that it is long term and that it focuses on skills and supervised practice. The first day of any training focuses on introductions as well as doing a pre-test questionnaire to later evaluate the training's impact.

The scheduling of this day is quite unfortunate, as it coincides with a *Bhandha*. Such a general strike, especially when called by the *Maoists,* entails a complete shutdown of the country. It does not hamper our day too much as the training is residential, but the effects of such a day are appalling in terms of economic and social damage for this country.

Before the end of the day I still have to review a planned needs assessment on the public health impact of the war in far-away Jumla district, a survey that should incorporate information from the local traditional healers (*Dhami Jankris*).

Thursday

The morning is dedicated to a clinical supervision class of the students of another ongoing internship course (as described under Wednesday). This course, for 10 students, is in its final month and focuses on psychosocial counseling for children affected by armed conflict. In the daily clinical supervision session (during the practical placements) of two hours the students discuss yesterday's cases. Today one student raises the question on how to deal with an adolescent boy who is reluctant to talk in the sessions but who does indicate that he wants to continue seeing the counselor. Another issue was raised on how to deal with confidentiality when the NGO management asks the counselor to relay client's information.

In the afternoon I continue with making plans for the registration and inception of Healthnet-TPO Nepal. This new NGO aspires to carry out community-based psychosocial care programs in the conflict-affected areas (such as the one described under Tuesday) and should, in collaboration with CVICT, boost the level of expertise in the area. It is within the same vision that Healthnet-TPO Nepal and CVICT will jointly operate the Post Graduate Diploma course (as described under Monday). Besides such strategic planning, the registration proves to be greatly bureaucratic (though luckily not overtly corrupted) and the process of organizational development a challenge – especially due to ever-lacking funding for mental health programs and a visible *brain-drain* by the INGO community or Western countries.

Friday

Today I am facilitating a training course for field monitors of the World Food Program (WFP) on issues of coping with distressing situations. WFP field monitors, working in rebel-controlled areas, are frequently exposed to stressful situations and are also at risk for secondary distress through the stories of their beneficiaries. This short training course was developed to create awareness on the possible psychosocial impact of conflict, self-identification of distress as well as individual coping styles and additional self-help techniques.

Fortunately, this evening is full moon, which is beautifully celebrated with music in the temple courtyard of *Kirateswhor* – a good interlude from NGO life in Nepal.

Mark Jordans, MA, psychologist, working with a Nepali NGO

Addressing the scarcity of mental health professionals

Between 1973 and 1997 disasters caused each year, on average, more then 84 000 deaths and affected the lives of 144 million people, with the majority of victims in developing countries (IFRC, 1999). The ratio of disaster victims in low- and middle-income versus high-income countries is estimated at 166:1, and the ratio of morbidity and mortality in low-income to high-income countries at 10:1 (De Girolamo & McFarlane, 1996; World Health Organization, 2002a).

The bulk of the 35 million refugees and internally displaced people worldwide reside in countries that on average have less than one psychiatrist or psychologist per 100 000 people (World Health Organization, 2001). Even the 500 000 people estimated to need some form of psychological support after the attack in New York on September 11, 2001 exceeded the service capacity, despite the fact that New York has the highest density of mental health professionals in the world (Herman & Susser, 2003). India, which has suffered from several typhoons and ethnic-religious clashes over the past years, has an estimated 4000 psychiatrists, representing a ratio of approximately 1 psychiatrist for 250 000 people (World Health Organization, 2001). This rate varies hugely between urban and rural areas, and between more developed and less developed states. Thus, in some states the ratio falls to one psychiatrist for more than one million people. The number of other mental health professionals, such as psychologists or psychiatric nurses, is even lower: there is 1 nurse for every 10 psychiatrists and 1 psychologist for every 20 (Patel & Saxena, 2003). With the exception of Singapore, other southeast Asian countries such as Birma, Thailand, Cambodia, Vietnam or Indonesia show a similarly bleak picture. In Africa, conflict and disaster-ridden countries such as Angola, Burundi, Eritrea, Guinea Bissau, Mozambique, Sierra Leone, Somalia and Rwanda have one indigenous psychiatrist, who may even work outside the mental health sector. The availability of psychologists and psychiatric nurses is hardly any better. If available, the majority of psychiatrists and psychologists work in urban areas and do not have access to survivors who in general reside in more peripheral areas. Government expenditure on mental health is extremely low. Whereas the burden of neuropsychiatric disorder is estimated to be 13%, most countries spend about 2% of their health budget on mental health. National mental health plans are an exception rather than a rule and sometimes rather paper tigers demanded by donors or UN agencies. Within this context of disinterest in mental health, local professionals cannot sustain themselves by designing and implementing a public mental health policy. Therefore, they are often obliged to survive in the private sector where a substantial proportion of health care is delivered; some estimates put this at 50% to 75% of all health consultations in countries such as Afghanistan or India (Patel & Saxena, 2003). Psychiatric hospitals put an additional strain on the limited available mental health capacity. Most hospitals are decayed and outdated remnants of the colonial past, and often the quality of care has been found to violate basic human rights (de Jong, 2001; National Human Rights Commission, 1999). Salaries are minimal and even before disaster strikes, many mental health professionals have left their country. For example, war- and tsunami-affected Sri Lanka has 28 psychiatrists, with approximately tenfold that number residing in the UK and 20-fold in the United States. To compound the human resource problem, complex emergencies, insecurity, genocide and terrorism may cause an exodus or even the extermination of intellectuals. The persecution of intellectuals by government, rebel or terrorist groups may become the final blow to the mental health infrastructure as shown in countries such as Algeria, Cambodia, Indonesia, Mozambique or Rwanda. Therefore, as the boxes in this chapter show, human resource capacity building is one of the major tasks of mental health professionals in the NGO and the government sector.

Box 4: Working through a local NGO in Sri Lanka: a difficult start

After 10 years of experience as a psychiatrist in Holland and finishing a Masters in Public Health I got a position with a local NGO in Jaffna, Sri Lanka. The job is an interesting mix of training, supervision in counseling and clinical work, management support, development of community mental health programs and possibly some research.

September 2003 I visited Jaffna for an assessment. Unfortunately it then still took another year and a half before our proposal was approved. Shortly before my departure I was informed that in the mean time two Volunteer Service Overseas (VSO) staff had joined the organization: a social worker with management experience and a clinical psychologist. December 2004 I was ready to go, but my flight was delayed at the last minute because of a visa problem. Two days later the Sri Lankan coastline was devastated by Tsunami and at once my delay felt like a narrow escape.

The NGO Shantiham I work with was established in 1987 to provide psychological help for victims of torture. Over the years the organization has shown tremendous power to survive bombing, shelling, a continuous brain drain, personal threats and displacements. By now it has developed into a training centre for counselors and psychosocial trainers in community mental health. It is a nonreligious NGO, but the present management is formed by dedicated Hindus and is a strongly hierarchical structure following principles that are not always easy to comprehend for an outsider. After Tsunami the NGO was actively involved in providing Psychological First Aid for the affected people. Demands poured in to give training in basic psychosocial principles and trauma reactions to local workers of different national and international NGOs. The available psychosocial trainers and counselors worked nonstop. The two psychiatrists provided supervision, and were involved in organizational issues and handling the many offers of help. Foreign experts and consultants started streaming in, for a short visit to the coast often followed by some training on PTSD and grief.

It is at this stage that I arrive. In the first two months I hardly see my two Sri Lankan colleagues due to their overload of work. For my information I am referred to the two VSO staff. By the end of the first month I have a brief meeting with my main Sri Lankan counterpart. I try to explain what my expectations and ideas are, but we have only 10 min and it will take another month before I meet him again. I use this time to familiarize myself with the organization, the existing mental health facilities and other local NGOs. I get involved in organizing a training for counselors. I discuss the possibility of taking over clinical work to set my Sri Lankan colleagues free for other activities, but there is no money for a translator. I try to write proposals for the offers that are pouring in, but the information I get is too fragmented to make any progress. Computer and email facilities are poor and often failing. Staff of the organization are getting exhausted by the overload of work. Meetings are very much ad hoc and internal communication is poor. Amidst this chaos I try to find myself a position. My presence at management meetings is discussed and agreed upon, which will help me to build up more of a relationship with the management. However, in practice, meetings take place and I am never informed. After confronting the management they promise to inform me next time, but they keep "forgetting." I try to arrange a visit to the Tsunami-hit areas: but again, the car just left or they went yesterday. I express my interest in assisting in their efforts to set up new community mental health programs, but again I am passively being kept out.

The implicit message seems to be: first we need to get to know you, before we let you in. It is difficult to grasp the fact that here I am, an experienced professional, in a post-Tsunami country crying out for psychiatrists, and there is hardly any work I can put my hands on.

After 20 years of civil war the Tamil society in the North East of Sri Lanka is showing features of collective trauma. My Sri Lankan colleague listed these features as mistrust and suspicion, conspiracy of silence, deterioration in morals and values, poor leadership, dependency and superficial, short-term goals. I start realizing that, being part of this society, my NGO has taken on many of these features. Apart from the different Asian communication pattern, where true relationships are often more important than truth, I see myself facing a wall of mistrust, disinterest and ad hoc decision making. I have to win the trust of my two Sri Lankan counterparts, who, due to the hierarchical structure, are the key to any activity. However, they are hardly available for any discussion and, if they are, they often say yes, but rarely follow things up. Also, there are differences of opinion between my two counterparts and because I hardly ever manage to see them together I am stuck in the middle.

I am now six months down the line and finally got a budget for a translator, which gives me a voice, ears and some independence. I can now take up the challenge to overcome the suspicion of my colleagues, making it clear that I came as a friend to assist them, not as an intruder intending to take over control of their NGO.

Marianne van der Veen, Psychiatrist/MPH Association for Health and Counseling, Jaffna, Sri Lanka

---

Box 5: Riots in Jalalabad, Afghanistan

On May 10, 2005, Jalalabad, a provincial capital in Eastern Afghanistan, was the scene of violent eruptions of anti-Western sentiments. HNI-TPO has been present in Afghanistan since 1994.

At the shrine of Mialisaheb in Samarkhel village I introduce two visiting psychologists to the traditional islamic healers who take care of the schizophrenic patients in this sanctuary. It is around 9.30 in the morning. We are waiting for the healer to make us a protective amulet with Koranic verses (one never knows) when my satellite phone rings. It's Munir, our Afghan office manager. He sounds worried. There is trouble in the city. Thousands of people demonstrate against the alleged desecration of the Quran at the American detention center in Guantanamo Bay. The village mullah offers us refuge, while the office sends us an old rented car to pick us up. It is better to keep a low profile and not to travel with an NGO car in this sitation.

At the outskirts of Jalalabad we get stuck in an exodus of hundreds of cars and rikshaws trying to escape the city. I see thick black smoke above the city. When we hear shooting nearby we seek refuge in the house of Roghman, an Afghan doctor who works with HNI-TPO. Without questioning we are led inside the visitors' room and supplied with cake and green tea. At least for this moment we are safe within the thick walls of this old family house. Outside are the sounds of more gunshots. The incoming phone calls inform us about yet other offices of UN organizations and INGOs that are set aflame. My colleagues come from the guest house to tell me that they are safe too.

When it seems to get quiet again in the afternoon we slip into the car and drive to our house. On the streets we see the remains of burned tires and broken windows, but the angry crowds have dispersed. At home we meet with our colleagues and share the stories of today. We are in continuous contact with our head offices in Kabul and Amsterdam who have arranged for evacuation.

Late afternoon we depart for the airstrip. Expatriates from other organizations tell us that they have lost all their properties. We realize how lucky we have been. When the first rumors of the riots reached the office our staff took all signboards down and removed the dish-antenna from the roof. The hundreds of men who filled the street in front of our office were told by neighbors that there was no NGO here. They proceeded to the nearby UNICEF office which was badly damaged. We are relieved when it is our turn to enter one of the eight-seat planes which shuttle between Kabul and Jalalabad.

After a short flight we reach Kabul and inform family, head office, and embassies about our safe arrival. BBC World and CNN show images of familiar streets in Jalalabad filled with exalted crowds. How could this have happened? HNI-TPO supports a network of more than 20 clinics and hospitals in the province. I never felt unsafe in Jalalabad, and did not notice that people objected to the health and psychosocial work that we did. The Afghans I speak with are ashamed about what happened. They say that the people are stirred up by anti-government elements. It shows me once more how working in Afghanistan is like walking on a tight rope.

Peter Ventevogel, psychiatrist, Previous Coordinator Mental Health Program HealthNet-TPO, Jalalabad, Afghanistan

Handling the complementarity between allopathic "western" and local healing methods

In view of this scarcity of mental health professionals, local populations use health services that are outside the purview and understanding of the dominant medical system. Complementary and traditional medical services are juxtaposed to conventional treatments. Almost half of the populations in many industrialized countries regularly use some form of T (traditional medicine) and CAM (complementary and alternative medicine).[1] Scotton & Batista (1996) assert that "70%–80% of the American public is so dissatisfied with the limited scientific model of current medical practice that they have used alternative healing practices within the last year." There also exists considerable use in low-income countries, ranging from 40% in China to 80% in African countries (World Health Organization, 2002a). Thus, a vast informal healthcare sector exists in all countries, and no comprehensive picture of this sector exists as yet in any country (Bodeker, 2000). In view of the above-mentioned scarcity of mental health professionals, healers provide an important contribution to psychosocial care. From a public health perspective traditional healers often have the advantage that they are easily accessible from a cultural and geographic point of view. For example, in Ghana 1% of the population is engaged as a healer or a shrine-holder. Among the Yoruba in Nigeria, healers form 10% of the adult population in rural areas, and about 4% in urban areas (Ademuwagun, 1979). In Guinea-Bissau there is 1 healer for 475 inhabitants, and in the Philippines and Mozambique there is 1 healer for every 200 people (de Jong, 1987; Northridge, 2002; Tan, 1985). Traditional healers are culturally and linguistically similar to their clients, share the cosmology of their clients, and generally have a holistic approach to healing especially useful to conflict-affected populations who may suffer a variety of traumatic impacts and symptoms, including emotional, psychological, physical/somatic, social and spiritual ones. Many healers work part-time as a healer while continuing their work in the communities to which they belong.

While more than a thousand quantitative studies on the outcome of psychotherapy have been carried out, there exist only a few studies that purport to evaluate the treatment effects of traditional healing. In comparison with accepted minimum standards of psychotherapy evaluation (Lambert *et al.*, 1998) one can be very critical about the methodology used for the evaluation of healing. Cross-cultural differences exist in disease expression, help-seeking behavior, and the aims of healing practices and treatment. Standardized instruments are useful for evaluating outcomes in relation to standard psychosocial interventions, but they may not encompass local constructions of mental distress, reasons for seeking traditional healing, or definitions of successful treatment, which may be grounded in spiritual cosmologies (Patel *et al.*, 2005). Despite these methodological shortcomings, several scholars found interesting results among healers. For example, Crapanzano's qualitative study (1973) attributes the greatest success to a Moroccan possession cult in psychosomatic and hysterical cases. Finkler (1985) in her study in Mexico concludes that healing attenuates symptoms associated with generalized anxiety or (pain associated with) depression in about 25% of patients. Kleinman's (1980) figures on Taiwan suggest a maximum positive treatment outcome for half of neurotic patients. (However, neither Finkler nor Kleinman provides clear figures about treatment effects for specific categories of patients.) In a later study in Taiwan, Kleinman and Gale (1982) compared a group of patients treated by shamans with patients treated by physicians. More than three-quarters of all patients improved. Regarding the effect of healing in the prevention and treatment of alcohol and drug abuse, Jilek (1994) cites a study that found 1-year post-therapy abstinence rates among opiate addicts ranging from 8% to 35% in the clientele of different healers. A 1-year follow-up study on Naikan therapy among alcohol addicts in Japan found that 49% were abstinent after 1 year (Takemoto *et al.*, 1979). It was found that 44%

of chronic alcoholics treated by *curanderos* in Peru had post-therapy abstinence periods of over 6 years (Jilek, 1994). Alcohol abstinence after joining a healing church in Malawi was 2.8 years (Peltzer, 1987).

Compared to allopathic mental health professionals, there apparently exists a high density of healers around the globe. These healers are often the main source of help for local populations. Despite the methodological flaws in outcome studies among these local practitioners, the results of their treatment are not largely discrepant with the results of western therapies, especially in the domain of substance abuse. Mental health workers have to be able to accept the complementarity of the "modern" and the "traditional" healing sectors. They should preferably understand the rationale of some form of collaboration. Convulsions are a domain that may provide an example of collaboration or mutual referral between the allopathic and the local healing sectors. In crisis situations in low-income countries one often sees the classical dissociative phenomena described by Janet or Freud during their time in the Salpêtrière in Paris. In situations of massive stress, a number of people show symptoms of dissociation varying from individual possession as an "idiom of distress" to classical fugue states and epidemics of medically unexplained or mass psychogenic illness with or without psychogenic fits (de Jong, 1987; Van Duijl *et al.*, 2005; Van Ommeren *et al.*, 2001). While setting up services, one has to consider which healthcare sector is best equipped to deal with the high prevalence of all kinds of convulsions, whether neurologic and/or dissociative in origin. Epilepsy has a high prevalence in many low-income countries and, due to a lack of neurological services, is often dealt with by psychiatry. In some areas of Africa and Asia, the prevalence of epilepsy is as high as 3.7%–4.9% and it is often presented to psychiatric and primary healthcare services during or after the help-seeking trajectory through the traditional healing sector (Adamolekum, 1995; de Jong, 1987). Offering treatment to those with epilepsy is a feasible option. A total of 95% of a sample of West African patients with generalized epileptic convulsions were correctly diagnosed and treated with phenobarbital by primary healthcare workers who received a couple of hours of training; the average seizure frequency decreased from 16 to 0.34 per month in Guinea-Bissau, from 5.33 to 0.22 in Burundi, and from 5.8 to 0.55 in Cambodia (de Jong, 1996, 2004). Dealing with the equally highly prevalent dissociative states, however, often requires sophisticated and psychotherapeutic skills, which – as we have seen – are often not available. In many cultures, adequate management for both groups implies triage of the epileptic patients and referral of those with dissociative states to the local healers, healing churches or possession cults who often are able to deal adequately with various dissociative states in a few individual or group sessions.

To conclude the previous paragraphs, the mental health professional that aspires to get involved in crisis work has to be able to function in a complex sociocultural political context. The large numbers of people with mental health problems after crises surpass the capacities of existing allopathic mental health services. These services are concentrated in urban centers, often provide outdated asylary care, and tend to occupy the scarce human resources that are available. The shortage of human resources is compounded by the geographic distribution of survivors who often reside in peripheral areas that are not covered by modern mental health services. Survivors have recourse to omnipresent local healers whose healing idioms fit with the survivors' idioms of distress and their spiritual cosmology. For the mental health professional this has several consequences. (S)he has to accept to somehow get involved in rehabilitating and deinstitutionalizing old-fashioned asylary care while straddling the development of a public mental program for disaster survivors. (S)he also has to accept that healers provide an important source of help and are part and parcel of coping styles developed in the local culture. This requires a modest attitude, even though in some domains healers may indeed do harm – like the possible transmission of HIV through scarifications (de Jong, 2001; Hiegel, 1996). It also implies some form of

collaboration with healers, for example by mutual referrals.

Taking specific characteristics of the survivors into account

In developing services for survivors one has to realize that survivors often belong to a different ethnic or socioeconomic group from those who seek to offer help.

They express their plight in a specific discourse and use a variety of explanatory models. Modern mental health services, even if they are community oriented, tend to exclude specific groups. There are several reasons for this. First, many mental health professionals are not adequately trained to deal with people who have suffered from chronic consequential traumatic stressors. Second, apart from the common stigma of mental disorder, many survivors are prejudiced due to attitudes or taboos in the local culture to seek help, either in the local or in the allopathic healthcare sector. A third reason is that mental health professionals may lack expertise to deal with certain disaster-related problems. An example of a cultural taboo that professionals may find difficult to address is the unspeakable trauma of rape. According to our experience rape sometimes can be mitigated by addressing key figures or with the help of rituals in an African context, but it may be extremely hard to address in for example Asia or the Balkans. Mental health professionals may be reticent to address the issue because they share cultural (counter) transference issues, because they feel a lack of expertise, or because they consider exposure techniques to be culturally inappropriate for such a traumatic event. Another cultural taboo is dealing with perpetrators instead of victims, even though in countries such as Burundi, Cambodia or Rwanda it is hard to differentiate between victims or perpetrators because these roles have often interchanged over time. Another example of a psychosocial problem where our profession lacks expertise in providing (short) treatment is family violence, which has an estimated prevalence of 60%–90% in countries such as Afghanistan or Pakistan.

A fourth reason why some groups are excluded from care is that many survivors are too poor to pay for services or too afraid to travel to access services, for example in countries such as Nepal or Palestine where survivors feel intimidated at road blocks. A fifth reason is that many survivors do not trust or understand the rationale of modern psychosocial or mental health support. As mentioned before, traditional services may offer support to survivors but do not always break through social stigmas, and can be expensive, although within the local cultural context that is an exception rather than a rule. The sixth reason why certain types of problems tend to be excluded from care is the lack of professionals in specialized areas of psychiatry or psychology. Except from a few academic centers in some LIMA countries, the numbers of specialists in the fields of child psychiatry, substance misuse, gerontology, sexuology, or forensic psychiatry are extremely limited. The same applies to local research capacity. A seventh rather logistic and often temporary reason why certain categories of patients are excluded is a lack of consistent availability of drugs, even if they are produced or imported at low costs.

These considerations have consequences for mental health professionals who prepare themselves to get involved in postdisaster work. Most importantly, the mental health professional should develop expertise in cultural psychiatry and psychology and be able to work with explanatory models (Kleinman, 1980). (S)he should be able to apply the explanatory model concept in four ways: (1) to specify semantic networks linking the experience of patients, healers, and other concerned parties; (2) to refer to perceived causes of illness; (3) to look at the "cognitive distance" between patients and practitioners, including allopathic services (Weiss, 2001); and (4) to integrate the explanatory models – both at a population level and at an individual level – into designing an intervention program. In addition, the mental health professional needs to develop expertise in developing services for highly vulnerable groups. Finally, a mental health professional working in these settings must realize that (s)he needs generic expertise in most subspecializations. In postdisaster and postconflict settings comprehensive textbooks of psychiatry, psychotherapy, traumatic stress syndromes, public health, methodology and statistics are important assets.

Box 6: Research capacity building in Burundi, Sudan, Sri Lanka, and Indonesia

I am coordinating a research project on the efficacy of a school-based psychosocial intervention for children affected by armed conflict in four countries (Burundi, Sudan, Sri Lanka, and Indonesia). Following the philosophy of HealthNet-TPO, my focus in this research project has been on capacity building; to train and support research teams in local partner organizations to independently implement research activities. The study consists of a qualitative pre-phase followed by a randomized controlled trial (RCT).

What follows is an account of excerpts of days within a 1-month qualitative research training program, for the research teams in Sri Lanka, Indonesia, and Burundi. In this qualitative pre-phase we are: (1) assessing the public mental health relevance of a psychosocial approach, (2) getting to know context-specific thinking on child development, conflict, and child mental health, and (3) preparing the RCT, through ethnographic techniques. Each day portrayed is preceded by a small background description of the setting and our partner organization.

Sri Lanka

The Tsunami of December 25, 2004 resulted in immense loss of life and destruction of infrastructure. It also reminded the world of an ethnic conflict between Hindu Tamils and Buddhist Sinhalese since 1983. Most Tsunami-affected areas were also conflict-affected areas and many internally displaced people have to face the recurrence of intense loss and fear on top of their involvement in a long history of war. Our long-term partner organization in the North of Sri Lanka, Shantiham, has been providing mental health services, since the start of the conflict, through a community-based approach.

Wednesday June 1: Sri Lankan Training Program – Day 5

It is already a hot day, when I leave my hotel at eight o'clock in the morning. A short bicycle ride reminds me that the city of Jaffna has been at the center of indiscriminate shelling campaigns by the army.

Today we will practice the methodology of *Focus Group Discussions* that we discussed yesterday. A team member volunteers to facilitate and chooses her own topic; "gender inequality in the Jaffna peninsula." A lively discussion follows, in which my translator forgets that he should not participate, but only translate. We appear to have a mixed group of people, with opinions falling in between the extremes of "I would like my wife to be a simple woman. If she works she would disgrace my position as a caretaker," and "We have to emancipate our women! There is too much inequality and suppression." One of the female participants hesitates initially, but eventually joins the discussion. It is this team member who later stops her employment with us, because a very good "proposal" (invitation for an arranged marriage) has come in and her new husband does not like her to work.

After several more practice rounds on different topics, with different facilitators, the working day ends. I decide to go for some running in the Jaffna Stadium, not far from the hotel. The sun sets beautifully over the barbed-wired seaside, and in the center of the running track children are playing soccer.

Indonesia

Our partner organization in Indonesia, Church World Service (CWS), has been present in the country since 1964 providing mainly relief services to vulnerable populations. The Tsunami of December 25 has had the most severe effects in Aceh, a conflict-affected province where CWS is active. The psychosocial intervention for children on which research will take place, however, will be another of CWS' working areas: the islands of Sulawesi. Central Sulawesi has been suffering the effects of a religious conflict between Christians and Muslims since the fall of Suharto in 1998, which has killed 1 000 and displaced about a 100 000 people. Even though there has been a peace deal since 2002, tensions have not subsided, partly because some parties appear to be profiting from the instability in a region rich in resources (cacao, wood).

Monday July 25: Indonesian Training Program – Day 12

Today we have planned the first of several *Community Meetings* to introduce the project and to ask permission for our field research activities. After a one and a half hour scenic drive we reach a village with an impressive church on a hilltop overlooking a monotonous collection of houses painted in Indonesia's national colors. Only later I learn that these houses have been rebuilt for the third time after the village had been completely burnt down twice.

After talking with one of the community leaders during a quick tour of the surroundings, we proceed to the open air community space designated for communal festivities, e.g., the traditional *Dero* dancing for which Central Sulawesi is well known. Here we meet the village headmaster, a teacher, the priest, a midwife, and a group of around 20 farmers, both men and women. They listen intently to our presentations and are happy to provide information and suggestions. The priest thinks it would be good for their homogenous Christian community to have more contact with the Muslim community, in order to facilitate reconciliation and to avoid further bloodshed and damage.

Burundi

Burundi is full of hope after the installation of the first elected president since the massacres of 1993. The head of the biggest former Hutu rebel group is leading a carefully balanced mixed Hutu–Tutsi government. His government's main tasks will be to engage the only rebel group that continues the guerilla warfare (the National Liberation forces or FNL) into peace negotiations and to target the all-pervasive poverty in this East-African nation. HealthNet-TPO Burundi started in 1999 and provides community-based psychosocial and psychiatric services for the population in 11 of Burundi's 16 provinces.

Thursday September 8: Burundian Training Program – Day 17

I start the day with breakfast in an internet café in the capital Bujumbura, which is crowded with United Nations' vehicles and soldiers. On the program for today is a visit to two of our four field researchers who have been practising Key Informant Interviews. We drive north of the capital to Bubanza, into the plains in which the FNL are present. A colleague points out the window and cautiously mentions that "there used to be villages from here to the airport in Bujumbura. People living here were killed during the 1993 massacre or were driven away."

The experience of the field researchers has been interesting. They have met with a nun working in an orphanage, the director of a vocational school, and a guardian in a center for war-affected, orphaned or separated children. We discuss amongst others that it has been difficult to gain trust with the Key Informants in such a short time, and that, to be able to flexibly adapt questions to different Key Informants, it is important to intimately know and practise the interview.

On the way back to Bujumbura the road is crowded with people on bicycles, some of them carrying big white food aid bags. We stop for food at a market place of a small town, and are quickly surrounded by curious children, some daring to touch my white skin. One of them asks a colleague: "Where did you find a human being like that?" (Wietse A. Tol, CTP Research Coordinator, HealthNet TPO, Ph.D. Candidate, VU Amsterdam)

REFERENCES

Adamolekum, B. (1995). The aetiologies of epilepsy in tropical Africa. *Tropical and Geographical Medicine*, **47**, 115–117.

Ademuwagun, Z.A. (eds.) (1979). *African Therapeutic Systems*. Waltham, Mass.: Crossroads Press.

Banerji, D. (1984). Primary health care: selective or comprehensive? *World Health Forum*, **5**, 312–315.

Bemak, F., Chung, R. & Borneman, T. (1996). Counseling and psychotherapy with refugees. In *Counselling Across Cultures*, 4th edn., eds. P.B. Pedersen, J.G. Draguns, W.J. Lonner & J.E. Trimble. Thousand Oaks, Calif.: Sage.

Berren, M.R., Beigel, A. & Ghertner, S. (1980). A typology for the classification of disasters. *Community Mental Health journal*, **16**, 103–111.

Bodeker, G. (2000) Planning for cost-effective traditional health services. In: *Traditional Medicine Better Science*. Proceedings of a WHO International Symposium, 11–13 September, Kobe, Japan. WHO: Kobe Centre.

Boehnlein, J.K. (1987). Clinical relevance of grief and mourning among Cambodian refugees. *Social Science and Medicine*, **25**, 765–772.

Carnegie Commission on Preventing Deadly Conflict. (1997). *Preventing Deadly Conflict: Final Report*. New York: Carnegie Corporation.

Clifford, T. (1990). *Tibetan Buddhist Medicine and Psychiatry*. York Beach, Me.: Weiser.

Corradi, J., Weiss Fagen, P. & Garreton, M. (1992). *Fear at the Edge: State Terror and Resistance in Latin America*. Berkeley, Calif.: University of California Press.

Crapanzano, V. (1973). *The Hamadsha*. London: University of California Press.

De Girolamo, G. & McFarlane, A.C. (1996). The epidemiology of PTSD: a comprehensive overview of the international literature. In *Ethnocultural Aspects of Posttraumatic Stress Disorder*, eds. A.J. Marsella, M.J. Friedman, E.T. Gerrity & R.M. Scurfield. Washington, D.C.: American Psychological Association.

de Jong, J.T.V.M. (1987). *A Descent into African Psychiatry*. Amsterdam: Royal Tropical Institute.

de Jong, J.T.V.M. (1996). A comprehensive public mental health programme in Guinea-Bissau: a useful model for African, Asian and Latin-American countries. *Psychological Medicine*, **26**, 97–108.

de Jong, J.T.V.M. (2001). Remnants of the colonial past: the difference in outcome of mental disorders in high- and low-income countries. *In Colonialism and Mental Health*, eds. D. Bhugra & R. Littlewood. New Delhi: Oxford University Press.

de Jong, J.T.V.M. (2002). Public mental health, traumatic stress and human rights violations in low-income countries: a culturally appropriate model in times of conflict, disaster and peace. In *Trauma, War and Violence: Public Mental Health in Sociocultural Context*, ed. J.T.V.M. de Jong. New York: Plenum-Kluwer.

de Jong, J.T.V.M. (2004). Public mental health and culture: disasters as a challenge to western mental health care models, the self, and PTSD. In *Broken Spirits: The Treatment of Asylum Seekers and Refugees with PTSD*, eds. J.P. Wilson & B. Drozdek. New York: Brunner/Routledge Press.

Epstein, M. (1995). *Thoughts Without a Thinker*. New York: Harper Collins/Basic Books.

Finkler, K. (1985). *Spiritualist Healers in Mexico*. New York: Praeger.

Hamburg, D.A., George, A. & Ballentine, K. (1999). Preventing deadly conflict: the critical role of leadership. *Archives of General Psychiatry*, **56**, 971–976.

Herman, D.B. & Susser, E.S. (2003). The World Trade Center attack: mental health needs and treatment implications. *International Psychiatry*, **1**, 2–5.

Hiegel, J.P. (1996). Traditional medicine and traditional healers. In *Mental Health of Refugees*, eds. J.T.V.M. de Jong & L. Clark. Geneva: WHO and UNHCR. Available at: http://whqlibdoc.who.int/hq/1996/a49374.pdf.

Hinton, D.E., Pham, T., Tran, M. et al. (2004). CBT for Vietnamese refugees with treatment-resistant PTSD and panic attacks: a pilot study. *Journal of Traumatic Stress*, **17**, 429–433.

IFRC (1999). *World Disasters Report 1999*. Geneva: International Federation of Red Cross and Red Crescent Societies.

Jilek, W.G. (1994). Traditional healing in the prevention and treatment of alcohol and drug abuse. *Transcultural Psychiatric Research Review*, **31**, 219–258.

Jordans, M.J.D., Sharma, B., Tol, W.A. & Van Ommeren, M. (2002). Training of psychosocial counselors in a non-Western context: the CVICT approach. In *Creating a Healing Environment: Psycho-social Rehabilitation and Occupational Integration of Child Survivors of Trafficking and Other Worst Forms of Child Labor*, ed. J. Fredericks. Geneva: United Nations International Labour Organization.

Jordans, M.J.D., Tol, W.A., Sharma, B. & Van Ommeren, M. (2003). Training psychosocial counseling in Nepal: content review of a specialized training program. *Intervention: International Journal of Mental health, Psychosocial Work and Counseling in Areas of Armed Conflict*, **1**, 18–35.

Kabat-Zinn, J. (2003). Mindfulness-based stress reduction (MBSR). Constructivism in the human. *Sciences*, **8**, 73–83.

Kleinman, A. M. (1980). *Patients and Healers in the Context of Culture*. Berkeley, Calif.: University of California Press.

Kleinman, A.M. & Gale, J.L. (1982). Patients treated by physicians and folk healers: a comparative outcome study in Taiwan. *Culture Medicine and Psychiatry*, **6**, 405–420.

Lambert, W., Salzer, M.S. & Bickman, L. (1998). Clinical outcome, consumer satisfaction, and ad hoc ratings of improvement. *Journal of Consulting and Clinical Psychology*, **66**, 270–279.

Lanjouw, S., Macrae, J. & Zwi, A. (1999). Rehabilitating health services in Cambodia: the challenge of coordination in chronic political emergencies. *Health Policy and Planning*, **14**, 229–242.

Lechat, M.F. (1990). The epidemiology of health effects of disasters. *Epidemiologic Reviews*, **12**, 192–198.

Linehan, M.M. (1993). *Cognitive-Behavioral Treatment of Borderline Personality Disorder*. New York: Guilford Press.

Messer, S.B. (2002). Empirically supported treatments: cautionary notes. *Medscape General Medicine*, **4**, 13.

Msuya, J. (2003). *Horizontal and Vertical Delivery of Health Services: What Are The Trade Offs?* Washington, D.C.: World Bank.

National Human Rights Commission (1999). *Quality Assurance in Mental Health*. New Delhi: NHRC.

Noji, E. K. (1997). *The Public Health Consequences of Disasters*. New York: Oxford University Press.

Northridge, M. E. (2002). Integrating ethnomedicine into public health. *American Journal of Public Health*, **92**, 1581.

Otto, M.W., Hinton, D., Korbly, N. B. *et al.* (2003). Treatment of pharmacotherapy-refractory posttraumatic stress disorder among Cambodian refugees: a pilot study of combination treatment with cognitive-behavior therapy vs. sertraline alone. *Behaviour Research and Therapy*, **41**, 1271–1276.

Patel, V. & Saxena, S. (2003). Psychiatry in India. *International Psychiatry*, **1**, 16–19.

Patel, V., Kirkwood, B., Weiss, H. *et al.* (2005). Chronic fatigue in developing countries: a population survey of women in India. *British Medical Journal*, **330**, 1190–1193.

Peltzer, K. (1987). *Some Contributions of Traditional Healing Practices Towards Psychosocial Health Care in Malawi*. Eschborn: Fachbuchhandlung fur Psychologie.

Quarantelli, E. (1994). *Future Disaster Trends and Policy Implications for Developing Countries*. Newark, Del.: Disaster Research Center.

Rifkin, S.B. & Walt, G. (1986). Why health improves: defining the issues concerning "comprehensive primary health care" and "selective primary health care". *Social Science Medicine*, **23**, 559–566.

Salama, P., Spiegel, P., Talley, L. & Waldman R. (2004). Lessons learned from complex emergencies over past decade. *Lancet*, **364**, 1801–1813.

Salimovich, S., Lira, E. & Weinstein, E. (1992). Victims of fear: the social psychology of repression. In *Fear at the Edge: State Terror and Resistance in Latin America*, eds. J. Corradi, P. Weiss Fagen & M. Garreton. Berkeley, Calif.: University of California Press.

Schreuder, B. & Kostermans, C. (2001). Global health strategies versus local primary health care priorities – a case study of national immunization days in Southern Africa. *South African Medical Journal*, **91**, 249–254.

Scotton, B. W. & Batista, J. R. (1996). *Textbook of Transpersonal Psychiatry and Psychology*. New York: Basic Books.

Silver, S. M. & Wilson, J. (1988). *Native American Healing and Purification Rituals for War Stress*. New York: Brunner/Mazel.

Strupp, H. H. (2001). Implications of the empirically supported treatment movement for psychoanalysis. *Psychoanalytic Dialogues*, **11**, 605–619.

Tan, M. L. (1985). Current state of research on traditional medicine in the Philippines. Research report no 2. AKAP research.

Teasdale, J.D. (1997). The transformation of meaning: the interactive cognitive subsystems approach. In *The Transformation of Meaning in Psychological Therapies: Integrating Theory and Practice*, eds. M. Power & C. R., Brewin. New York: Wiley.

Van Duijl, M., Cardeña, E. & de Jong, J. T. V. M. (2005). The validity of DSM-IV dissociative disorders categories in South-West Uganda. *Transcultural Psychiatry*, **6**, 219–241.

Van der Hart, O. (1983). *Rituals in Psychotherapy: Transition and Continuity*. New York: Irvington.

Van der Hart, O. (1988). *Coping with Loss: The Therapeutic Use of Leave-Taking Rituals*. New York: Irvington.

Van Ommeren, M., Sharma, B., Komproe, I. *et al.* (2001). Trauma and loss as determinants of medically unexplained epidemic illness in a Bhutanese refugee camp. *Psychological Medicine*, **31**, 1259–1267.

Watts, A.W. (1969). *Psychotherapy East and West*. New York: Ballantine Books.

Weiss, M.G. (2001). Cultural epidemiology: an introduction and overview. *Anthropology and Medicine*, **8**, 1–29.

World Health Organization (1978). *Primary Health Care: Report of the International Conference on Primary Health Care, Alma-Ata*. Health for All Series: number 1. Geneva: World Health Organization.

World Health Organization (2001). *Atlas Country Profiles of Mental Health Resources*. Geneva: World Health Organization. See http://mh-atlas.ic.gc.ca/

World Health Organization (2002a). Traditional medicine strategy 2002–2005. Available at: http//:www.who.int/medicines/organization/trm/orgtrmmain.shtml.

World Health Organization (2002b). *World Report on Violence and Health*. Geneva: World Health Organization.

NOTE

1 The term "traditional medicine" is used here to denote the indigenous health traditions of the world; "complementary and alternative medicine" primarily refers to methods outside the medical mainstream, particularly in industrialized countries; and "conventional medicine" refers to "biomedicine" or "modern medicine" (see *American Journal of Public Health*, October 2002).

PART IV

Special topics

11

Traumatic death in terrorism and disasters

Robert J. Ursano, James E. McCarroll, & Carol S. Fullerton

Terrorism and disasters are not infrequent occurrences in the present-day world. Common to these events is the likelihood of violent death and the presence of human remains – burned, dismembered, mutilated, or relatively intact.[1] Exposure to mass death as well as individual dead bodies is a disturbing and sometimes frightening event. The handling of the remains of the dead following combat, natural disasters, disasters of human origin, and terrorism, accidents, and other forms of traumatic death is known to cause distress. The nature of the stress of exposure to traumatic death and the dead and its relationship to post-traumatic stress disorder (PTSD) and other post-traumatic psychiatric illnesses is not well understood (Breslau & Davis, 1987; Lindy et al., 1987; Rundell et al., 1989; Ursano, 1987; Ursano & McCarroll, 1990).

The tasks of body recovery, identification, transport, and burial may require prolonged as well as acute contact with mass death. Recent research has shown that victims, onlookers, and rescue workers are traumatized by the experience or expectation of confronting death in disaster situations (Dyregrov et al., 1996; Jones, 1985; Miles et al., 1984; Schwartz, 1984; Taylor & Frazer, 1982). Exposure to abusive violence (Laufer et al., 1984) and to the grotesque (Green et al., 1989) significantly contributes to the development of psychiatric symptoms in war veterans, particularly intrusive imagery (Clohessy & Ehlers, 1999; Laufer et al., 1985; Lifton, 1973).

Initial studies on the effects of handling the dead were observational with few systematic descriptions of the differences that occur at various stages through the process, or group or individual differences in responses. Hersheiser and Quarantelli (1976) reported on how the dead were treated by the living following a flood. They observed increasing respect for the body through the phases of search, recovery, identification, and preparation for burial. About a third of the volunteers who recovered bodies from the Mount Erebus air crash in Antarctica experienced transient problems of moderate to severe intensity at 3 months and one-fifth continued to report high levels of stress-related symptoms (Taylor & Frazer, 1982).

In a survey of 592 US Air Force personnel involved in the recovery, transport, and identification of the bodies of the Jonestown, Guyana, mass suicide, youth, inexperience, lower rank, and greater exposure to the dead were associated with higher levels of emotional distress (Jones, 1985). Higher rates of dysphoria were also found in blacks compared to whites, possibly due to greater identification with the black victims by the black body handlers.

During the past two decades there have been a number of studies of the effects of handling remains on rescue workers recovering remains from the collapse of a hotel skywalk (Miles et al., 1984), police and firefighters (Bryant & Harvey, 1996; Fullerton et al., 1992; Regehr et al., 2000), disaster workers following the collapse of a freeway due to an earthquake

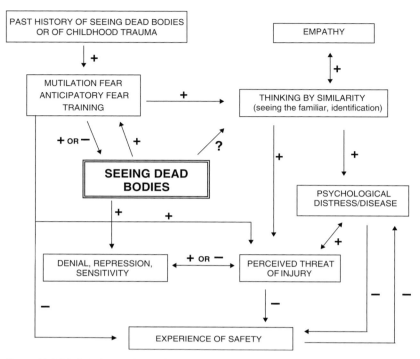

Figure 11.1 Model of cognitive and emotional processing of exposure to death and the dead by disaster workers

(Marmar *et al.*, 1996), ambulance service workers (Clohessy & Ehlers, 1999), divers recovering bodies from an airline disaster (Leffler & Dembert, 1998), and war (McCarroll *et al.*, 1993a, 1995b, 2001, 2002; Sutker *et al.*, 1994). In all these situations there are examples of the fact that regardless of profession or past experience, exposure to violent death can create psychological distress and contribute to psychiatric disorders. Figure 11.1 illustrates the inter-relationship of past experience, psychological, cognitive and environmental influences in disaster workers exposed to the dead.

Traumatic stressors associated with exposure to mass death

In order better to understand the nature of the stress experienced by exposure to traumatic death,

Table 11.1 Stressors in traumatic death

Anticipation of exposure to traumatic death
High levels of sensory stimulation
Types of remains (e.g., children, gruesome, intact)
Degree of exposure
Novelty, surprise, and shock
Personal effects

we compiled data from observations, interviews, and surveys from over 1 000 disaster remains handlers (Cervantes, 1988; Maloney, 1988a, 1988b; McCarroll *et al.*, 1993a, 1993c, 1995b, 1996; Robinson, 1988; Ursano & McCarroll, 1990; Ursano *et al.*, 1992, 1995). Commonly reported stressors associated with traumatic death are listed in Table 11.1. The conditions and events that may mediate or moderate those stressors are presented in Table 11.2.

Table 11.2 Mediators and moderators of stressors in traumatic death

---

Previous experience
Training
Volunteer status
Emotional involvement of the worker with the dead
Good supervision and management practices (food, water, rest breaks, work scheduling)
Outbriefing by supervisors
Knowledge of avenues of referral
Follow-up by supervisors

Anticipation of exposure

Anticipation of exposure to death is itself a potent stressor that can be debilitating and affect performance, behavior, and health. It is an important, but often overlooked, aspect of disaster and rescue work. The stress burden may begin before the actual exposure (McCarroll et al., 1993b, 1995c). The period prior to the exposure to remains provides an opportunity for predisaster training and intervention. Predisaster counseling may be effective in part through its effects on anticipated stress (Myers, 1989). Lower anticipated stress may come from training and previous experience, and result in improved performance and decreased fatigue and risk of adverse psychological effects.

The disaster worker anticipates the stress of upcoming work before it actually begins and may begin work with an already substantial stress burden. Ersland et al. (1989) reported that waiting time was a frequently reported stressor among professional firefighters. Disaster workers may wait minutes to days after notification before they actually begin their rescue work. In interviews of disaster workers, we have heard stories of extended periods of waiting and high levels of stress. For example, novice rescue workers recruited to remove bodies from a plane that had caught fire and burned after landing had to wait several hours while wooden supports were put under the wings of the plane so it would not collapse on them.

The stress of anticipation has important psychological and physiological effects. In a group of military personnel with no previous experience in handling remains, females had a significantly higher level of anticipated stress than males (Arthur, 1987; Mitchell et al., 1958; Susnowski, 1988). However, when experienced men and women were compared, there were no differences in anticipated stress (McCarroll et al., 1993d).

Military physicians who responded to the Pentagon bombing on September 11, 2001 described anticipating their reaction to what they might encounter, a lack of preparation concerning sensory stimuli, a fear of their own reaction to viewing the dead, and anticipation anxiety manifested as impatience and restlessness while riding to the disaster site (Keller & Bobo, 2002).

Sensory stimulation

Profound sensory stimulation is often an extremely bothersome aspect of handling the dead. The handler is assaulted through all the senses. The smell was often noted as the most bothersome aspect of the job, but visual and tactile sensitivity were also reported. One remains handler at Dover Air Force Base was concerned about not being able to "wash the smell away." He wondered if the odor was real or "in my head." Individuals who reported working with the bodies from the Jonestown mass suicide and those who worked with the Marine bodies from the Beirut bombing in 1985 were greatly disturbed by the overwhelming odor of these already decaying bodies. Workers will often try to mask the odor with burning coffee, smoking cigars, working in the cold or using fragrances such as peppermint and orange oil. However, such a strategy can backfire by associating yet another smell with the remains. Often such masking substances are not available and the fragrances can make some people sick. Mouth breathing is almost always effective in limiting the exposure to odors associated with mortuary operations.

The preparation and consumption of food was frequently difficult after exposure to traumatized bodies. Badly burned bodies were reported to look and smell like roast beef. After exposure to burned bodies many individuals, including some members of our research team, avoid eating meat for weeks and months following exposure to the dead. To one body handler, rice in brown gravy looked like maggots. Following the 1989 United plane crash in Sioux City, Iowa, one rescue worker reported that he had lost all sexual interest because he could not look at women's bodies without being reminded of the dead females he had recovered from the site of the crash. Security police guarding the dead at Sioux City felt great discomfort when the wind blew blankets off the dead exposing parts of the bodies.

One emergency medical service worker complained about the way the morgue workers handled the bodies of people she brought in. She was particularly disturbed by the loud sound of the head striking the surface of a hard examining table when a body was thrown onto it.

Other visual and tactile sensations associated with the dead were also reported. Many reported wearing gloves to handle the bodies, even rescue workers who were unlikely to touch bodies. This seemed to serve both a real and an imagined protective role. In some settings, the gloves also became a symbol of being a member of this special group – the body handlers.

Type of remains

Children

Some remains are troublesome to almost all recovery and mortuary workers. Handling or viewing the bodies of children is uniformly stressful regardless of the age or sex of the body handler or whether that individual has children. Children's bodies were reported as difficult because they appeared innocent, or they had "untimely deaths." Other descriptions were: "They were complete victims. They had not yet lived. They had no control over it." Pathologists described increased stress associated with doing autopsies on children.

Natural

Some workers also reported natural looking bodies and those with no apparent cause of death as being disturbing. Bodies that were fully clothed and with no apparent cause of death were described as "eerie."

I would say that it was probably more difficult for me to deal with remains that had a single gunshot wound or single penetration that we knew were going to go home viewable; more so than an air crash where the remains were severely charred or decomposed. I think we key on the face of that person. If there isn't a face or a head, it seemed like the whole focal point of expression was gone. In the case of —, who had a single shrapnel wound to the neck, we knew he was going home, out of the war, because of a little damn piece of metal, a fragment. I think it probably bothered me to see how sensitive life is to foreign objects compared to a hell of a crash or an explosion, which tears you up.

Pine (personal communication, 1988) reported that in cases of the "untouched, but dead, everybody stops." A young woman who had died in a plane crash appeared natural to a recovery worker. However, her feet had been underneath the seat rack and were torn off leaving only two stumps.

Historic

Remains of long-dead service members or other victims of trauma are often recovered through accidental means or through searches based on access to the former battlefield or new information. For example, remains are still being returned from the Pacific theater in World War II and, particularly, from the Vietnam War. The recovery and identification of these remains is generally much less stressful to mortuary workers than those from a recent war or tragedy. The workers who recover such remains usually have a great sense of pride and accomplishment, particularly when the result fills a missing piece in a family's life (Sledge, 2005). The deceased are treated with special care and there is sometimes a sense of awe among the workers as they feel they are privileged in being the first to see a hero after a long rest. Feelings of exhilaration and excitement are often reported when there is a forensic puzzle to be solved. However, responses to historic remains are not uniformly positive. The handling of personal effects of Holocaust victims and survivors has been seen as disturbing, especially to young, inexperienced workers (McCarroll *et al.*, 1995a).

Nonhuman

Even a nonhuman body can produce discomfort. Pine (personal communication, 1988) reported a person who was very distressed at finding a dead pet dog in the luggage compartment of a commuter aircraft crash. The person said that he "could not handle" the dead dog and was distressed because he knew others would not take it seriously.

Commonly encountered and idiosyncratic reactions to remains

Many types of remains are difficult to handle, but the amount of distress associated with them is not uniform. For some, gruesome remains may not resemble a person and may cause less distress than an intact body. Badly burned bodies, bodies that had lain in water for a long time, and decapitated bodies were also vivid in people's memory. Burned bodies have a strong smell and bodies that have been in water will swell and skin will come off, making them difficult to handle physically. Disassociated body parts can also be difficult to handle, particularly hands. In addition to these general categories, which could be considered to be high-risk categories, each person is usually vulnerable to different types of remains. Supervisors should not only be aware of the potential for distress due to the types of bodies that are commonly considered stressful, but also listen for what might trouble the individual that is different from others.

Degree of exposure

The duration (or degree) of exposure to the dead is an important predictor of post-traumatic stress

reactions. When volunteers are assigned to escort a body through the identification process, they are exposed to many more bodies. The sight of so many remains at one time and place increases the level of exposure and contributes to the stress of the experience. Some volunteers, including those who had prior experience with traumatic death in police or emergency service work, described the sight of a large number of remains as "overwhelming." One man reported, "The bodies just kept coming and coming. It felt like you were surrounded." Another said, "It's hard not to look when you are surrounded. You are too tense to be bored."

Two studies involving body handlers longitudinally found significantly higher levels of intrusion and avoidance symptoms at 3–5 months and 13–15 months after the war than in the comparison group (McCarroll *et al.*, 1993a, 1995b). The forensic dentists who identified the remains of the Branch Davidians in Waco, Texas had significantly higher distress, related to the hours of exposure to the remains (McCarroll *et al.*, 1996). Symptomatic distress in emergency service workers was related to the degree of exposure to the traumatic incident, the severity, and type of activities including working with dead bodies (Weiss *et al.*, 1995).

In the only study examining pre and post responses of mortuary workers to handling bodies, intrusion and avoidance symptoms were measured in four groups of workers based on their degree of exposure to the remains (McCarroll *et al.*, 2002). When age, sex, volunteer status, and experience were controlled, postexposure intrusion symptoms increased significantly for all groups exposed to the dead, and avoidance symptoms increased in the two groups with the most exposure. Importantly, even after controlling for symptoms expressed in anticipation of exposure to the dead, exposure itself increased post-traumatic symptoms.

Novelty, surprise, and shock

In addition to the raw, offensive sensory stimulation, surprise, shock and fear of the unexpected are disturbing aspects of handling dead bodies. When we asked a group of experienced military body handlers how they would train a group of inexperienced people to retrieve bodies if they only had a day to do so, we were told, "Tell them the worst. Make it so there are no surprises. Let them know what they are in for."

The surprise and shock of seeing the victim's face when the body bag is opened was described by one subject: "When our soldiers open that bag, they don't know what they are going to see!" Another man who handled bodies in Vietnam recalled that he was always upset when bodies were lying face down in body bags. The back of the head is very strong and usually intact regardless of the condition of the face. He was always frightened of what he might see when he turned the body over. Pathologists at Dover Air Force Base X-rayed the body bags before opening them in order to lessen the initial shock and surprise. They reported that seeing bodies at a crime scene was generally more difficult than seeing the same bodies in a laboratory where the setting was familiar and surprises were unlikely.

The opening of the first body bag at the mortuary after a disaster is nearly always a quiet, anxiety-filled event. One group of inexperienced body handlers during Operation Desert Storm physically moved 15–20 feet away from the body when the bag was opened without anyone having spoken a word. When the body bag was fully open and there were no surprises, they moved closer. One individual described having to recover a child's body for burial. When he initially picked up the body, he was surprised by the way it felt in his arms because it reminded him of recently carrying one of his own children.

Rescuers may consciously avoid coming into contact with a dead body. A police harbor unit diver recalled his first underwater contact with the foot of a body:

I hoped it was just a sneaker … feeling the ankle I thought, "let it be just a boot" … feeling the leg, "please, God, let it just be a wader."

This concern was also expressed by a fireman.

A lot of firemen do not want to recognize a dead infant. One fireman went into a room full of smoke and felt around, touched the dead infant, and said it was a dog.

Personal effects

Among the most difficult jobs for mortuary workers is handling the personal effects of the dead. This is often surprising to inexperienced managers of a temporary mortuary or collection site. It is usually believed that gruesome remains are more disturbing to workers and, as a result, inexperienced persons are sometimes assigned to handle personal effects. In general, regardless of the state of the remains, personal effects have the power to humanize the deceased. They provide a link between the dead and the worker than is often not present until the remains acquires a name or otherwise begins to take on human properties, which can occur when personal effects are associated with the deceased. Almost invariably, mortuary workers will remark about a watch that continues to run after the person is dead or a watch that stopped running at the moment of impact. Identification cards, rings, pictures, wallets, and letters are among the strongest reminders of the deceased's humanity. As contact with personal effects becomes more intimate and prolonged, the likelihood of disturbance for the worker, at least temporarily, is increased.

During the Vietnam war, handling the personal effects of the dead was more stressful for some soldiers than processing the remains for shipment home. As in other wars, some soldiers carried extensive collections of letters and photographs from loved ones and other personal material. Military graves registration personnel had to screen these items for objectionable material and the presence of blood or body fluids before they could be sent home. In reading letters of the deceased, the feeling of knowing the family bothered some workers, particularly the fact that they knew the soldier was dead and the family back home did not. Graves registration personnel who had worked in Vietnam provided anecdotes:

In Vietnam, we lost more of our people who dealt with personal property that had to read the letters and screen the personal effects, than the ones who actually worked with the hands-on side of it … with human remains. That's something that a lot of people find hard to believe, but after you explain it to them, that a guy would sit there day after day reading those letters from a loved one. That would probably be more of a mental stress than those who worked with the deceased human remains from combat.

Say a guy got zapped after 11 months; he had 11 months worth of letters. Somebody had to sit down and physically read every one of those letters because they would be sent back to the next of kin. Those guys who worked on the personal property side, they would have to sit there and do that day after day, month after month, and finally, for some of them, the stress of getting emotionally involved with those people ... anybody could. You know, you sit there day after day and read through a guy's stuff, especially if you've got children and if you've got any kind of feeling within you whatsoever. But some of them just couldn't cope with it. Some had to be sent back to the mortuary side and some had to be put back for reassignment.

We were just taking the personal effects off the remains and we had the soldier's billfold in our hands and here was a picture with his wife and two children. You know the impact that had on me! It just stopped me cold and I said something to the men. I said "Isn't this God-awful that we know this soldier is dead and his wife and children are going to get that news in a matter of hours or days."

Identification or emotional involvement with the deceased may produce a high degree of distress. Many subjects described identification, a sense of kinship with the body, in different ways. Some reified identification in a magical way with guidance of how to act: in the same way that a body handler took care of a body from the battlefield, someone would take care of him. A common reaction was, "It could have been me." Children's bodies often stimulated a sense of emotional involvement. The viewers frequently reported thoughts such as, "I remember when my kids were about that age."

Other examples of emotional involvement that are disturbing to body handlers are the bodies of friends and acquaintances and "brothers in uniform." Pathologists had an unwritten rule that they would not do an autopsy on a friend. "I wanted to remember him the way he was." An officer in charge of a large graves registration facility in Vietnam reported, "I always feared seeing somebody I knew." A fireman said

What makes the biggest impact is seeing a dead firefighter – it brings it home. You have to deal with the realities: you're here and he is not.

A body handler who participated in the Grenada operation reported

Most of us had horrendous nightmares about escorting a friend or family member home in a casket.

A senior police official told us

I had a cop die in my arms. I still cannot get it out of my head. I didn't know him. He got shot in the back five times. I took him off the roof and got him down to the sixth floor and he died in my arms. I still can't get that out of my mind, still think about it once in awhile, if I hear a name or something comes out. But, I won't dwell on it. I just didn't like the idea that a brother I had worked with died in my arms.

At Dover Air Force Base, one group of body handlers became very upset after working for weeks with the personal effects of one victim. They developed the fantasy that they knew the victim and his family. Another group became anxious when they saw features of a body (soot in throat, posture), which they thought indicated the individual had been alive after the crash. Experienced personnel, professionals and nonprofessionals, cautioned newcomers against becoming emotionally involved. Most experienced workers could describe how they avoided emotional involvement. These body handlers gave tips to new personnel such as "Don't look at the face. Don't get emotionally involved. Don't think of it as a person."

At Sioux City, rescue workers reported distress when they saw handwritten materials in the wreckage. "It meant someone wrote it. They had been alive." Young workers, learning to work with the personal effects of Operation Desert Storm casualties, gingerly went through the personal effects, relaxing only when a more senior worker made it a standard routine with forms to complete.

In the Gander, Newfoundland, US Army plane crash prior to Christmas week, 1985, the discovery of toys in the wreckage sent waves of anxiety and concern through the disaster workers as they worried that children had been on the plane. None, in fact, were on board.

Previous experience and training

Previous experience (see Table 11.2) with a stressful event has been shown to reduce the effects of the stressor. In studies of parachute jumpers (Fenz & Epstein, 1967) and pilots (Drinkwater *et al.*, 1968; Mefferd *et al.*, 1971), those with less experience reported higher levels of fear and anxiety than experienced persons. The relationship between experience and psychological responses in disaster workers has been documented; however, the mechanisms underlying this relationship have not been closely examined. Experienced disaster workers consistently show lower stress following a disaster than inexperienced workers. A higher proportion of nonprofessional rescuers than professionals reported poor mental health 9 months after recovering victims from an oilrig collapse at sea (Ersland *et al.*, 1989). The more experienced rescuers were less likely to have poor mental health than the less experienced rescuers.

Weisaeth (1989) observed that a high level of disaster training or experience was significantly correlated with optimal behavior during the disaster. Firefighters experienced in mass disasters had lower stress responses after the event than did nonprofessional firefighters (Hytten & Hasle 1989). The long-term effects of past experience and training are less clear. During the first week after a disaster, professional rescue workers had significantly greater unpleasant feelings than nonprofessionals; however, the reverse was true 9 months after the disaster (Lundin, 1990). Weisaeth's (1989) study of disaster behavior among survivors of an industrial explosion suggested that training and experience were extremely powerful variables in predicting health outcome. Persons who had experienced severe flooding in southeastern Kentucky had fewer symptoms than those who had not experienced floods (Norris & Murrell, 1988). These findings were interpreted as evidence for stress inoculation and emphasized the advantages of prior experience with a stressor.

Inexperienced voluntary workers who recovered the bodies of children from a bus accident reported significantly more intrusion and avoidance at 1 month and more avoidance at 13 months than the professional workers (Dyregrov *et al.*, 1996).

For forensic dentists working with the remains of the Branch Davidians, co-worker support was significantly higher for experienced dentists than for those who were inexperienced in handling remains (McCarroll *et al.*, 1996). Interestingly, spouse support was significantly related to lower levels of stress symptoms in the inexperienced dentists but not in those with more experience. These findings challenge the belief that highly trained professionals are immune from the post-traumatic stress of body recovery and identification.

Volunteer status and emotional involvement with the dead

Volunteer status was related to lower psychological distress and intrusive and avoidance symptoms in military personnel anticipating working with the dead of the Persian Gulf War (McCarroll *et al.*, 1995c). Emotional involvement, sometimes experienced as identification with the dead, is an important mechanism in the stress–illness relationship (Ursano *et al.*, 1999). In research on mortuary workers who handled remains from the USS Iowa explosion, three types of identification in mortuary workers were examined: identification with the self ("It could have been me"), identification with a friend ("It could have been a friend"), and identification with a family member ("It could have been a family member"). Interestingly, those who identified with the deceased as a friend were more likely to have PTSD, had more intrusive and avoidant symptoms, and somatization.

Good supervision and management practices

Some studies show few or no negative effects from handling remains (Alexander & Wells, 1991; Tucker *et al.*, 2002). Organizational and managerial practices may serve a prophylactic role in preventing adverse post-traumatic reactions in experienced police body handlers (Alexander, 1993). Thompson and Solomon (1991) speculated that the management of the participants affected the relative lack of adverse outcomes in a sample of police officers. The officers were well trained and prepared for the task and were monitored throughout the procedure and thereafter, showing concern of management for their welfare.

Close supervision is important for monitoring the welfare of the worker as well as the accomplishment of the many tasks associated with recovery and identification of the dead following a disaster. To decrease fatigue and distress, workers should be provided with food, water, opportunities for sleep (when the site is remote), changes of clothing, hygienic conditions for washing and bathing, and rest breaks away from the recovery site or morgue.

Outbriefing by supervisors, referral, and follow-up

The manner in which the recovery and mortuary operations are completed can have an effect on the worker's feelings about what has gone before. In many disasters, workers are simply told they are no longer needed and sent on their way. At a minimum, there should be a "thank you" from a senior official. When workers come and go as a group, it is helpful for a senior official to describe the totality of the event for people, such as the number of remains recovered, supplies used, support rendered by outside agencies, and other timely information that will help the worker put the event in perspective. Workers who desire a spiritual message at the end of an operation sometimes request a memorial service. While mental health debriefings are not required or advised, it is helpful for workers to know if assistance can be provided once they leave the scene. Finally, if possible, supervisors may personally contact or telephone the worker some weeks after the event to inquire about that worker's welfare. While such later contact is, at minimum, a considerate and courteous act, it also will help the supervisor obtain information that may be helpful to management in the future.

Specific stresses of exposure to death and the dead in war

Death from friendly fire

The death of a soldier caused by an error of comrades is termed death by friendly fire. For example, during ground combat, the assault force may call in artillery fire to hit a target that is very close. The artillery fire may fall short of the target and hit the assaulting troops. Aircrews are never perfectly accurate in the engagement of their targets. Bombs can misfire or friendly forces be mistaken for enemy. Military commanders and troops generally realize that friendly fire deaths are an unavoidable part of war. Such deaths occasionally also occur in civilian police work. However, that does not remove the shock, remorse, and trauma of the experience.

During Operation Desert Storm, body handlers reacted to friendly fire deaths as they would to deaths resulting from combat with the enemy. The dead were comrades who had fallen in battle. A military officer who supervised body handlers at Dover Air Force Base during Operation Desert Storm was angry because he believed that personnel killed by friendly fire did not receive the Purple Heart upon their death. His assumption expressed his feelings of the wastefulness of the death. In fact, these men did receive the Purple Heart. In other friendly fire deaths, troops had been clearly marked by clothing, position, or vehicles and the deaths "should not have happened." The remains handlers reacted to these deaths with great anger and dismay.

Death of women

The deaths of American military women in the Persian Gulf War of 1990–1991 stirred disquiet among the body handlers and supervisors. On looking back on the experience, one body handler remarked, "The first woman casualty was the hardest to handle." The remains handlers had seen her interviewed on TV, which made her more real. Her personal belongings were kept separate from those of the men and were not handled through the usual procedures. Supervisors insisted that a woman be present when the body of a dead female soldier was being identified. This angered the male remains handlers. The remains of females were kept completely wrapped and the number of personnel involved in the identification procedures was kept to a minimum. The bodies of men, although always treated with respect, were not required to have a male escort and their remains were left uncovered during the identification procedures.

The body of a pregnant woman killed in Panama in 1989 was kept separate from the other dead. Remains handlers treated her wooden casket as special. It was placed to the side and no other bodies or boxes were stacked on top.

Accidental deaths

Accidental deaths in war due to avoidable accidents or misconduct were termed "dumb deaths" by the observers. These deaths were reported to be particularly disquieting. The people had made it through combat and then were later killed while playing with munitions or handling weapons in an unsafe manner.

Enemy dead

American soldiers in Operation Just Cause in Panama reported few feelings about enemy dead. An exception was when several soldiers went through the wallet of a dead Panamanian soldier and saw pictures of family, children, and a First Communion. They broke down and cried and later went to see the chaplain to talk.

Personal threat to the body handler

In a study of the anticipated stress of handling remains, personal threat to the body handler was one of the significant clusters of concerns (McCarroll

et al., 1995d). In order to retrieve persons killed in combat, soldiers may have to endure hostile fire and remains may be booby-trapped.

In the response to the Pentagon attack, recovery workers were concerned about exposure to toxic materials such as jet fuel, dust, asbestos, and unknown contaminants. In addition to environmental contaminants, unexploded ordnance and other explosives, workers must contend with the possibility of the HIV virus and other known and unknown pathogens. As a result, more protective equipment must be available and worn at a disaster scene. The wearing and maintenance of protective clothing and equipment sometimes requires extensive training. Such clothing and equipment also add to the weight burden of rescuers and produce fatigue faster than would normally be the case.

Coping with exposure to the dead

Coping strategies vary in the different stages of exposure to traumatic death and with the degree of experience of the body handler (see Table 11.3).

Before exposure

Few organizations practise their response to a disaster although such events are expectable. Only the timing is unpredictable. In the case of the crash of United Airlines Flight 232 in Sioux City, Iowa, in July 1989, an air crash disaster drill had been performed prior to the crash and was reported to have been very helpful. Generally, inexperienced personnel who volunteer to help at a disaster site are rarely given more than a few hours to prepare for what they will see and do.

People often reported feeling frightened of their own reactions to the bodies, asking themselves, "Will I be able to handle it?" Those who volunteered in pairs or larger groups thought that they could help each other get through the experience. Initial preparation by a supervisor, usually by an inbriefing, is essential for inexperienced volunteers. Those we interviewed were unanimous in saying that before

Table 11.3 Coping strategies used in exposure to traumatic and disaster-related death

Stressor	Coping Strategy
Before exposure (waiting)	
Lack of information regarding tasks and roles	Training, preparatory briefing
Anticipating one's reaction to bodies	Inbriefing describing condition of remains
	Gradual exposure to the site with escort
During exposure (on site)	
Sensory overload	Avoidance or attenuation of strong stimuli
Handling victims' personal effects	Maintain emotional distance and emphasize the importance of the task
Fatigue and overdedication	Decrease and limit exposure to remains by work breaks, food, sleep, supervision
Intense personal feelings	Pairing with experienced personnel
	Supervisory support
	Humor
	Talking
	Maintain emotional distance and emphasize the importance of the task
Personal threat	Protective clothing, decontamination
	Information about possible risks
After exposure (postevent)	
Need for information	Outbriefing
	Education
Intense feelings (e.g., sadness, alienation)	Outbriefing
	Family and organizational support
	Awards
	Maintain personal perspective on events

volunteers enter a disaster scene they should be "told the worst" so as to minimize the surprises at the crash site or mortuary. In a recent disaster, a supervisor provided a sequence of short, staged preparation briefings in which he became more explicit as he moved volunteers from an initial assembly area to their eventual work site. This technique was reported afterwards to have been very helpful.

Experienced personnel expecting to be sent on an operation reported little psychological preparation. Nervousness was sometimes reported when they did not know what sort of trauma to expect, the condition of the bodies, or how difficult it would be to extract or identify the victims. One experienced dental pathologist reported that when he knew he would be the only professional on a recovery and

identification operation he had nightmares the night before. When he knew he was going with others, he slept soundly.

During exposure to the dead (on site)

Individuals defend against the multiple sensory stimuli associated with the dead: the sights of the bodies (grotesque, burned, and mutilated), the sounds during autopsy (heads hitting tables and saws cutting bone), the smells of decomposing and burned bodies; and the tactile stimuli experienced as bodies are handled.

Workers often reported that they did not see badly damaged bodies as human. Supervisors facilitated this process of decreasing emotional involvement (disidentification) by telling inexperienced volunteers, "Don't think of it as a body. Think of it as a job." Natural looking bodies were often seen as all too human. Such remarks as, "He can't be dead. He hardly has a scratch on him" were common. People reported many internal, automatic strategies by which they distanced themselves from the bodies, such as not looking at faces.

As mentioned previously, many people attempted to mask odors by burning coffee, smoking cigars, working in the cold and using fragrances such as peppermint oil and orange oil inside surgical masks (Cervantes, 1988). Most reported that such strategies did not help much in reducing the odors. Some olfactory adaptation did occur and workers generally dropped these strategies over time. Personnel who touch bodies or body parts almost always wear gloves. This decreases the tactile contact with the remains, which is particularly difficult with decomposed and burned bodies which are especially hard to handle due to the loss of tissue.

Past experience was frequently reported as helpful but it did not make one invulnerable. Even very experienced personnel could be shocked or surprised by the sight of the grotesque. An experienced pathologist reported extreme discomfort at the sight of a body whose shoulder girdle had been cleanly sliced by a helicopter blade. When he first saw the body, he did not recognize what had happened. When he did recognize the injury, he wondered whether the individual had felt the cut, suffered, or lived long after the injury. He continued to have intrusive images of this scene.

Physical fatigue was a frequent and significant stressor due to the long and irregular hours, little sleep, poor eating schedules, moving heavy loads, and minimal time to recuperate. The stress of the experience was reported to be reduced when the individual took frequent breaks or the supervisor acted to decrease the visual contact with bodies, such as by providing chairs that faced away from the bodies, or putting partitions between the identification stations. Overdedication contributed to the tendency to go on working under conditions that normally would not be tolerated. Even though breaks

were seen as desirable, at the Dover mortuary following the Gander air crash, for example, many individuals worked up to 20 h per day. Managers had to require some people to leave the area.

Some workers voluntarily left the scene because of nausea, fatigue or psychological discomfort. This did not always mean that the person was going to be ineffective. A senior noncommissioned officer reported:

I talked to some of the guys who worked Gander. There were days when they'd go in there and they would pick up an arm or a leg and they'd start thinking about what that arm used to be attached to and the fact that it was all burned up. They would have to walk outside of those plastic tents that they were working out of and sit down and have coffee, smoke a few cigarettes and just walk away for a day because on that particular day their psyche was not enough to deal with what they were seeing that day. The next day they were OK.

In general, grief and upset per se are not often observed on site because of feelings about one's public image. Most workers were concerned about how they would look in front of the other workers, both supervisors and subordinates. No one wanted to look like they "couldn't handle it." In response to the question of "What if the leaders are not able to be macho that day? Do you lose faith in them?" The answer from an experienced team leader was:

No, no, no! You can't lose faith in them. You have to talk to them and let them talk to you. "What was it that bothered you on that case?" Tell them that it's OK to get sick or say "Hey! I can't deal with it today." Because their psyche won't allow them to deal with that body that day, we can't think any less of them because tomorrow it might be our turn.

Unfortunately, such an attitude is not always present. We heard stories of supervisors laughing when someone said they "couldn't take it."

Everyone recognized humor as a substantial tension-reducer during and after operations. Humor was more common when the workers were out of public view. Most humor was still considered respectful. Some body handlers were frightened of black humor, feeling it reflected having gone over the edge, and becoming too hardened. The professional role identity of individuals who handled the dead also facilitated coping with the psychological stress. The professional role was usually well defined. For nonprofessionals, roles had to be defined and reinforced by others. Often, a good time to define roles was during the inbriefing where the importance of each person's job was emphasized. For most volunteers, the idea that they were performing an important service for the dead, the families of the dead, and the community was very important.

The role of the medical examiner is well defined and of recognized importance. Curiosity and a sense of detective work helped sustain the medical examiners. They were frequently cautioned against becoming emotionally involved in their cases because their objectivity might be questioned in court. Being objective also served a protective function. In some situations, however, they were not able to avoid emotional involvement. Most reported that they did not like to do autopsies on children, friends, family members or torture deaths in which the suffering of the individual was obvious.

The mortician strives to do everything right because of the families. He or she takes pride in the cosmetic treatment of the deceased. This goal reinforced the idea that something memorable would be given to the survivors. Working to provide something memorable for the survivors can decrease feelings of helplessness in the face of death (Cassem, 1977).

The fire, police, and emergency medical service personnel are strongly motivated by the opportunity to save lives. Deaths often caused them to question their competence. In a fire rescue company when occupants of a house were found dead the firefighters said to each other, "They were dead before the bells went off!" meaning that the victims had probably died before the fire alarm had even sounded and they were not to blame.

The leader and the work group were inevitably seen as sources of support during difficult operations. The professional work group was the primary source of support. The presence of an experienced co-worker, especially for the uninitiated, was important. A new individual could share the tasks and the feelings with an experienced partner and decrease the shock and surprise of the initial exposure.

A large urban search and rescue fire company reported a very high level of social support and unit cohesion. During each shift, about 12 people lived together in a room that served as a kitchen, a dining room, and a living room at the rear of the firehouse near the vehicles. They were proud of their comradery:

We're like a family! We provide psychological first aid to each other – reassurance. All he, the guy next to you on the line, needs is the reassurance of someone else nearby.

Workers always noticed the support or lack of support by senior leaders and the organization as a whole. Volunteer body handlers at Dover Air Force Base after the Gander disaster were alert to whether their supervisor visited or their senior commanders expressed support (Maloney, 1988b).

After exposure (post event)

Disaster workers often needed help in the hours or days shortly after exposure to the dead. During this time, volunteers reported high levels of discomfort, both physical and psychological. Fatigue, irritability and a need for a transition "back to the real world" were commonly expressed. Experienced persons described themselves as doing what they had to in their mortuary work in order to get the job done; however, it was often at a high personal cost. The experience of professional support frequently came from a critique of the technical aspects of the work. One fireman pointed out that this sort of discussion had

Two phases – an individual phase and a group phase. You find out months or years later that something had bothered someone and you never found out about it before – he never talked about it. You argue about what had been wrong.

For almost everyone, professional counseling or psychiatric assistance, even if available, was generally viewed as unacceptable. Often this was due to fears that the person would be fired, could not successfully testify in court, would be ridiculed by fellow workers, or would lose their job. Most said they did not really feel the need for counseling. However, almost all of those interviewed said they could have benefited from a brief talk about the experience, particularly if it involved the work group. Some wished it had even been mandatory.

Events occurring outside the mortuary often triggered intense feelings in the volunteer body handlers. While viewing a memorial service on television one man reported

I felt the grief they [the families] were going through. They started naming names – when they came to mine [the body he had escorted through the identification process], I went in the bathroom and cried and cried.

Another reported

Memorial services interfere with coping. At that point, it's no longer a job; it gets to be a name, a human being. You can't do both at the same time. You associate everything you do with each person. It all comes together.

Spouses of the body handlers were frequently unwilling to hear about the workers' experiences. At other times the workers themselves decided not to talk to their spouses about their disaster work. One man reported that his wife required him to take his clothes off at the door and shower after working with remains. Others described the stress of their first (and sometimes only) attempt at sharing feelings about their work with their spouses. Some said that they were unlikely to repeat the experience.

Somatic symptoms are common after exposure to death and the dead (Ursano et al., 1995). Interestingly, somatic symptoms were not explained by depressive symptoms present before exposure in a group of remains handlers (McCarroll et al., 2002). Military remains handlers working in the mortuary after the USS Iowa gun turret explosion in 1989 showed intrusive and avoidant symptoms elevated at 1, 4, and 13 months but these symptoms decreased over time (Ursano et al., 1995). Probable PTSD was present in 11% at 1 month, 10% at 4 months, and 2% at 13 months while depression was not increased.

The return to work was difficult for many, particularly when co-workers were not sympathetic or sensitive. Most workers appreciated some time off after the job was over. Some wanted to have time with their families; others wanted time alone. There was generally a feeling that those who had not been at the site could not fully understand the experience. This contributed to the difficulty of talking about the experience. People who came by the mortuary for only a visit were called "turistas."

Consistent with other reports (Maloney, 1988a, 1988b; Robinson, 1988) in the aftermath of an incident alcohol use was widely reported. Some workers reported that large amounts were consumed without intoxication while others reported that "getting smashed" was normal at the end of each day of an operation. Drinking also provided a social context for the work group and an opportunity to receive and provide support to each other. Some military workers reported that when the troops were restricted to one beer per evening, the restriction did not apply to body handlers. When several individuals were ordered away from a disaster site for rest, they reported returning to their rooms and drinking alcohol.

Discussion

Exposure to traumatic death is common in natural and manmade disasters and is a significant psychological stressor that can make victims of rescuers. The rescue worker is traumatized through the senses: viewing, smelling and touching, experiencing the grotesque, the unusual, the novel and the untimeliness of the death. The stress of body handling begins prior to the exposure with the anticipation. Nonvolunteers and those with no previous experience appear to experience more distress during this time. The extent and intensity of the sensory properties of the body such as visual grotesqueness, smell, and tactile qualities are important aspects of the stressor. It may be heuristically useful to consider exposure to human remains as a special category of toxic exposure in which such dimensions as the type of agent, frequency, intensity and duration of exposure all add to the risk of later stress reactions

(Bartone *et al.*, 1989), breakdown, disease or even psychological growth. Exposure to a child's mutilated body appears to be extremely toxic regardless of the age of the remains handler or whether that person has children.

There is often a paradox in people's reactions to traumatic material. Reactions tend to be both idiosyncratic and common. That is, one can predict that which is disturbing to most people (e.g., children's bodies, personal effects such as pictures, and a sense of revulsion at putrid smells), but there is also usually a personal reaction that is unique to the person. People will notice certain aspects of exposure to the dead that are not common. For example, an experienced forensic pathologist was somewhat bothered by a reaction to the bodies of victims that had been wrapped in gauze due to the fact that they would not be viewable by the family. When workers carried them, the wrapped remains reminded him of rag dolls, but he knew that they were not. Another person, upon seeing the distended jaws of dead victims who had had their jaw muscles cut for dental identification, thought that their faces looked like the faces of clowns.

Although all sensory modalities are involved in contact with a body, odor may have the greatest potential to re-create significant past episodes in a person's life. The strength of memory appears to vary with the special involvement a person has with the odor (Engen, 1987). The amount of forgetting of olfactory recognition memory, both long and short term, is very small and, thus, the accurate recognition of odors when encountered again is very high (Engen, 1987; Engen *et al.*, 1973). While odors are easily recognized, they are impossible to recall at will, which is fortunate for most persons exposed to the smells of death. One can easily remember the color and shape of an apple, but cannot conjure up its smell. There is a need for those who prepare food to be aware of the power of olfactory memory to vividly re-create a scene and to induce the reliving of some portion of the experience. Even though the recall of olfactory memory is relatively poor, we were informed of two cases of individuals who had served as remains handlers at

the Jonestown disaster who later received medical discharges from the military for PTSD. A complaint common to both individuals was waking up at night with a vivid recollection of the smells of the bodies at Jonestown (Orman, personal communication, 1989).

The meaning or social context of a death is an additional dimension of the stress felt by the individual body handler. The body itself as well as the memories of the individual (or group) can take on connotations not attributed to them in life. This change in the view of the dead by survivors has been termed the "social identity" of the dead (Sledge, 2005). For example, people who die in war can be identified as heroes when no heroics were involved in their death. On the other hand, the death of a drug dealer arouses less sympathy among policemen or medical examiners regardless of the manner of death or the condition of the body. The innocent, who are seen as victims, almost never fail to arouse feelings among those who deal with the remains. Interviewees who were body handlers during the Vietnam war talked about the stress of handling a large number of bodies of soldiers killed in action in an unpopular war. Deaths caused by friendly fire were similarly stressful. The deaths of these soldiers often seemed to have been a tremendous waste, which contributed to feelings of depression and hopelessness among the disaster workers.

The role of identification and emotional involvement in the production and resolution of the stress of handling dead bodies requires further study. Working with personal effects is an infrequently recognized, but powerful stimulus for the emotional involvement of the remains handler and subsequent distress. Such emotional involvement (for example, feelings of knowing the dead) appears to heighten the trauma of the experience. On the other hand, it may serve to eliminate the unfamiliar and the unknown qualities of the dead – changing what is new and novel into something familiar and part of the past (Ursano & Fullerton, 1990). The switching on of these cognitive mechanisms – identification, personalization, and emotional involvement – from the trauma of association with dead bodies requires further study. Whether certain individuals are more prone to this perceptual style or whether it represents a basic biological mechanism that all individuals activate to varying degrees is unknown. Ways of decreasing identification and emotional involvement may be effective preventive measures.

The coping strategies used by rescue personnel differ in the before, during and after stages of disaster work. An informative and role-setting inbriefing is critical to the adjustment of the volunteer and will also be helpful to orient the experienced worker. This briefing helps form the context for much of what is later felt and seen. When it is not provided, volunteers may have greater difficulty adjusting to the scene and the work, and may fare poorly. However, no matter how well workers are briefed, there is always some shock to the reality of the situation.

The overwhelming nature of the sensory stimulation usually leads participants, particularly volunteers, to develop cognitive and behavioral distancing (avoidance) strategies. Failure to protect against emotional involvement with the victim is recognized by most workers as putting a person at risk for psychological distress. Scheduling is the job of the supervisor. Before fatigue sets in, which can contribute to emotional vulnerability, it is essential that managers establish schedules and ensure that rescue workers follow them. While there is little that supervisors can do about alcohol abuse off site, they can inform participants that the potential for alcohol abuse is high following exposure to trauma.

Transition out of the rescue work after exposure appears to be facilitated by an outbriefing where the workers can ask questions and information can be provided about the event, the body identification process, and community reactions. Statements of appreciation and recognition made at this time aid recovery. Family and organizational support is central during the transition period. When both the family and the primary work group show sensitivity and caring, the participant appears more likely to verbalize his or her feelings regarding what has been seen and done.

The personal experience of trauma is usually private and personal. Often it does not result in an outpouring or any expression of feelings at all. Such reactions are often personal and unobserved (McCarroll *et al.*, 1995a). As a result, people often will not attend debriefing groups voluntarily or consult a mental health provider. Many rescue workers and volunteers will not share everything with people who were not present with them through the ordeal. Research has failed to consistently demonstrate that debriefing prevents postevent distress (Deahl, 2000; Gist *et al.*, 1997; National Institute of Mental Health, 2002). There have been several reviews of the literature and summaries of the current status of debriefing in the array of techniques to help persons who have faced traumatic situations (Raphael & Wilson, 2000; Raphael & Wooding, 2004). Alexander (1993) cautions that while support groups are important, careful consideration must be given to the aims, methods, and composition. Along with the possibility of a positive effect, improperly run groups may have harmful effects (Kenardy, 2000). Groups with mixed exposure levels may be more likely to produce increased symptoms by exposure of those less exposed persons to the stories of those who were more exposed. It is important that outcomes other than PTSD be examined in debriefing studies (e.g., depression, substance abuse, work absences, and disability).

Numerous strategies are used to cope with the stresses of body handling. Most appear to be effective in the short run; however, which are more effective and their long-term consequences are unclear. Avoidance strategies appear to be effective during initial exposure to dead bodies. We do not know the effect of using such strategies over a longer time period. Reports from volunteers and experienced personnel indicate that at some point they can no longer avoid reminders of previous disasters. For example, names of the victims, the sight of an object, or a smell may bring the experience back. Such an experience may be helpful or harmful. The triggering of memories may help to work through the experience. On the other hand, the recall of unwanted memories can be disturbing and interfere with the present tasks. It remains an open question when and under what circumstances the individual should be encouraged to talk or think about aspects of the disaster that were previously avoided.

Spouses of disaster workers need to be educated about their loved ones' experiences. Many workers claimed that they wished their spouses had been informed of the nature of their work. Information can be provided to spouses in order to allay their concerns and may reinforce this naturally occurring support system. Brief informational groups held for spouses can also be a useful intervention.

Inexperienced workers may be at higher risk for acute effects than experienced personnel. The latter, however, are not immune from suffering the same psychological discomforts as the volunteers. Some experienced personnel reported becoming somewhat calloused through repeated exposure, but no one believed it possible to be totally desensitized.

Additional research of this powerful stressor is needed to further describe its components and better understand the role of sensory stimulation in recall, particularly in PTSD, and the normal working through of traumatic events. Finally, not all results of disaster rescue work are negative. Volunteers almost unanimously report that they would volunteer again if another disaster occurred. People were proud of their contribution and of having done an important job that others either could not do or would never have the opportunity to do. It has been previously reported that most people do quite well following exposure to massive trauma. An important theoretical as well as practical question is how people use trauma to move toward health (Ursano, 1987).

REFERENCES

Alexander, D. A. (1993). Stress among police body handlers. *British Journal of Psychiatry*, **163**, 806–808.

Alexander, D. A. & Wells, A. (1991). Reactions of police officers to body-handling after a major disaster: a before and after comparison. *British Journal of Psychiatry*, **159**, 547–555.

Arthur, A. Z. (1987). Stress as a state of anticipatory vigilance. *Perceptual and Motor Skills*, **64**, 75–85.

Bartone, P. T., Ursano, R. J., Wright, K. M. & Ingraham, L. H. (1989). The impact of a military air disaster on the health of assistance workers: a prospective study. *Journal of Nervous and Mental Disease*, **177**, 317–328.

Breslau, N. & Davis, G. C. (1987). Posttraumatic stress disorder – the stressor criterion. *Journal of Nervous and Mental Disease*, **175**, 255–264.

Bryant, R. A. & Harvey, A. G. (1996). Posttraumatic stress reactions in volunteer firefighters. *Journal of Traumatic Stress*, **9**, 51–62.

Cassem, N. (1977). Treating the person confronting death. In *Harvard Guide to Modern Psychiatry*, ed. A. M. Nicholi, Jr., pp. 599. Cambridge, Mass.: Belknap Press of Harvard University Press.

Cervantes, R. (1988). Psychological stress of body handling. Part II and Part III: debriefing of Dover AFB personnel following the Gander tragedy and the body handling experience at Dover AFB. In *Exposure to Death, Disasters and Bodies*, eds. R. J. Ursano & C. Fullerton, pp. 125–162 (DTIC: A 203163). Bethesda, Md.: F. Edward Hebert School of Medicine, Uniformed Services University of the Health Sciences.

Clohessy, S. & Ehlers, A. (1999). PTSD symptoms, response to intrusive memories and coping in ambulance service workers. *British Journal of Clinical Psychology*, **38**, 251–265.

Deahl, M. P. (2000). Debriefing and body recovery: war grave soldiers. In *Psychological Debriefing*, eds. B. Raphael & J. P. Wilson, pp. 108–130. New York: Cambridge University Press.

Drinkwater, B. L., Cleland, T. & Flint, M. M. (1968). Pilot performance during periods of anticipatory physical threat stress. *Aerospace Medicine*, **39**, 944–999.

Dyregrov, A., Kristoffersen, J. I. & Gjestad, R. (1996). Voluntary and professional disaster-workers: similarities and differences in reactions. *Journal of Traumatic Stress*, **9**, 541–555.

Engen, T. (1987). Remembering odors and their names. *American Scientist*, **75**, 497–503.

Engen, T., Kuisma, J. E. & Eimas, P. D. (1973). Short-term memory of odors. *Journal of Experimental Psychology*, **99**, 222–225.

Ersland, S., Weisaeth, L. & Sund, A. (1989). The stress upon rescuers involved in an oil rig disaster, "Alexander L. Kielland" 1980. *Acta Psychiatrica Scandinavica Supplementum*, **80**(355), 38–49.

Fenz, W. D. & Epstein, S. (1967). Gradients of physiological arousal in parachutists as a function of an approaching jump. *Psychosomatic Medicine*, **29**, 33–51.

Fullerton, C. S., McCarroll, J. E., Ursano, R. J. & Wright, K. M. (1992). Psychological responses of rescue workers: fire fighters and trauma. *American Journal of Orthopsychiatry*, **62**, 371–378.

Gist, R., Lohr, J., Kenardy, J. *et al.* (1997). Researchers speak out on CISM. *Journal of Emergency Medicine*, **22**, 27–28.

Green, B. L., Lindy, J. D., Grace, M. C. & Gleser, G. C. (1989). Multiple diagnosis in posttraumatic stress disorder. The role of war stressors. *Journal of Nervous and Mental Disease*, **177**, 329–335.

Hersheiser, M. R. & Quarantelli, E. L. (1976). The handling of the dead in a disaster. *Omega*, **7**, 195–208.

Hytten, K. & Hasle, A. (1989). Fire fighters: a study of stress and coping. *Acta Psychiatrica Scandinavica Supplementum*, **355**, 50–55.

Jones, D. J. (1985). Secondary disaster victims: the emotional effects of recovering and identifying human remains. *American Journal of Psychiatry*, **142**, 303–307.

Keller, R. T. & Bobo, W. V. (2002). Handling human remains following the terrorist attack on the Pentagon: experiences of 10 uniformed health care workers. *Military Medicine*, **167**, 8–11.

Kenardy, J. (2000). The current status of psychological debriefing. *British Medical Journal*, **321**, 1032–1033.

Laufer, R. S., Gallops, M. S. & Frey-Wouters, E. (1984). War stress and trauma. *Journal of Health and Social Behavior*, **25**, 65–85.

Laufer, R. S., Brett, E. & Gallops, M. S. (1985). Dimensions of posttraumatic stress disorder among Vietnam veterans. *Journal of Nervous and Mental Disease*, **173**, 538–545.

Leffler, C. T. & Dembert, M. L. (1998). Posttraumatic stress symptoms among U.S. Navy divers recovering TWA Flight 800. *Journal of Nervous and Mental Disease*, **186**, 574–577.

Lifton, R. J. (1973). *Home From the War*. New York: Simon & Schuster, Inc.

Lindy, J. D., Green, B. L. & Grace, M. C. (1987). The stressor criterion and posttraumatic stress disorder. *Journal of Nervous and Mental Disease*, **175**, 269–272.

Lundin, T. (1990). The rescue personnel and the disaster stress. In *Proceedings of the Second International Conference on Wartime Medical Services*, eds. J. E. Lundeberg, U. Otto & B. Rybeck, pp. 208–216. Stockholm, 25–29 June. Sweden: Frsvarets forskningsanstalt-FOA.

Maloney, J. (1988a). The Gander disaster: body handling and identification process. In *Exposure to Death, Disasters and Bodies*, eds. R. J. Ursano & C. Fullerton, pp. 41–66 (DTIC: A 203163). Bethesda, Md.: F. Edward Hebert School of Medicine, Uniformed Services University of the Health Sciences.

Maloney, J. (1988b). Body handling at Dover AFB: the Gander disaster. In *Individual and Group Behavior in Toxic and Contained Environments*, eds. R. J. Ursano & C. Fullerton, pp. 97–102 (DTIC: A 203267). Bethesda, Md.: F. Edward Hebert School of Medicine, Uniformed Services University of the Health Sciences.

Marmar, C. R., Weiss, D. S., Metzler, T. J., Ronfeldt, H. & Foreman, C. (1996). Stress responses of emergency services personnel to the Loma Parieta earthquake Interstate 880 freeway collapse and control traumatic incidents. *Journal of Traumatic Stress*, **9**, 63–85.

McCarroll, J. E., Ursano, R. J. & Fullerton, C. S. (1993a). Symptoms of posttraumatic stress disorder following recovery of war dead. *American Journal of Psychiatry*, **150**, 1875–1877.

McCarroll, J. E., Ursano, R. J., Fullerton, C. S. & Lundy, A. (1993b). Traumatic stress of a wartime mortuary: anticipation of exposure to mass death. *Journal of Nervous and Mental Disease*, **181**, 545–551.

McCarroll, J. E., Ursano, R. J., Wright, K. M. & Fullerton, C. S. (1993c). Handling of bodies after violent death: strategies for coping. *American Journal of Orthopsychiatry*, **63**, 209–214.

McCarroll, J. E., Ursano, R. J., Ventis, W. L. *et al.* (1993d). Anticipation of handling the dead: effects of experience and gender. *British Journal of Clinical Psychology*, **32** (Pt 4), 466–468.

McCarroll, J. E., Blank, A. S. & Hill, K. (1995a). Working with traumatic material: effects on Holocaust Memorial Museum staff. *American Journal of Orthopsychiatry*, **65**, 66–75.

McCarroll, J. E., Ursano, R. J. & Fullerton, C. S. (1995b). Symptoms of PTSD following recovery of war dead: 13–15 month follow-up. *American Journal of Psychiatry*, **152**, 939–941.

McCarroll, J. E., Ursano, R. J., Fullerton, C. S. & Lundy, A. C. (1995c). Anticipatory stress of handling remains of the Persian Gulf War: predictors of intrusion and avoidance. *Journal of Nervous and Mental Disease*, **183**, 698–703.

McCarroll, J. E., Ursano, R. J., Fullerton, C. S. *et al.* (1995d). Gruesomeness, emotional attachment, and personal threat: dimensions of anticipated stress of body recovery. *Journal of Traumatic Stress*, **8**, 343–347.

McCarroll, J. E., Fullerton, C. S., Ursano, R. J. & Hermsen, J. M. (1996). Posttraumatic stress symptoms following forensic dental identification: Mt. Carmel, Waco, Texas. *American Journal of Psychiatry*, **153**, 778–782.

McCarroll, J. E., Ursano, R. J., Fullerton, C. S., Liu, X. & Lundy, A. (2001). Effect of exposure to death in a war mortuary on posttraumatic stress symptoms. *Journal of Nervous and Mental Disease*, **189**, 44–48.

McCarroll, J. E., Ursano, R. J., Fullerton, C. S., Liu, X. & Lundy, A. (2002). Somatic symptoms in Gulf War mortuary workers. *Psychosomatic Medicine*, **64**, 29–33.

Mefferd, R. B., Hale, H. B., Shannon, I. L., Prigmore, J. R. & Ellis, J. P. (1971). Stress responses as criteria for personnel selection: baseline study. *Aerospace Medicine*, **42**, 42–51.

Miles, M. S., Demi, A. S. & Mostyn-Aker, P. (1984). Rescue workers' reactions following the Hyatt Hotel disaster. *Death Education*, **8**, 315–331.

Mitchell, J. H., Sproule, B. J. & Chapman, C. B. (1958). The physiological meaning of the maximal oxygen intake test. *Journal of Clinical Investigation*, **37**, 538–547.

Myers, D. G. (1989). Mental health and disaster. In *Psychosocial Aspects of Disaster*, eds. R. Gist & B. Lubin, pp. 198. New York: John Wiley & Sons.

National Institute of Mental Health (2002). Mental health and mass violence: evidence based early psychological intervention for victims/survivors of mass violence. A workshop to reach consensus on best practices. NIH Publication No. 02–5138. Washington, D.C.: US Government Printing Office.

Norris, F. H. & Murrell, S. A. (1988). Prior experience as a moderator of disaster impact on anxiety symptoms in older adults. *Journal of Community Psychology*, **16**, 665–683.

Raphael, B. & Wilson, J. P. (2000). *Psychological Debriefing*. New York: Cambridge University Press.

Raphael, B. & Wooding, S. (2004). Debriefing: its evolution and current status. *Psychiatric Clinics of North America*, **27**, 407–423.

Regehr, C., Hill, J. & Glancy, G. D. (2000). Individual predictors of traumatic reactions in firefighters. *Journal of Nervous and Mental Disease*, **188**, 333–339.

Robinson, M. (1988). Psychological support to the Dover AFB body handlers. In *Exposure to Death, Disasters and Bodies*, eds. R. J. Ursano & C. Fullerton, pp. 68–74 (DTIC: A 203163). Bethesda, Md.: F. Edward Hebert School of Medicine, Uniformed Services University of the Health Sciences.

Rundell, J. R., Ursano, R. J., Holloway, H. C. & Silberman, E. K. (1989). Psychiatric responses to trauma. *Hospital and Community Psychiatry*, **40**, 68–74.

Schwartz, H. J. (1984). Fear of the dead: the role of social ritual in neutralizing fantasies from combat. In *Psychotherapy of the Combat Veteran*, ed. H. J. Schwartz, pp. 253–267. New York: Spectrum Publications.

Sledge, M. (2005). *Soldier Dead*. New York: Columbia University Press.

Susnowski, T. (1988). Patterns of skin conductance and heart rate changes under anticipatory stress conditions. *Journal of Psychophysiology*, **2**, 231–238.

Sutker, P. B., Uddo, M., Brailey, K., Vasterling, J. J. & Errera, P. (1994). Psychopathology in war-zone deployed and non-deployed Operation Desert Storm troops assigned graves registration duties. *Journal of Abnormal Psychology*, **103**, 383–390.

Taylor, A. J. W. & Frazer, A. G. (1982). The stress of post-disaster body handling and victim identification work. *Journal of Human Stress*, **8**, 4–12.

Thompson, J. & Solomon, M. (1991). Body recovery teams at disasters: trauma or challenge? *Anxiety Research*, **4**, 235–244.

Tucker, P., Pfefferbaum, B., Doughty, D. E. *et al.* (2002). Body handlers after terrorism in Oklahoma City: predictors of posttraumatic stress and other symptoms. *American Journal of Orthopsychiatry*, **72**, 469–475.

Ursano, R. J. (1987). Commentary. Posttraumatic stress disorder: the stressor criterion. *Journal of Nervous and Mental Disease*, **175**, 273–275.

Ursano, R. J. & Fullerton, C. S. (1990). Cognitive and behavioral responses to trauma. *Journal of Applied Social Psychology*, **20**, 1766–1775.

Ursano, R. J. & McCarroll, J. E. (1990). The nature of a traumatic stressor: handling dead bodies. *Journal of Nervous and Mental Disease*, **178**, 396–398.

Ursano, R. J., Fullerton, C. S., Wright, K. M. *et al.* (eds.) (1992). *Disaster Workers: Trauma and Social Support*. Bethesda, Md.: Uniformed Services University of the Health Sciences.

Ursano, R. J., Fullerton, C. S., Kao, Tzu-Cheg & Bhartiya, V. R. (1995). Longitudinal assessment of posttraumatic stress disorder and depression after exposure to traumatic death. *Journal of Nervous and Mental Disease*, **183**, 36–42.

Ursano, R. J., Fullerton, C. S., Vance, K. & Kao, T. C. (1999). Posttraumatic stress disorder and identification in disaster workers. *American Journal of Psychiatry*, **156**, 353–359.

Weisaeth, L. (1989). A study of behavioral responses to an industrial disaster. *Acta Psychiatrica Scandinavica Supplementum*, **80**, 13–24.

Weiss, D. S., Marmar, C. R., Metzler, T. J. & Ronfeldt, H. M. (1995). Predicting symptomatic distress in emergency services personnel. *Journal of Consulting and Clinical Psychology*, **63**, 361–368.

NOTE

1 Many people are sensitive about the words used to refer to the dead. "Remains" is considered the more respectful term. "Bodies" is more informal and occurs frequently in the medical literature. The terms are used interchangeably here.

12

Weapons of mass destruction and pandemics: global disasters with mass destruction and mass disruption

Robert J. Ursano, Carol S. Fullerton, Ann E. Norwood, & Harry C. Holloway

Some disasters, such as those resulting from weapons of mass destruction (WMD) and pandemics, have the potential for global reach because of the nature of their destructive forces and their effects on individual and community sense of vulnerability, safety and social cohesion. The use of WMD by terrorists gained international attention after the Japanese cult Aum Shinrikyo released sarin gas in the Tokyo subway system in 1995. Concern was heightened when it was learned that the group had also (unsuccessfully) released anthrax and had attempted to obtain the Ebola virus. In the United States, the terrorist attacks of September 11, 2001, and the letters containing anthrax spores that were mailed to media outlets and government officials in October that same year shattered Americans' belief that they were immune from such events. More recently, bombings in London and Madrid and the ongoing suicide attacks in the Middle East are reminders of the psychological and behavioral effects on individuals and communities of terrorism. Although the WMD attacks are often circumscribed, the psychological impact is widespread, as the altered sense of safety and the future resonates to distant sites. Because the ultimate goal of terrorism is to disrupt the social cohesion, values and social capital of a society, protecting and repairing mental health is an important aspect of community preparedness and response planning.

Pandemics also have a potential global reach of mass destruction and historically have been more

devastating than any other type of disaster. The history of the influenza pandemic – occurring about every 10–30 years – has marked the global reach and concern for mass death. In centuries past, this concern has included the plague, polio and smallpox. The estimated 20–40 million people who died from the Spanish influenza pandemic of 1918–1919 (more people than died in World War I) are a reminder of the deadly potential of this global disaster (http://virus.stanford.edu/uda/). The outbreaks of severe acute respiratory syndrome (SARS) in Asia and Canada also caused global concern and highlighted the mental health concerns that are relevant to a pandemic outbreak. More recently, concern about avian influenza has dramatically increased with 244 cases and a nearly 60% fatality rate (WHO, 2006).

There are virtually no empirical data on the mental health impacts of mass outbreaks of infectious disease such as a pandemic. This is largely because few pandemic health threats in the last century have been studied by behavioral scientists. Almost half of the community population exposed to the SARS outbreaks experienced increased stress during the outbreak, nearly 20% exhibited signs of traumatic stress, and many felt horrified and helpless (McAlonan *et al.*, 2005).

In this chapter, we review individual and community psychological and behavioral responses to these two types of disaster with global reach: WMD used by terrorists; and pandemics, outbreaks of infectious disease which span the globe.

Terrorism

Weapons of Mass Destruction are particularly important terrorist agents. There is no single definition of terrorism recognized by government agencies. Terrorism refers to a threat or action that creates terror or horror and is undertaken to achieve a political, ideological, or theological goal. Terrorism represents a special type of a disaster – one caused by human malevolence, which produces higher rates of psychiatric casualties than do natural disasters or technological accidents (North, 1995). Terrorists intend to disrupt society by creating intense fear and disorganization. They seek to violate basic expectations of everyday life by attacking sites of government, work, recreation, and worship. These acts shatter usual predictable routines, people's beliefs in a just world, and people's sense of personal and community safety.

Suicide attacks are often a part of terrorist WMD attacks, and ensure accurate delivery of the weapons, enable low-cost multiple widespread simultaneous attacks and lastly increase social disruption because of the cultural rules and expectations violated. Suicide attacks have been a tactic in violent struggles since ancient times. The effectiveness of such attacks depends upon the use of the well-trained, ideologically or religiously committed individual as a means of guiding an effective weapon to the chosen target. Such volunteers are recruited often from the young and ideological and not, as often assumed, from the disadvantaged. The effectiveness of suicide attacks – of human beings as deadly delivery systems – depends in part upon the ethnocentric and ill-conceived belief that people involved in deadly quarrels prefer self-survival to destruction of hated enemy, and the delivery of highly valued messages about the worthiness of their cause or belief. The willingness to sacrifice one's life demonstrates *sui*

generis that the cause is worthy of the ultimate commitment.

Suicide attacks have been utilized by national militaries in war (e.g., Japanese kamikaze and plans by Nazi Germany to attack New York City) and secular insurgents (e.g., Tamil Tiger assassination of Rajiv Gandhi). While the tactic is identified by many as a tool of Muslim extremists (e.g., Al Qaeda, Hamas and Hezbollah) it has been utilized by secular groups (e.g., Tamil Tigers) as well as religious groups. Its usefulness to terrorists who may not have access to sophisticated guidance systems is obvious. The sacrifice of the attacker may excite the interest of the community that supports the beliefs of the terrorist and enable the terrorist group to recruit and to raise funds to support them. However, armies as well as terrorist groups have long recognized the value of sending well-motivated well-trained soldiers on missions that will deliver destruction to the enemy but will not afford an opportunity for survival. The nerve gas attack in Tokyo and the attacks of September 11, as well as numerous other examples, illustrate that such tactics can be used to deliver WMD of several types (Atran, 2003).

Suicidal attackers may be of any gender, or come from a wide variety of cultural, political, and religious backgrounds. They are seldom psychiatrically ill. They require a good deal of psychological and material group support to carry out their mission. They must believe that the mission they are given is of critical importance and have the skills and commitment to carry it out. They may use various modes of transport and subterfuge to reach their target. The dramatic nature of their action nearly always interests the media (Cronin, 2003).

The primary goal of terrorism is to create terror. This simple but often forgotten element means that the target of terrorism is not only those who are killed, injured, or even directly affected. The target is an entire nation. Therefore, there are three populations of concern for mental health professionals: (1) those directly exposed, who may become ill with post-traumatic stress disorder

(PTSD), depression, and alcohol use; (2) those who were vulnerable before the event and now must manage their lives with fewer resources (for example, the loss of child care or a much longer commute) – such losses of social supports may tip the vulnerable over the edge into illness; and (3) the potentially millions who experience an altered sense of safety and hypervigilance. All three of these populations require care but the tools for reaching the different groups and their needs are different.

Weapons of mass destruction

Although there have been thousands of terrorist attacks throughout the world using conventional weapons, the use of WMD – in particular chemical and biological agents – is a relatively new phenomenon. Chemical, biological, and radiological agents can produce mass destruction, but in the future they likely will be used more commonly as weapons of mass disruption. These weapons can be used in a manner that produces relatively few fatalities but that produces substantial psychological, social, and economic harm (Hyams *et al.*, 2002). The term *chemical, biological, radiological, nuclear, and high-yield explosive* (CBRNE) agents is now used by many to designate the agents of interest without conjecture about their impact.

CBRN agents (that is, CBRNE agents excluding explosives) possess a number of unique characteristics that make them especially effective at creating terror. Conventional weapons produce immediate and tangible health consequences. In the immediate aftermath of a CBRN attack, however, one often cannot determine whether or not one has been injured. Most CBRN agents are invisible and odorless. Many produce delayed illness and can be detected only by the use of special equipment.

These weapons have special psychological implications because they are imperceptible. The experience of feeling threatened or safe depends heavily on the information provided by the government and scientific experts. Most of this information is obtained through the mass media. Risk communication and news coverage revealing the relative efficacy of the efforts to manage consequences of a CBRN attack play a central role in how groups and individuals react: whether or not they perceive themselves at high or minimal risk, whether they have confidence in the government and medical response, and their determination of what protective actions should be taken.

The medical community and society in general have little experience with illnesses caused by these agents. This lack of familiarity heightens fear and apprehension, because it can be difficult to predict who will become ill and how the illness will evolve, especially when agents found in nature may have been modified.

These weapons are characterized by their potent traumatic stressors, which are associated with increased psychiatric morbidity. Some agents produce disfiguration, which amplifies fear and increases the psychological impact of the weapons. For example, the burns caused by vesicant agents such as mustard gas and the pustules resulting from smallpox are disquieting. Threat to life has been shown to be one of the most potent of psychological stressors, and all of these weapons have the potential to create morbidity and mortality on a grand scale. For many of these agents, the availability of medical treatment is limited, and in many cases the effectiveness of treatment is uncertain because of the possibility that the agent has been modified. Biological agents that can be transmitted from person to person, such as those that cause plague and smallpox, can create widespread fear and anxiety because of rapid and broad dissemination in an age of global travel.

The weapons of terrorism also evolve. The novelty this produces can itself increase terror. Suicide bombings, shoes that explode, and trucks carrying high explosives create new hypervigilance. The use of jetliners as tools of terror as in September 11 was especially effective because it entailed the novel use of the familiar and the element of surprise.

Although high-yield explosives produce physical effects similar to those of conventional explosives, the psychological and social consequences are increased by an order of magnitude. The September 11 attacks on the World Trade Center in particular, because of the scale of destruction and the large numbers of dead, had profound consequences, not just for those directly affected, but internationally. The London and Madrid bombings, although with less explosive power, magnified their community disruptive power by targeting normal and "expected to be safe" modes of transportation for everyday life.

CBRNE agents are special forms of disasters. They raise new and important considerations in first aid, triage, management of contaminated casualties, movement restrictions or evacuation, and separation from loved ones with shelter in place (DiGiovanni, 1999; Pfefferbaum & Pfefferbaum, 1998; Ursano et al., 1995). Mental health providers require familiarity with these public health interventions and their roles in support of them (see Table 12.1). In addition, understanding the psychological and behavioral responses of adults and children to these threats and requirements for safety is generally new and not familiar to mental healthcare providers and planners.

Table 12.1 Roles of mental healthcare providers in CBRNE

- Community consultation for preparedness
- Hospital disaster response planning
- Consultation to leadership
- School system preparedness
- Triage patients
- Consultation to healthcare providers
- Consultation to first responders
- Educate and advise media communication
- Identify high-risk groups for surveillance and intervention
- Treat acute and longer term psychiatric sequelae
- Manage behavioral responses to public health interventions

Psychiatric morbidity in the wake of events involving CBRNE agents

Terrorist attacks using conventional weapons such as guns and bombs have well-known psychiatric sequelae. PTSD was seen in roughly half of the patients 6 months after the 1987 Enniskillen bombing in Northern Ireland (Curran et al., 1990). In a study of French survivors of terrorist attacks, 18% of survivors were diagnosed with PTSD and 13% with major depression (Abenhaim et al., 1992). In a study of direct survivors of the Oklahoma City bombing in the United States, 34% had PTSD and 22% had major depression; 55% had no diagnosis, and nearly 40% of those with PTSD and depression had no previous psychiatric illness. The incidence of new cases of illness in those with no previous diagnosis is highest in those directly exposed (North et al., 1999).

Like other kinds of disasters, it is expected that events involving CBRNE agents will result in psychiatric morbidity for some. People who are directly exposed may experience psychological distress. In addition, because of the uncertainty regarding who has been exposed and who may be attacked next; many unexposed individuals may also experience such distress. For most, these acute psychological reactions will resolve over time. However, for some, the reactions will not resolve and instead develop into symptoms of psychiatric disorders. Acute stress disorder (ASD), PTSD, depression, phobias, alcohol and nicotine abuse, and complicated bereavement will likely be encountered, as will somatic concerns.

For most individuals, post-traumatic psychiatric symptoms following CBRNE terrorism are transitory. These early symptoms usually respond to receiving education, obtaining enough rest, and maintaining biological rhythms (e.g., sleeping at the same time, eating at the same time). Media exposure can be both reassuring and threatening. Limiting such exposure can minimize the disturbing effects, especially in children (Pfefferbaum et al., 2001). Providing education to spouses and significant others of those distressed can help in treatment as well as in identifying the worsening or persistence of symptoms. Those who are indirectly exposed to ongoing threats of terrorism may experience significant symptoms (Shalev *et al.*, 2006).

Post-traumatic stress disorder is not uncommon after terrorist events. Acute stress disorder and early PTSD may be more like the common cold – experienced at some time in life by nearly all. If they persist, they can be debilitating and require psychotherapeutic and pharmacological intervention. However, PTSD is neither the only trauma-related disorder nor even perhaps the most common (Fullerton & Ursano, 1997; Norris, 2002; North *et al.*, 1999; Ursano, 2002). People exposed to terrorism are at increased risk for developing depression, generalized anxiety disorder, panic disorder, and increased substance use (Breslau *et al.*, 1991; Kessler *et al.*, 1995; North *et al.*, 1999, 2002). After a terrorist event, the contribution of the psychological factors to medical illness can also be pervasive – from heart disease (Leor *et al.*, 1996) to diabetes (Jacobson, 1996). It is important to note that injured survivors often have psychological factors affecting their physical condition (Kulka *et al.*, 1990; North *et al.*, 1999; Shore *et al.*, 1989; Smith *et al.*, 1990; Zatzick *et al.*, 2001).

Traumatic bereavement (Prigerson *et al.*, 1999; Shear *et al.*, 2005); unexplained somatic symptoms (Engel & Katon, 1999; Ford, 1997; McCarroll *et al.*, 2002); depression (Kessler *et al.*, 1999); sleep disturbance; increased alcohol, caffeine, and cigarette use (Shalev *et al.*, 1990); and family conflict and family violence are not uncommon after traumatic events. Anger, disbelief, sadness, anxiety, fear, and irritability are expected responses. In each, the role of exposure to the traumatic event may be easily overlooked by a primary-care physician. Anxiety and family conflict can accompany the fear and distress of new terrorist alerts, toxic contamination, and the economic impact of lost jobs and company closure or relocation. Medical evaluation that includes inquiring about family conflict can provide reassurance, can begin a discussion for referral, and can be a primary preventive intervention for

Table 12.2 CBRN: areas of special concern

- Overwhelming of medical facilities
- Mass sociogenic illness
- Panic
- Responses of hospital staff and first responders

children whose first experience of a disaster or terrorist attack is mediated through their parents.

Behavioral responses to CBRN agents: areas of special concern

Behavioral responses to CBRN agents represent several areas of special concern including the overwhelming of medical facilities, mass sociogenic illness, panic and responses of hospital staff and first responders (see Table 12.2).

Overwhelming of medical facilities

Case example 1

After Iraq's invasion of Kuwait in 1990, Israeli officials began to prepare the public for missile attacks. Gas masks and autoinjectors of antidotes against nerve gas were distributed to the entire population (Karsenty *et al.*, 1991). Israelis were advised to select a room in their homes and seal all its openings except an entrance door (Karsenty *et al.*, 1991). The population was instructed to enter the sealed room and put on their gas masks if an alarm was sounded. Residents had between 4 and 5 min of warning between the sounding of the missile alarm and any impact. Between January 18 & February 28, 1991, there were 23 missile attack alerts, of which 5 proved to be false alarms. A total of 39 Iraqi missiles landed in Israel. A total of 1059 people presented to Israeli emergency rooms in response to the alarms (including false alarms). Of these, 234 individuals (22%) were direct casualties of the missile explosions (232 people injured and 2 killed by the missile explosions), and the remaining 78% were behavioral and psychiatric casualties. These indirect casualties included 544 patients (51%) with acute anxiety; 230 patients (22%) who had autoinjected atropine without exposure to agent; 40 (4%) who were injured while running to the sealed rooms; and 11 who died (1%) – 7 who suffocated due to leaving the filter closed on their gas masks and 4 who died of intercurrent myocardial infarctions (Karsenty *et al.*, 1991). The number of patients presenting with anxiety or unnecessary injections of atropine were highest after the initial missile attack alarms and decreased over time (Karsenty *et al.*, 1991). Another finding was that psychological reactions were found to be almost twice as high when the patient was alone or with only one other person in the sealed room (Karsenty *et al.*, 1991). The use of a bedroom as the sealed room was also associated with a lower frequency of psychological reactions (Karsenty *et al.*, 1991). The Israeli experience with the threat of the use of chemical weapons is consonant with the Japanese findings of substantial symptoms of anxiety and autonomic arousal following actual exposure or belief of exposure to chemical weapons.

Case example 2

The Aum Shinrikyo cult launched two successful attacks using sarin gas. In June 1994, sarin was used in Matsumoto, Japan, resulting in 7 deaths and more than 200 injuries. On March 20, 1995, 5 2-person teams placed plastic pouches hidden in newspapers on three subway lines that were converging at major subway stations in Tokyo (Tucker, 1996). The pouches contained liquid sarin, an organophosphate nerve agent, which evaporated slowly after the terrorists punctured the bags with sharpened umbrella tips (Tucker, 1996). Passengers overcome by the fumes exited trains at 16 different stations along the three subway lines (Tucker, 1996). The attack killed 11 people (passengers, firefighters, subway workers, and police

officers) and resulted in more than 5500 casualties (Bowler *et al.*, 2001; Ohbu *et al.*, 1997). In total, 1046 people were admitted to 98 different hospitals because of visual symptoms, nausea, headache, cough, dyspnea, cardiac symptoms, and neuropathy (Bowler *et al.*, 2001).

Events involving CBRN agents highlight the importance of the psychology of individual risk perception and how decisions to seek medical evaluation are made. Conventional terrorist weapons, such as explosives or guns, produce immediate and visible health consequences. Healthcare systems have a great deal of experience in managing these incidents on a small scale. There is little direct experience in the management of CBRN terrorism in the United States.

Based on the experiences in Israel and Japan, there is a concern that medical facilities may be initially overwhelmed by people seeking care, many of whom will not have actually been exposed. Belief that one has been exposed leads to the seeking of healthcare. One of the commonalities among events involving CBRN agents is the high proportion of people seeking medical assistance who are concerned that they have been exposed, but for whom no etiology for their symptoms is found. In Tokyo, for example, a very high proportion of the 5000 patients who sought care were not admitted and had no signs of exposure (Ohbu *et al.*, 1997). Many misattributed the signs and symptoms of anxiety and autonomic arousal to intoxication by sarin.

The rapid influx of noninjured as well as injured patients is a major concern, because the number of patients may overwhelm capacity. Triage to distinguish those who may be distressed from those who are injured is a critical first step in emergency care. Planners have struggled to devise a nonpejorative term to describe individuals who fear that they are ill but prove not to be. This group has been referred to using terms such as *psychological casualties*, *the worried well*, and other terms that are stigmatizing. The use of terms such as these may result in inappropriate care, for example determining through triage that individuals are psychological casualties before performing an adequate medical assessment.

Mass sociogenic illness

Case example 3

In 1987 in Goiânia, Brazil, two individuals who were scavenging for items to sell removed approximately 20 g (1500 Ci) of cesium-137 from an old radio-therapy machine in an abandoned medical clinic. The machine was taken apart at the shop of a local junk dealer. The isotope attracted attention because it glowed in the dark, and it was given to friends and family members in the immediate vicinity (Collins & Bandeira de Carvalho, 1993). A total of 249 people were contaminated internally or externally, and 4 died. All were relatives or neighbors of those who lived near the yard where the source had been disassembled or were employees or owners of the two junkyards to which pieces of the teletherapy unit had been taken (Brandao-Mello *et al.*, 1991). Only those people in the four-block epicenter were exposed to radiation (Collins & Bandeira de Carvalho, 1993), yet approximately 113 000 Goiânia residents (10% of the city) sought screening. Of interest in planning triage, 11% of the 113 000 exhibited classic symptoms of radiation exposure (nausea, reddened skin, etc.) before being assessed (Collins, 2002). After they were given a clean bill of health, their symptoms dissipated within a few hours (Collins, 2002).

The occurrence of mass sociogenic illness in the wake of an attack with CBRN agents is a major concern for planners, who worry about the strain it will place on an already overburdened medical system. Mass sociogenic illness, also referred to as mass psychogenic illness and epidemic hysteria, is a social phenomenon in which two or more people share beliefs about a constellation of symptoms for which no identifiable etiology can be found (Boss, 1997). This illness is typically triggered by an environmental event, often an odor or perceived odor, for which there is a robust emergency response. Individuals with unexplained symptoms

attribute their illness to the environmental incident. These epidemics involve otherwise healthy people. In some instances, there may be group members with actual illness who are witnessed by individuals who then develop similar symptoms but without demonstrable pathology. Outbreaks of mass socio-genic illness have been reported after nuclear and chemical releases, incidents of excessive smog, and contamination of a water supply (Boss, 1997). In the wake of September 11 and in a climate of fear of additional attacks, a series of outbreaks of mass sociogenic illness were reported. On September 29, 2001, paint fumes in a Washington state middle school triggered a bioterrorism scare in which 16 students and 1 teacher were medically evaluated (Wessely *et al.*, 2001). On October 3, 2001, rumors of bioterrorism received on a short text service prompted more than 1000 students in Manila, Philippines, to deluge clinics with complaints of flu-like symptoms (Wessely *et al.*, 2001). Outbreaks of itchy red rashes that have occurred in more than two dozen elementary and middle schools across the United States since fall 2001 are also thought to represent mass sociogenic illness (Talbot, 2002).

Panic

The word *panic* is often used to describe psychological responses to terrorism involving CBRNE agents. *Panic* refers primarily to a group phenomenon in which intense, contagious fear causes individuals to think only of themselves. They become paralyzed by fear or seek escape by any means necessary – "every man for himself." *Panic* also refers to an individual response that is characterized by the loss of rational thought due to overwhelming terror. A major goal of preparation for and response to events involving CBRNE agents is the prevention of panic and the preservation of individual, group, and community function.

Although panic does occur after disasters, it is rare (Aguirre, 2005; Mawson, 2005). Surprise and novelty are risk factors for panic. Other factors include the belief that there is a small chance of escape; seeing oneself as being at high risk of becoming ill; limited resources that are available on a first-come, first-served basis; a perceived lack of effective management of the catastrophe; and loss of credibility by authorities (Holloway *et al.*, 1997).

The assumption that people will panic or become irrational after an attack with CBRNE agents has negative consequences. At times, authorities have provided inaccurate information and unfounded reassurances across a wide range of emergencies, including the recent anthrax attacks, motivated in part by a wish to calm the public. Ultimately, however, misleading statements and lying undermine credibility and contribute to even greater fear. The panic myth may also lead to neglect of the public's role in planning and responding to these events and missed opportunities to capitalize on the resourcefulness of non-professionals and civic organizations (Glass & Schoch-Spana, 2002). The community helps itself and gains psychological well being by its self actions to respond and recover.

Responses of hospital staff and first responders

In the United States, medical professionals have little experience in managing casualties resulting from releases of chemical, radiological, and biological agents. In the short term, physicians and other health professionals may experience fear, shock, anger, helplessness, and worries about their families and friends. Absenteeism is a major concern. In the 1994 outbreak of pneumonic plague in Surat, India, for example, 80% of the private physicians fled the city (Garrett, 2000). An anonymous survey was conducted on the 41st day of the Persian Gulf War in 42% of Israeli general hospitals. The questionnaire presented a scenario in which a spokesman for the Israel Defense Forces has announced that there has been a chemical warfare missile attack and has requested that hospital personnel report to duty. Questionnaires were distributed among all levels of hospital staff: 42% indicated that they would be willing to return to work (Shapira *et al.*, 1991). For those unwilling to

return to work, 75% cited concerns about personal safety as their primary reason (Shapira *et al.*, 1991). Demoralization is also a concern if there are high mortality rates and an inability to provide adequate care for advanced illness. Familiarity with chemical and biological agents and training before the attack may enhance performance by the medical staff and help prevent breakdown. A realistic and well-rehearsed plan for dealing with events involving CBRNE agents will also help minimize feelings of helplessness and guilt about matters that could have gone more smoothly. Mental health consultation to hospital personnel can help ameliorate short-term distress and sustain functioning. Noncompliance with guidelines for use of personal protective equipment can create a significant health problem after CBRNE attacks (Fullerton & Ursano, 1990).

Risk communication

Enlisting the cooperation and participation of the public after a WMD attack is a goal of public education and risk communication in particular. Multiple studies confirm that people assess risk and threat based on their feelings of control and their level of knowledge and familiarity with an event (MacGregor & Fleming, 1996). Therefore, peanut butter is not sufficiently recognized as a risk to health and air travel is seen as overly risky (Slovic, 1987). In addition people can only learn or understand a small amount of information at a time and have difficulty understanding any additive effects of risk. Widespread fear, uncertainty, and stigmatization are common after terrorist attacks and disasters. These fears require education about the actual risk and instruction in how to decrease risk, whether the risk is falling buildings in an earthquake or infection from a biological weapon. Instruction in active coping techniques can increase feelings of control and efficacy. In particular, fears of biological contagion or exposure to other contaminants can decrease community cohesion and can turn neighbor against neighbor as one tries to feel safe by identifying those who are exposed or ill as "not me."

The fear of exposure to toxic agents – including biological, chemical, and radiologic agents – can lead hundreds or even thousands to seek care, overwhelming hospitals and the healthcare system. Belief that one has been exposed to chemical and biological weapons leads individuals to seek healthcare and to change life patterns regardless of actual exposure.

Clear, accurate, timely, and consistent information exchange is needed between healthcare professionals, government and local leaders, and the general public in times of a disaster. The public wants to know and can best join in response and recovery when they are told what is known, what is not known, what is being done and when they will hear more information (U.S. Department of Health and Human Services, 2002). For medical and public health care professionals, explaining and describing risk is probably the most challenging situation for communicating with nonscientists. Key challenges include difficulties in translating scientific information, conflicts in risks and messages, and disagreements on the extent of the risk and how it should be assessed. Physicians have the ears of their community in their medical offices, at schools and community functions, and through the media; therefore, they are an important natural network for educating about risk and prevention.

Medical and behavioral health personnel should participate in the development of public information plans. Information from official and unofficial sources before, during, and after a disaster will shape expectations, behaviors, and emotional responses (Holloway et al., 1997). The delivery of consistent, updated information across multiple channels by way of widely recognized and trusted sources diminishes the extent to which misinformation can shape public attribution (Peters et al., 1997).

Special issues associated with bioterrorism

Healthcare providers and the healthcare system are first responders in bioterrorism events. Bioterrorism differs from natural disasters in a number of fundamental ways. The microbial world is invisible and mysterious, and it can be frightening and unknown to many, including leaders, members of the media, and the general public. Bioterrorism is an act of human malice intended to injure and kill civilians and is associated with a higher rate of psychiatric morbidity than are so-called acts of God. A hurricane is usually an isolated event with consequences. Bioterrorism – due to the incubation period of microorganisms, and evolving echoes of exposure, fear, and possible spread of contagion – is a process trauma with consequences spread widely over time. In addition, there is the threat of further attacks, announced or covert. Bioterrorism is unbounded by time and space. Global travel can spread infected, asymptomatic individuals widely and quickly. The agents responsible for infectious diseases cannot be discerned by the unaided senses, which creates uncertainty and a sense of vulnerability and fear.

Bioterrorism can produce unfamiliar diseases that present challenges in diagnosis and treatment. The modern medical community has limited experience with the diseases produced by bioterrorism agents such as anthrax and the smallpox virus. Naturally occurring outbreaks of infection may be difficult to distinguish from intentional attacks. Patient presentations and the at-risk populations differ in a terrorist attack from naturally occurring outbreaks because of the different routes of dissemination and possibly altered microorganisms.

Quarantine, movement restrictions, forced evacuation, mandatory vaccination, and mandated treatment would curtail many civil liberties. In addition, the belief that one has been exposed to a toxic or infectious agent determines healthcare seeking, not actual exposure. After the anthrax attacks on the United States capitol about 31% of those not in the "hot zone," i.e., the contaminated area where exposure was possible, thought they had been exposed (North, 2005). In contrast, nearly 46% of those who were placed in prophylactic antibiotic treatment for anthrax failed to complete the entire course of treatment (Reissman *et al.*, 2004).

The tendency to use draconian measures increases as fear and anxiety increase. The demand for these actions as well as the failure to use them may contribute to community conflict and erode the public's confidence in the government. Careful analysis of the costs (including social costs) and benefits of these measures is needed.

Fear of contagion can have devastating consequences for all aspects of daily life after a bioterrorism event. The result may be that some communities become isolated and unable to obtain food and supplies. The lack of personnel due to infection or fear of infection can cripple basic community functions and financial institutions. After one year more than half of those who sustained an anthrax infection had not returned to work and showed increased psychological symptoms (Reissman *et al.*, 2004).

It is important to realize that the economic and mental health impacts of bioterrorism occur in different sequences and phases than they do in natural disasters. Fear of contamination (warranted or unwarranted) creates second- and third-order effects such as the collapse of tourism and the flight of businesses soon after an event. Terrorist attacks will specifically target basic societal infrastructure such as transportation, mail delivery, and communication.

For all of these reasons, the mental health and behavioral effects of bioterrorism present substantial challenges for the healthcare system. The public health and mental health infrastructures have eroded to the point that they can barely meet requirements under normal circumstances. Many hospitals run short of beds during an average flu season. Ambulances are frequently diverted from urban emergency departments that have reached capacity. Changes in healthcare delivery have resulted in fewer hospital beds and just-in-time inventories, which have severely limited surge capacity for mass casualty events. Clinical care has been degraded because of the focus on episodic care rather than infrastructure development. The nationwide nursing shortage also hampers effective responses. The limited availability of treatment resources such as vaccines and antibiotics is also an impediment to a successful medical response to bioterrorism and to decreasing fear and anxiety. Normal care for hospital patients will necessarily be critically modified in a major bioterrorism attack, and elective treatments will be suspended entirely. Emergency care will be provided using a triage model that maximizes the efficient provision of care and bed utilization.

If contagious agents are used, many hospitals may have to close their doors to noninfected patients needing emergent care. Absenteeism can result from the conflicted loyalties of the hospital staff, divided between caring for their own families and taking care of patients. Developing plans to ensure that employees' families are cared for in the wake of a bioterrorism attack may diminish this absenteeism. Hospital bioterrorism response plans require provisions for supporting staff and for managing both expected and unexpected volunteers. Hospital staff, police, and security personnel must be prepared to manage secure access to the hospital.

Sophisticated terrorists will understand that the agents that cause diseases in livestock and agriculture constitute important weapons that can produce devastating economic and psychological consequences. As seen in the United Kingdom, foot-and-mouth disease can rapidly spread to livestock in a wide geographic region, resulting in millions of dollars of losses. Bioterrorism attacks on livestock and agriculture will disproportionately affect the mental health of rural populations. Recent experiences with depopulation and carcass disposal after the outbreak of foot-and-mouth disease in the United Kingdom underscore the importance of integrating mental health into the veterinary response. Agricultural preparedness and response should specifically incorporate psychological and behavioral expertise. For example, an important mental health preventive intervention can be working with veterinarians to encourage farmers and ranchers to freeze genetic materials so that important strains of plants and animals can be rebuilt after bioterrorism or a natural outbreak of disease. Mental health outreach to farmers and ranchers can be critical in coping with the losses caused by a bioterrorism attack.

Mental health intervention is a prompt and effective medical response to a bioterrorism attack. Early detection, successful management of casualties, and effective treatments bolster the public's sense of safety and increase confidence in institutions. Because the overriding goal of terrorism is to change people's beliefs, sense of safety, and behaviors, mental health experts are an essential part of planning and responding.

After a bioterrorism attack, the mental health needs of three populations are of concern: (1) those who are directly exposed and develop traditional psychiatric disorders, (2) those with pre-existing mental illness that may be reactivated or exacerbated, and (3) those with limited support systems and resources (see Figure 12.1). The traditional airplane crash and natural disaster models of providing mental health services have limited applicability in bioterrorism. New models of monitoring shifting community mental health needs in real time, as well as innovative models for delivering care, are required. In these extreme environments, the use of telephone conferences, video teleconferences, and other technologies for providing mental health intervention can conserve limited resources and diminish disease transmission. Experts should help determine the skills needed for effective mental health preventive strategies and interventions. These skills can then be taught and refreshed across the medical training and education levels.

Communication, a core principle of mental health and behavioral care, is central to consequence management after a bioterrorism attack. The initial detection of disease begins a period of uncertainty in which the source of exposure, the scope of the outbreak, the number of people exposed, and the possibility of other agents being used are not fully known. The public's primary concern is about safety. Because biological agents are imperceptible, the public actively seeks information to gauge whether they are at risk and what steps they can take to protect themselves. There is a pressing need to hold repeated retreats with journalists, risk communication experts, and infectious disease specialists to craft consistent and practical educational messages for the public. These retreats can facilitate candid exchanges and establish ongoing relationships critical to responding effectively to a bioterrorism attack. These meetings can develop a common strategy for controlling the spread of false rumors, scapegoating, and conspiratorial theories.

Public mental health response to pandemic flu

Since the highly lethal pandemic outbreak of influenza in 1918, there have been only a few global threats from infectious agents. SARS and avian influenza have brought worldwide attention to the possibility of a pandemic spreading across the globe. The outbreaks of SARS in Asia and Canada, which caused global concern but fortunately did not result in large-scale outbreaks or a global pandemic, gives us the most recent data on the mental health concerns that are relevant in a pandemic outbreak situation.

The migration of animals – birds in the case of Avian flu – and people are a growing public health

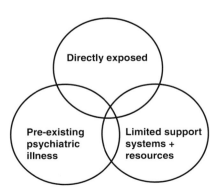

Figure 12.1 Populations at risk

concern. The mobility of people in the modern world is one of the major vectors for the rapid spread of any infectious agent. For example at the time of the Hajj each year in the 12th month of the Islamic (lunar) calendar, over one million people travel to Mecca – nearly half from non Arab countries. Similarly, for the smaller ritual Umrah, over 2.5 million traveled in 2004 to Mecca. This mass migration raises potential for major public health and infection control problems (Ahmed *et al.*, 2006). Other times of human migration – holidays and vacations – and the "human migratory patterns" are routes of transmission.

In the SARS outbreak nearly 40% of the community population experienced increased stress in family and work settings during the outbreak; 16% showed signs of traumatic stress; and high percentages of the population felt helpless, apprehensive, and horrified by the outbreak (McAlonan *et al.*, 2005). About 30% of the community thought they would contract SARS, while only a quarter believed they would survive if they contracted the disease, despite an actual survival rate of 80% or more. Such a high rate of perceived risk might have preceded widespread distress and disruption had the outbreak been either more widespread or more lethal (Lau *et al.*, 2005). Community residents were diligent in adopting person-to-person transmission precautions. However, precautions were adopted differentially based upon anxiety levels and perceived risk of contracting the disease, indicating the importance of stress and anxiety, as well as baseline mental health, on the public's response willingness and ability to take necessary precautions (Lau *et al.*, 2005).

Front-line health workers may be particularly vulnerable to negative mental health sequelae of treating outbreak victims. Nurses who treated SARS patients reported high levels of stress and about 11% had traumatic stress reactions, including depression, anxiety, hostility and somatization symptoms (Chen *et al.*, 2005).

While there have been relatively few large outbreaks in recent times to inform an appropriate response to a potentially pandemic flu, the exist-

Table 12.3 Similarities and differences in WMD, natural disaster, and pandemic

Dimension	WMD[a]	Natural disaster[b]	Pandemic[c]
Altered sense of safety	++++	+++	++++
Intentional	+++		
Unpredictable	+++	++	++
Localized geographically		+++	
Local fear	+++	+++	+++
National fear	+++		+++
National bereavement	+++	+	+++
Consequences spread over time	+++	++	+++
Loss of confidence in institutions	+++	+	+++
Community disruption	+++	+++	+++
Target basic societal infrastructure	+++		
Overwhelm healthcare systems	++++	+++	+++
Hoaxes/copycats	+++		

[a] WMD – chemical, biological, radiologic, nuclear, explosive.
[b] Natural disaster, e.g., hurricanes, tornados, earthquakes.
[c] Pandemic – infectious epidemic that is not localized and can span the globe.

ing data on infectious disease outbreaks, data from WMD, natural disasters, and public mental health principles can be brought to bear on the planning for a response (see Table 12.3). Public mental health measures must address numerous areas of potential distress, health risk behaviors, and psychiatric disease. In anticipation of significant disruption and loss, promoting health protective behaviors and health response behaviors is imperative. Special attention is needed for: (1) risk communication; (2) safety communication through public/private collaboration; (3) psychological, emotional, and behavioral responses to public education, public health surveillance and early detection efforts; (4) psychological responses to community containment strategies (quarantine, movement restrictions, school/work/other community closures); (5) healthcare service surge and continuity; and (6) responses to mass prophylaxis strategies using vaccines and antiviral medication.

Response to a pandemic flu outbreak is divided into four phases: preparedness, early outbreak response, later response and recovery, and mental health intervention planning. The first step in fostering health enhancing psychological, emotional, and behavioral responses is an effective public health program of risk assessment and communication, public health prevention measures, and consequence management. These require effective political and community leadership, appropriate pre-event organization, and staffing and funding.

The inter-relationship between psychological, emotional, and behavioral responses and the other elements of the response plan is important to consider. While planning can be based on the assumption that public health efforts will be successful, planning for failure, e.g., failure mode analysis, is critical to enable behavioral and consequence management for all outcomes. Community and behavioral crisis can result from lack of support and services, absence of a vaccine and ineffective therapies.

Preparedness for pandemic

Preparedness for a pandemic includes educating the public, preparation of leadership, and sustaining preparedness and training leadership. Public education must begin before a pandemic occurs, and be embedded in existing disaster public education campaigns, resources, and initiatives (e.g., Department of Homeland Security, www.ready. gov, Red Cross, CDC public education and preparedness www.hhs.gov/pandemicflu/plan/, and Health and Human Services www.pandemicflu. gov). Education focuses on facts, including what is known, what is not known, and how individuals, communities, and organizations can prepare for a potential outbreak. Public education can alter threat awareness, e.g., "Is there a risk to me?",

threat assessment, e.g., "How great is the risk to me?", and preparedness behaviors in every phase of an event. Public education in advance of an outbreak addresses various threats, those of low risk and those of high risk.

Leadership preparation includes understanding which members of the population will be most vulnerable and who will need the highest level of health services, including mental health services. This will include those at greatest risk for problems related to contagion, such as those with psychiatric illness, children, elderly, homeless, and those with losses, who must be considered when planning.

If responses are under-supported and fail, the community anger and lowered morale may complicate the ability of a community to respond to an outbreak, as well as recover once an outbreak has ended. Sustaining preparedness requires maintaining motivation, capital assets, equipment, and funding in order to continue preparedness efforts over the long term, not just to focus on immediate needs.

Planning leadership functions requires identifying community leaders, spokespersons, and natural emergent leaders who can affect community and individual behaviors and who can endorse and model protective health behaviors. It is often forgotten that the workplace is a resource as well as a population at risk. Corporations have public education resources to reach large populations. The media and celebrity groups are also important leaders in most modern societies and have a critical role in providing communication.

Early pandemic response

Communication and information dissemination are important first responses to an actual or believed pandemic outbreak of infectious disease. Wide dissemination of uncomplicated, empathically informed information on normal stress reactions can serve to normalize reactions and emphasize hope, resilience, and natural recovery. Recommendations to prevent exposure, infection, or halt disease transmission may be met with skepticism, hope, and fear. These responses vary based on the individuals' and the local community's past experiences with government agencies. In addition, compliance with recommendations for vaccination or medication treatment or prophylaxis will vary greatly and will not be complete. The media can either amplify skepticism or promote a collaborative approach. Interactions with the media will be both challenging and critical. The public must clearly and repeatedly be informed about the rationale and mechanism for distribution of limited supplies (e.g., Tamiflu®). Leadership will find it difficult but extremely important to adhere to policies regarding such distribution. Abuses of policy will undercut public safety and public adherence to other government risk-reduction recommendations.

Tipping points, events which dramatically increase or decrease fear and helpful or health-risk behaviors, will occur. Deaths of important or particularly vulnerable individuals (e.g., children), new unexpected and unknown risk factors, and shortages of treatments are typical tipping points. The behavioral importance of community rituals (e.g., speeches, memorial services, funerals, collection campaigns, television specials) can help manage community-wide distress and loss.

The public health system must be prepared for surges in demands for healthcare, especially in the early stages of a pandemic. Those who believe they have been exposed (but actually have not) may and often do outnumber those exposed. The care demand can quickly overwhelm a community's medical response capacity. Planning for the psychological and behavioral responses which accompany the health demand surge, the community responses to shortages, and the early behavioral interventions after identification of the pandemic and prior to availability of vaccines are important to public health preparedness.

Later pandemic response and recovery

Later response and recovery includes sustaining and rebuilding community function. Community social supports – formal and informal – are very important. Providing tasks for community action can supplement needed work resources, decrease helplessness and instill optimism. In-person social supports may be hampered by the need to limit movement or contact due to concerns of contagion. Virtual contact – via web, telephone, television, and radio – will be particularly important at these times. At other times local gathering places – religious, schools, post offices, and shops – can be points of access for education, training, and distribution. As much as reasonable, instilling a sense of normalcy can be effective in fostering resiliency. This includes planning for return to work, and for children to school, when conditions allow. In addition, observing rituals and engaging in regular activities can decrease community and organizational distress and untoward behaviors. Keeping families and members of a community together is important (especially in any required relocations). If fear and anxiety persist, over time, the management of racial and social conflicts may take on added significance. Stigma and discrimination may also marginalize and isolate certain groups, thereby impeding their return to optimism, hope and access to resources.

Mass fatality and management of bodies, as well as community responses to mass deaths are difficult and challenge planners. The human aspects of mourning, ritual, religion and family are important resources to incorporate in to the logistical plan. Containment measures related to bodies may be in conflict with religious rituals of burial, and the usual process of grieving. Local officials need to be aware of the potential negative impact of disrupting normal funeral rituals and processes of grieving in order to adhere to safety precautions. Public health announcements should include (if known) how long the virus or "infection" remains in the corpse and what should be done with bodies. In a pandemic, funeral resources will be overwhelmed and mortuaries may not be willing to handle contaminated bodies. To facilitate long-term grief recovery as well as practical needs, careful identification of bodies must be ensured, and appropriate and accurate records maintained.

Table 12.4 Intervention planning for pandemic

Increase health protective and response behaviors
Plan for risk communication
Plan for safety communication
Public education for threat management and recovery
Facilitate community-directed efforts
Psychological First Aid
Care for first responders to maintain their function and
   workplace presence
Mental health surveillance

Table 12.5 Principles of Psychological First Aid

- Establish safety; identify safe areas and behaviors
- Maximize individuals ability to care for self and family and provide measures that allow individuals and families to be successful in their efforts
- Teach calming skills and maintenance of natural body rhythms (e.g., nutrition, sleep, rest, exercise)
- Maximize and facilitate connectedness to family and other social supports to the extent possible (this may require electronic rather than physical presence)
- Foster hope and optimism while not denying risk.

Mental health intervention planning for pandemic

Mental health planning for a pandemic must address basic principles (see Table 12.4). Efforts to increase health protective behaviors are a priority in planning interventions. Individuals under stress, first responders in particular and caregivers in families, need reminders to take care of their own health and limit potentially harmful behaviors. This includes taking medication, giving medications to the elderly and children, and when to go for vaccinations. Communication of risk should follow basic risk communication principles. Interactions with the media will be both critical and challenging. Good safety communication involves promoting clear, simple, and easy-to-do measures that are effective in helping individuals to protect themselves and their families.

Educating the public not only informs and prepares them, but it also enlists them as partners in the process and plan. Education and communication must address fear of contagion, danger to family and pets, and mistrust of authority and government. The tendency to expect or act as if these are not present can delay community-wide health protective behaviors. Facilitating community-directed efforts involves organizing communal needs and directing action toward tangible goals. This action-oriented, hopeful group behavior can foster the inherent community resiliency and recovery.

Using evidence-informed principles of Psychological First Aid – fostering safety, hope, connectedness, self efficacy, and calming – are important components of the response to a pandemic (see Table 12.5). First responders comprise a diverse population, from medically trained personnel to volunteers with no experience. Care must be provided to help first responders maintain their function and workplace presence. This requires ensuring the safety and care of their families.

Mental health surveillance is important for directing services and funding. This requires ongoing population-level estimates of mental health problems and determinations of who is at greatest risk. Surveillance for PTSD, depression and altered substance use as well as psychosocial needs (e.g., housing, transportation, schools, employment) and loss of critical infrastructure necessary to sustain family and community function is needed.

Conclusion

New and old disasters can now affect the world as a whole and large populations that span the globe. WMD and pandemic infection frighten people, disrupt communities and are little known or considered by most, adding to their stressful mental health burden. Planning for these types of disaster requires modifications of natural disaster plans and awareness of the importance of new and different disaster behaviors. Health-protecting and health risking behaviors, as well as psychiatric illness and distress must be planned for, anticipated, and included in field exercises and resource planning.

REFERENCES

Abenhaim, L., Dab, W. & Salmi, L.R. (1992). Study of civilian victims of terrorist attacks (France 1982–1987). *Journal of Clinical Epidemiology*, **45**, 103–109.

Aguirre, B.E. (2005). Emergency evacuations, panic and social psychology. *Psychiatry Journal of Interpersonal and Biological Processes*, **68**(2), 121–129.

Ahmed, Q.A., Arabie, Y.A. & Mernish, Z.A. (2006). Health risks at the Hajj. *The Lancet*, **367**, 1008–1115.

Atran, S. (2003). Genesis of suicide terrorism. *Science*, **299**, 1534–1539.

Boss, L.P. (1997). Epidemic hysteria: a review of the published literature. *Epidemiologic Reviews*, **19**, 233–243.

Bowler, R.M., Murai, K. & True, R.H. (2001). Update and long-term sequelae of the sarin attack in the Tokyo, Japan, subway. *Chemical Health and Safety*, **1–3**, 2001.

Brandao-Mello, C.E., Oliveria, A.R., Valverde, N.J., Farina, R. & Cordeiro, J.M. (1991). Clinical and hematological aspects of 137Cs: the Goiânia radiation accident. *Health Physics*, **60**, 31–39.

Breslau, N., Davis, G.C., Andreski, P. & Peterson, E. (1991). Traumatic events and posttraumatic stress disorder in an urban population of young adults. *Archives of General Psychiatry*, **48**, 216–222.

Chen, C.S., Wu, H.Y., Yang, P. & Yen, C.F. (2005). Psychological distress of nurses in Taiwan who worked during the outbreak of SARS. *Psychiatric Services*, **56**, 76–79.

Collins, D.L. (2002). Human responses to the threat of or exposure to ionizing radiation at Three Mile Island, Pennsylvania, and Goiânia, Brazil. *Military Medicine*, **167** [Suppl. 2], 137–138.

Collins, D.L. & Bandeira de Carvalho, A. (1993). Chronic stress from the Goiânia ^{137}Cs radiation accident. *Behavioral Medicine*, **18**, 149–157.

Cronin, A.K. (2003). *Terrorists and Suicide Attacks.* Washington, D.C.: Congressional Research Service; The Library of Congress.

Curran, P.G., Bell, P., Murray, A. *et al.* (1990). Psychological consequences of the Enniskillen bombing. *British Journal of Psychiatry*, **156**, 479–482.

DiGiovanni, C.J. (1999). Domestic terrorism with chemical or biological agents: psychiatric aspects. *American Journal of Psychiatry*, **156**, 1500–1505.

Engel, C.C. & Katon, W.J. (1999). Population and need-based prevention of unexplained symptoms in the community. In *Strategies to Protect the Health of Deployed U.S. Forces: Medical Surveillance, Record Keeping, and Risk Reduction.* Washington, D.C.: National Academy Press.

Ford, C.V. (1997). Somatic symptoms, somatization, and traumatic stress: an overview. *Nordic Journal of Psychiatry*, **51**, 5–13.

Fullerton, C.S. & Ursano, R.J. (1990). Behavioral and psychological responses to toxic exposure. *Military Medicine*, **155**, 54–59.

Fullerton, C.S. & Ursano, R.J. (1997). *Posttraumatic Stress Disorder: Acute and Long-Term Responses to Trauma and Disaster.* Washington, D.C.: American Psychiatric Press.

Garrett, L. (2000). *Betrayal of Trust: The Collapse of Global Public Health.* New York: Hyperion.

Glass, T.A. & Schoch-Spana, M. (2002). Bioterrorism and the people: how to vaccinate a city against panic. *Clinical Infectious Diseases*, **34**, 217–223.

Holloway, H.C., Norwood, A.E., Fullerton, C.S., Engel, C. C. Jr. & Ursano, R.J. (1997). The threat of biological weapons: prophylaxis and mitigation of psychological and social consequences. *Journal of the American Medical Association*, **278**, 425–427.

Hyams, K.C., Murphy, F.M. & Wessely, S. (2002). Responding to chemical, biological, or nuclear terrorism: the indirect and long-term health effects may present the greatest challenge. *Journal of Health Politics, Policy, and Law*, **27**, 273–291.

Jacobson, A.M. (1996). The psychological care of patients with insulin-dependent diabetes mellitus. *New England Journal of Medicine*, **334**, 1249–1253.

Karsenty, E., Shemer, J., Alshech, I. *et al.* (1991). Medical aspects of the Iraqi missile attacks on Israel. *Israel Journal of Medical Sciences*, **27**, 603–607.

Kessler, R.C., Sonnega, A., Bromet, E., Hughes, M. & Nelson, C.B. (1995). Posttraumatic stress disorder in the National Comorbidity Survey. *Archives of General Psychiatry*, **52**, 1048–1060.

Kessler, R.C., Barber, C., Birnbaum, H.G. *et al.* (1999). Depression in the work place: effects of short-term disability. *Health Affairs*, **18**, 163–171.

Kulka, R.A., Schlenger, W.E., Fairbank, J.A. *et al.* (1990). *Trauma and the Vietnam War Generation: Report of*

Findings from the National Vietnam Veterans Read-justment Study. New York: Brunner/Mazel.

Lau, J.T., Yang, X., Pang, E. *et al.* (2005). SARS-related perceptions in Hong Kong. *Emerging Infectious Diseases*, **11**, 417–424.

Leor, J., Poole, W.K. & Kloner, R.A. (1996). Sudden cardiac death triggered by an earthquake. *New England Journal of Medicine*, **334**, 413–419.

MacGregor, D.G. & Fleming, R. (1996). Risk perception and symptom reporting. *Risk Analysis*, **16**, 773–783.

Mawson, A.R. (2005). Understanding mass panic and other collective responses to threat and disaster. *Psychiatry Journal of Interpersonal and Biological Processes*, **68**, 95–113.

McAlonan, G.M., Lee, A.M., Cheung, V., Wong, J.W. & Chua, S.E. (2005). Psychological morbidity related to the SARS outbreak in Hong Kong. *Psychological Medicine*, **35**, 459–460.

McCarroll, J.E., Ursano, R.J., Fullerton, C.S., Liu, X. & Lundy, A. (2002). Somatic symptoms in Gulf War mortuary workers. *Psychosomatic Medicine*, **64**, 29–33.

Norris, F.H. (2002). 60,000 disaster victims speak. Part I: An empirical review of the empirical literature, 1981–2001. *Psychiatry*, **65**, 207–239.

North, C.S. (1995). Human response to violent trauma. *Baillière's Clinical Psychiatry*, **1**, 225–245.

North, C.S. (2005). Anthrax attack on the US Capital. Paper presented at Complex Global Health Conference, Italian Embassy, Washington, D.C.

North, C.S., Nixon, S.J., Shariat, S. *et al.* (1999). Psychiatric disorders among survivors of the Oklahoma City bombing. *Journal of the American Medical Association*, **282**, 755–762.

North, C.S., Tivis, L., McMillen, J.C. *et al.* (2002). Psychiatric disorders in rescue workers after the Oklahoma City bombing. *American Journal of Psychiatry*, **159**, 857–859.

Ohbu, S., Yamashina, A., Takasu, N. *et al.* (1997). Sarin poisoning on Tokyo subway. *Southern Medical Journal*, **90**, 587–593.

Peters, R.G., Covello, V.T. & McCallum, D.B. (1997). The determinants of trust and credibility in environmental risk communication: an empirical study. *Risk Analysis*, **17**, 43–54.

Pfefferbaum, B. & Pfefferbaum, R.L. (1998). Contagion in stress: an infectious disease model for posttraumatic stress in children. *Child and Adolescent Psychiatric Clinics of North America*, **7**, 183–194.

Pfefferbaum, B., Nixon, S.J., Tivis, R.D. *et al.* (2001). Television exposure in children after a terrorist incident. *Psychiatry*, **64**, 202–211.

Prigerson, H.G., Shear, M.K., Jacobs, S.C. *et al.* (1999). Consensus criteria for traumatic grief: a preliminary empirical test. *British Journal of Psychiatry*, **174**, 67–73.

Reissman, D.B., Whitney, E.A., Taylor, T.H. Jr. *et al.* (2004). One-year health assessment of adult survivors of *Bacillus anthracis* infection. *Journal of the American Medical Association*, **291**, 1994–1998.

Shalev, A.Y., Bleich, A. & Ursano, R.J. (1990). Posttraumatic stress disorder: somatic comorbidity and effort tolerance. *Psychosomatics*, **31**, 197–203.

Shalev, A., Tuval, R., Frenkiel-Fishman, S., Hadar, H. & Eth, S. (2006). Psychological responses to continuous terror: a study of two communities in Israel. *American Journal of Psychiatry*, **163**, 667–673.

Shapira, Y., Marganitt, B., Roziner, I. *et al.* (1991). Willingness of staff to report to their hospital duties following an unconventional missile attack: a state-wide survey. *Israel Journal of Medical Sciences*, **27**, 704–711.

Shear, K., Frank, E., Houck, P.R. & Reynolds, C.F. (2005). Treatment of complicated grief. A randomized controlled trial. *Journal of theAmerican Medical Association*, **293**, 2601–2608.

Shore, J.H., Vollmer, W.M. & Tatum, E.L. (1989). Community patterns of posttraumatic stress disorders. *Journal of Nervous and Mental Disease*, **177**, 681–685.

Slovic, P. (1987). Perception of risk. *Science*, **236**, 280–285.

Smith, E.M., North, C.S., McCool, R.E. & Shea, J.M. (1990). Acute postdisaster psychiatric disorders: identification of persons at risk. *American Journal of Psychiatry*, **147**, 202–206.

Talbot, M. (2002). Hysteria hysteria. *New York Times*, June 2, p.42.

Tucker, J.B. (1996). Chemical/biological terrorism: coping with a new threat. *Politics and the Life Sciences*, **15**, 167–183.

Ursano, R.J. (2002). Post-traumatic stress disorder (editorial). *New England Journal of Medicine*, **346**, 130–131.

Ursano, R.J., Fullerton, C.S. & Norwood, A.E. (1995). Psychiatric dimensions of disaster: patient care, community consultation, and preventive medicine. *Harvard Review of Psychiatry*, **3**, 196–209.

U.S. Department of Health and Human Services. (2002). *Communicating in a Crisis: Risk Communication*

Guidelines for Public Officials. Washington, D.C.: Department of Health and Human Services.

Wessely, S., Hyams, K.C. & Bartholomew, R. (2001). Psychological implications of chemical and biological weapons. *British Medical Journal*, **323**, 878–879.

WHO (2006). Epidemic and Pandemic Alert, World Health Organization. http://www.who.int/csr/disease/avian_influenza/country/cases_table_2006_09_08/en/index.html

Zatzick, D.F., Kang, S.M., Hinton, L. *et al.* (2001). Post-traumatic concerns: a patient-centered approach to outcome assessment after traumatic physical injury. *Medical Care*, **39**, 327–339.

13

Workplace disaster preparedness and response

Nancy T. Vineburgh, Robert K. Gifford, Robert J. Ursano,
Carol S. Fullerton, & David M. Benedek

Introduction

In the United States and countries throughout the world, natural and human-made disasters have affected the workplace, resulting in extensive psychological, behavioral, and health consequences for workers, families, and communities (Ursano et al., 2006). Natural disasters such as the Kobe earthquake, the Asian Tsunami, and Hurricane Katrina destroyed businesses, large and small, and disrupted the livelihood, health, and social supports of large populations. Human made disasters resulting in similar consequences range from industrial accidents, the worst occurring in 1984 in Bhopal, India, claiming some 20 000 lives due to lethal gas exposure (Dhara & Dhara, 2002), to violent acts of disgruntled employees, to the effects of terrorism and bioterrorism. In some instances, the workplace has been the intentional target of traumatic events, such as the US Kenya embassy bombing, the Oklahoma City bombing, the events of September 11 and the anthrax attacks on the United States Postal Service (Stith Butler et al., 2003; Ursano et al., 2003; Vineburgh et al., 2005a, 2005b, 2005c). Disasters also affect people on their way to work, as happened in the subway sarin gas attacks in Tokyo and the transportation terror bombings in Madrid (Miguel-Tobal et al., 2006) and London (Rubin et al., 2005).

Work is a central organizing factor in most lives, providing economic survival, a sense of identity, social connectedness, and purpose (Levinson, 1965; McLean, 1973). Employed individuals spend more than a third of their day at work (Institute of Medicine (IOM), 2003), and work is most often the source of one's health and mental health benefits (Schouten et al., 2004). After September 11, more than two times as many individuals experiencing persistent distress accessed information at work rather than from a medical practitioner, and over three times as many sought information and counseling at work rather than from a community-based mental health provider (Stein et al., 2003). There is increasing evidence that workplace health-promotion activities and programs can change behavior and psychosocial risk factors for individual employees and the collective risk profile of the employee population (IOM, 2003).

The resilience of industry, which is essential for sustaining the economy, health, security, and defense of nations, requires a resilient workforce led by informed leadership and management (Ursano et al., 2004a, 2004b). Many workplaces, especially corporations, utilize crisis management teams to assess the risk of critical incidents and to implement response strategies. These teams and plans are often operationally focused with an emphasis on business continuity as opposed to organizational and human continuity (Mankin & Perry, 2004). To address the impact of disasters on employee health and safety, industry must possess knowledge and resources for responding to the psychological and behavioral consequences of critical incidents including terrorism and bioterrorism (Fullerton *et al.*, 2003; Ursano *et al.*, 2006; Vineburgh *et al.*, 2005a, 2005b, 2005c).

This chapter will describe the evolution of the workplace as an environment responsive to the mental health of employees; the kinds of traumatic incidents that occur in workplaces requiring planning and on-site interventions; and the roles and opportunities for health and mental health providers to assist organizations in planning, responding to and recovering from critical incidents.

The chapter will conclude by providing a conceptual framework for mental health and occupational health providers to join with corporate professionals (corporate security, medical, employee assistance, human resources, and communications) and workplace stakeholders in the public sector in developing, integrating and implementing disaster psychiatry principles and evidence-based interventions that can protect and help sustain the United States' economic and social capital in the face of disasters and terrorism in the twenty-first century.

Historical overview: work, work hazards, and health

Recognition of the link between work, work hazards, and physical and emotional health dates back to antiquity. In a passage in *Oeconomicus* attributed to Socrates, manual labor in Ancient Greece compelled workers to be sedentary before a fire for a full day resulting in "physical degeneration" and "deterioration of the soul" (Gochfeld, 2005a). The Industrial Revolution of modern times and the labor movement that grew out of it brought attention, both in literature and government reform, to the hazardous working conditions in factories of overcrowding, exploitation of children and women, and disease. Public health, which came into being in the mid 1800s, addressed many of the social conditions resulting from industrialization, but not the actual work hazards.

Table 13.1 Selected history of workplace trauma and disasters

Eighteenth century	Health and safety laws for workers
1818	Dupont
Nineteenth century	Occupational medicine
Early twentieth century	Industrial psychiatrist/ psychologist/ social workers
1920s	Hawthorne Plant Study
1935	Alcoholics Anonymous
1940s	Macy's company – emotional first-aid stations
1940s	World War II
1980s	Depression in the workplace

The United States lagged a century behind England and Europe in enacting legislation to protect the health and safety of its workers (Gochfeld, 2005a).

In the absence of labor laws, some American employers developed their own employee protective measures. An example occurred in 1818 when Dupont experienced its second and most serious explosion. Forty employees lost their lives and workers fled not just the factory, but their jobs (Kinnane, 2002). The incident was attributed to the plant foreman's drinking, which was an expectation and routine part of the eighteenth and early nineteenth century workday akin to our coffee break (Trice & Schonbrunn, 1981) (see Table 13.1).

Dupont put an end to on-the-job drinking, instituted overtime and night pay, savings accounts, and widow's pensions. Importantly, the Dupont families worked alongside their employees and lived amongst them near the mills (Kinnane, 2002). These interventions, which resulted in a return to work, enabled leadership to demonstrate that employees mattered, and modeled courage and commitment to work in risky environments. Mattering (Rosenberg & McCullough, 1981) and leadership visibility in the face of workplace trauma (Dutton *et al.*, 2002; Greenberg, 2002) are important disaster mental health interventions discussed later in this chapter.

Occupational mental health: the context for addressing workplace trauma

Psychiatry in industry

The context for addressing workplace trauma and disasters evolved from and most often occurs within the domain of occupational mental health. Occupational mental health is a broad term that has encompassed the work and contributions of psychiatry, psychology, and social work (McLean, 1973), as well as the field of occupational medicine through the role of the corporate medical director, the occupational nurse, and wellness and work/life professionals. Occupational medicine and the safety profession emerged in the late nineteenth and early twentieth centuries primarily to address the hazards of heavy industry such as steel (Gochfeld, 2005a, 2005b). The field of industrial psychiatry followed, but was mainly in the service of corporate human resources (Anderson, 1944; McLean, 1973; Southard, 1920). The successes of psychological testing in the Army during World War I encouraged a number of American employers to hire psychiatrists to enhance their organization's personnel process (Anderson, 1944; Lott, 1946; McLean, 1973; Southard, 1920). In 1924, R. H. Macy and Company retained the services of Dr. V.V. Anderson (1944) who set up a mental health clinic and conducted surveys on the high accident rate of Macy's well-known delivery service (McLean, 1973). The clinic, run as part of the medical department with psychologists and psychiatric social workers, found the so-called troubled employee was often the victim of poor job training or problems related to home that interfered with performance. Anderson felt the clinic, sometimes referred to as an emotional first-aid station (Lott, 1946), communicated a sense that management was, "alive to the needs and possibilities of each employee," (Anderson, 1944). The transportation surveys of Macy's delivery service revealed that 70% of those with an accident record had mental disorders or drinking problems (Anderson, 1944). A new selection method was devised that lowered the rates of accidents, insurance coverage, and employee turnover.

Anderson's work, as well as the work of a number of pioneering psychiatrists in industry of the period (McLean, 1973; Trice & Schonbrunn, 1981), established a model in which the industrial psychiatrist functioned as a consultant to or employee of industry working as part of an integrated team. The team included psychologists and social workers who reported to medical, human resources or senior management (Southard, 1920). A primary role of the industrial psychiatrist, as part of social psychiatry, was preventive expanding beyond treatment of an individual's mental disorder to encompass and address the social conditions and health of communities and the nation (Southard, 1920).

The work of Dr. George Elton Mayo (1934), a psychologist who was a professor of industrial research at the Harvard Business School advanced the social significance of work and its application to industrial psychiatry. In the late 1920s, Mayo conducted 20 000 employee interviews and closely observed small working groups at the Hawthorne Plant of Western Electric in Chicago (McLean, 1973). The Hawthorne studies concluded that industry has two functions: economic and social. Productivity was seen as a form of social behavior, and the plant's activity as an interaction between structure, culture, and personality. Employee reactions to stress occur when there is resistance to change, when there are faulty control and communication systems, and in the adjustment of the individual worker to the structure of his work environment. An important paradigm in disaster mental health consultation and intervention described at the end of this chapter is based upon the relationship between organizational structure, culture, and employee health.

The role of alcohol in workplace trauma, health, and safety

World War II represented a turning point in the way employers viewed the psychological and behavioral health of employees and workplace

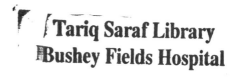

safety (Vineburgh, 2006). The reintegration of a large military population (many with alcohol problems), in addition to a large population of marginalized workers brought into industry during wartime to meet production demands, focused attention on alcoholism and its link to workplace accidents and employer productivity (Trice & Schonbrunn, 1981). Workman's compensation, which was enacted in the first two decades of the twentieth century and had become more strongly enforced, held employers liable for workplace injuries, furthering the incentive to reduce workplace accidents caused by drinking problems. Importantly, a promising intervention for rehabilitation and recovery had become available in the form of Alcoholics Anonymous (AA) (Henderson & Bacon, 1953).

The Yale Center for Alcohol Studies, founded in 1940, created a business case linking problem drinking and employee productivity. The Yale Center estimated that alcoholism cost employers over one billion dollars annually with the problem drinker losing an average of 22 days of work a year. A number of companies including unions utilized the services of recovering alcoholics who worked with corporate medical directors to identify and confront employees suspected of alcohol misuse. Dr. Gehrmann, a leading occupational health advocate in the medical community and medical director of Dupont, reported that he had struggled to little or no avail for 28 years to help alcohol-dependent drinkers before the existence of AA. Over a 5-year period in which he referred employees to AA, he got a 65% recovery rate (Trice & Schonbrunn, 1981). The Yale Plan educated business leadership and management that alcoholism was a disease and recommended AA as a community-based intervention or through the formation of chapters within industrial plants and settings (Henderson & Bacon, 1953; Steele, 1989). The problems of alcoholism in industry during this period gave rise to numerous employee assistance provider (EAP) programs that exist today. The EAP programs are described in depth in the section, "Workplace trauma: incidents and resources for responding."

Executive health, education and leadership training

During the 1950s and 1960s occupational mental health through industrial psychiatry and psychology was focused on the development and growth of the executive and management (see Table 13.2). Institutions such as the Menninger Foundation in collaboration with universities such as Cornell, the National Association for Mental Health and the American Psychiatric Association advanced the training of psychiatrists, industrial physicians, and executives (McLean, 1973). Occupational mental health now included a number of disciplines and topics, and reflected the fact that the worker had become increasingly identified by his/her workplace (McLean, 1973). A renowned occupational psychologist and consultant to industry leadership (Levinson, 1965) wrote, "Instead of a geographical orientation point, many now have developed a corporate orientation point. They identify themselves with an organization – a company, church, university, or government department. The work organization frequently provides the thread of continuity for a family moving from one area to another and may become a psychological anchor point for it. Often a man's social friendships arise from his work associations. Old Navy men have long had a ready bond of friendship, and two strangers who work for a nationwide organization are likely to have much in common" (see Table 13.2).

Table 13.2 Occupational mental health disciplines

- Occupational medicine
- Social, clinical, and industrial psychology
- Cultural anthropology
- Social psychiatry
- Psychiatry proper

The impact of depression on workplace mental health

With the advent of a new class of pharmacologic interventions for depression, selective serotonin reuptake inhibitors (SSRIs), in the late 1980s, there developed a growing body of literature on the economic burden of depression in the workplace (Birnbaum et al., 1999; Greenberg et al., 1990; Stewart et al., 2003). Many large employers became interested in its early identification and treatment, and SSRIs provided a relatively straightforward form of treatment that could be prescribed by physicians who were not trained in psychiatry. It is important to consider the role of pharmaceutical companies in this phase of occupational mental health. Many of the studies, education programs for the workplace and the general public, as well as intervention programs nationally and internationally were funded by manufacturers of depression medications (Miller, 1993). While this funding from the pharmaceutical industry has made new medications available, it has also raised concerns such as the potential for exploitation of research participants (Angell, 1997; Nundy & Gulhati, 2005) and selective reporting of results (De Angelis et al., 2005).

Economic burden of mental and behavioral disorders in the workplace

While alcohol and depression are but spokes in the wheel of occupational health and psychiatry, both disorders have shaped and sustained enormous visibility and utilization of occupational mental health programs for over a half a century. Importantly, both depression and alcohol misuse are common mental and behavioral disorders resulting from exposure to traumatic events. In addition to the emotional costs on individuals, families and communities, these disorders continue to exert a significant economic burden on industry and business. It is estimated that depression costs employers $44 billion annually in lost productivity (Birnbaum et al., 2000; Stewart et al., 2003).

Depressed people report an average of 5.6 h per week in reduced performance or absenteeism as compared to 1.5 h weekly among nondepressed. Of this lost time, 81% is attributable to reduced performance while at work, a phenomenon referred to as *presenteeism* (Bender, 2003). Alcoholism and alcohol abuse cost employers from $33 billion to $68 billion per year (Mangione et al., 1998). Alcohol is a major factor in injuries, at home, at work, and on the road. Absenteeism is estimated to be 4 – 8 times greater among alcoholics and alcohol abusers. Family members of alcoholics also have greater rates of absenteeism (retrieved at www.opm.gov/ehs/alcohol.asp).

Disaster mental health: a public health strategy to manage workplace trauma

Epidemiology of workplace disaster mental health

Knowledge of the psychological sequelae of disasters drawn from population-based studies of affected communities, in combination with knowledge of the economic burden of mental disorders in the workplace, supports the need for disaster mental health interventions in occupational settings. From studies of affected communities, we know that individuals exposed to trauma have been found to increase their use of alcohol, tobacco, and other drugs. This is especially the case for those with pre-existing alcohol abuse or other psychiatric difficulties (Galea et al., 2002; North et al., 1999; Pfefferbaum & Doughty, 2001; Ursano et al., 2003; Vlahov et al., 2002). People exposed to terrorism and disaster are at increased risk for depression, generalized anxiety disorder and panic disorder, increased substance use and post-traumatic stress disorder (PTSD) (Fullerton et al., 2003; North et al., 1999, 2002).

With recognition of the traumatic effects in the workplace of those exposed to the terrorist events of September 11 on the World Trade Center in New York City and in Washington, D.C., disaster mental health has become of increased interest to mental health and occupational health professionals (Gochfeld, 2005b).

Most acts of terrorism in the United States have occurred where and when people work, and because corporations and the workplace are identified high-value targets of international terrorism. Therefore, it is essential that interventions for preparedness, response, and recovery occur in occupational settings (Fullerton *et al.*, 2003; Ursano *et al.*, 2004a; Vineburgh, 2004). Terrorism is associated with a greater negative impact on mental health than other disasters because of its malicious intent (Stith Butler *et al.*, 2003; Ursano *et al.*, 2003). Whether in close proximity to or far from the affected site, people exposed to terrorism are at increased risk for a range of health-related responses. These include distress as well as mental illness and changes in behaviors that have health and community and corporate economic consequences. Exposure to terrorism also results in changes in perceived safety, and can lead to unwillingness to travel or unwillingness to come to work. Similarly altered trust in leadership and disrupted work performance due to depression or family concerns are only a few of the potentially costly workplace responses that can be anticipated.

Workers and the workplace experience both short-term and long-term health consequences from exposure to terrorism. A significant population experiencing persistent distress 2 months after September 11 reported (Stein *et al.*, 2003) that the distress disrupted work (65% reported accomplishing less), social life (24% avoided public places) and led to increases in behavior that posed health risks (38% using alcohol, medication or other drugs to relax, sleep, and reduce terrorism-related worries). A study of Pentagon employees 13 months following September 11 found those with acute stress disorder, depression and increased rates of alcohol use also had a decreased sense of safety at home and in travel (Grieger *et al.*, 2003). A study of this same population conducted a year later found that there were persisting effects of distress and mental disorder (Grieger *et al.*, 2005). Terrorism is now classified as the most extreme

form of workplace violence (Bowie *et al.*, 2005) furthering the imperative for disaster consequence management in industry (Vineburgh *et al.*, 2005a, 2005b, 2005c).

Resilience

It is important to recognize that resilience, the ability of most people to recover and return to normal life, is the documented and therefore expected outcome in all studies of disaster (North, 2003; Ursano, 2002; Ursano *et al.*, 2003). Resilience is a growing topic of interest in mental health and mental health promotion (American Psychological Association Help Center, 2004; Vineburgh, 2004). Resilience is also a growing topic of interest in the workplace. It bridges the health and continuity of the organization and its people (Coutu, 2002; Ursano, 2002). Resilience language and concepts can reframe discussions with and education of employers and employees around disaster and terrorism preparedness (Vineburgh, 2004). The concept of resilience in the face of trauma or disaster has been noted for many years. Military psychiatrists in World War I developed treatments for combat stress that were based on the notion that most people would recover and should not be treated as if they had a devastating disease. However, even though the concept has been around for many years, resilience seems to be a phenomenon that is discovered, then forgotten and rediscovered by the mental health community (Artiss, 1963).

A public health model for disaster consequence management

An Institute of Medicine (IOM) report: *Preparing for the Psychological Consequences of Terrorism: A Public Health Strategy*, identifies the workplace as an important setting in which to address public health planning for the psychological consequences of terrorism (Stith Butler *et al.*, 2003). Because most acts of terrorism in the United States have occurred where and when people work, it is essential that interventions for preparedness, response, and recovery occur in occupational settings. Sustaining our workforce – its organizational health and the well-being of workers – sustains our communities and important national resources and services. The work of organizations must continue, as evidenced by the Pentagon's post September 11 strategic planning despite the high level of anxiety and possible future threat, and the continuation of the United States Postal Service network regardless of the risk of exposure during and after the anthrax attacks.

The public health approach to the psychological consequences of terrorism focuses on prevention and health promotion, as well as treatment (Stith Butler *et al.*, 2003). Lessons learned from preparing for the psychological consequences of terrorism serve additional benefits that can be applied to a variety of other violent events and critical incidents.

A review for the National Institute of Occupational Safety and Health (NIOSH) to determine the present knowledge of the efficacy and effectiveness of interventions for mass traumatic events in occupational settings (Fullerton *et al.*, 2003) found the workplace a forgotten and important venue for mental health outreach around disaster. The NIOSH report offered several recommendations that underscore the significance of workplace disaster preparedness: workplaces must develop comprehensive strategies that encompass interventions before, during and after trauma; research in this area must be expanded; lastly, there is a need to broaden the range of trauma outcomes examined to include not just PTSD, but depression, substance use and abuse, violence, physical health, anger, and interpersonal functioning (Ursano *et al.*, 2003).

Occupational health providers, including employee assistance professionals, corporate medical directors, and occupational health and wellness professionals, can play an important role in integrating principles of disaster mental health because their work is often structured within this three-dimensional public health model: health promotion, prevention, and treatment/treatment referral. A public health model consists of health promotion (raising awareness of the risk), prevention (interventions to mitigate the risk) as well as treatment, and conceptualizes interventions for the pre-event, event and postevent phases of disaster. With disaster mental health training, workplace professionals can make a significant contribution to the delivery of disaster-related interventions (Stith Butler *et al.*, 2003; Ursano *et al.*, 2003). Because the United States' federal response to disaster is geared to local, immediate need in the aftermath of disaster, workplace health programs can provide pre-event training and respond to short- and long-term consequences, from distress to more serious mental disorder. A public health approach to disaster consequence management can be applied to natural disasters affecting the workplace, workplace violence, and industrial accidents, not just terrorism (Stith Butler *et al.*, 2003).

Workplace trauma: incidents and resources for responding

Workplace trauma encompasses a range of critical incidents or issues whose effect(s) on one or more employees has the potential to undermine the individual or collective safety (perceived or actual), health, performance, and morale of the exposed and/or affiliated worksites. A critical incident can occur within or outside of the workplace. Examples of incidents occurring within a workplace include an act of violence wrought by a disgruntled employee, an industrial explosion or workplace injury at a plant, threat of or actual exposure to an infectious disease such as severe acute respiratory syndrome (SARS), to a terrorist attack like September 11 or a bioterrorist attack, e.g., anthrax, which targets and affects employees at one or more worksites. Other incidents, occurring outside of the workplace, can also affect the workplace: serious accidents, homicide or kidnapping of an employee or employee's family that

Table 13.3 Workplace trauma

- Accidents
- Absenteeism
- Alcoholism
- Industrial health and occupational medicine
- Organized labor and the unions
- Leadership and supervision
- Motivation and incentives
- Industrial mental health programs
- Occupational roles and status
- Personality variables and the work setting
- Psychiatric illnesses (traumatic neurosis, psychosomatic reactions, organic brain syndromes)
- Rehabilitation of the physically and psychiatrically disabled
- Meaning of work
- Structure, function and environment of the work organization

affects co-workers, the experience of transportation terror on the way to work, or a natural disaster such as a hurricane, tornado or earthquake that affects an employee or group of employees and disrupts work or inhibits a return to work. Other critical incidents that affect employee morale and their health and mental health include massive downsizings (General Motors, Fall 2005) or workplace violations (Enron), which leave employees feeling helpless, threatened or mistrustful (see Table 13.3).

Studies have shown that employees exposed to workplace violence have suffered impaired psychological and physical health as well as productivity (Budd *et al.*, 2001; Rogers & Kelloway, 1997; Schat & Kelloway, 2000). Co-worker-initiated workplace violence is associated with negative effects on emotional well-being, while public-initiated workplace violence is associated with fear of future violence (LeBlanc & Kelloway, 2002). Numerous workplace-related agencies such as NIOSH, part of the Centers for Disease Control and Prevention of the US Department of Health and Human Services, provide annual statistics on workplace violence and workplace injuries as well as workplace trauma information that is industry-specific. Information

for management and occupational health providers on responding to specific types of critical workplace incidents have been developed (Blythe, 2002; Kahn & Langlieb, 2003; Wallace & Webber, 2004).

Employee assistance programs and providers (EAPs) can be particularly important for health and mental health consultants in working with corporations or behavioral heath providers around disaster mental health issues and events. Employee assistance programs are workplace mental health programs, which began after World War II to address problem drinking in the workplace. These programs expanded in the 1970s and 1980s to encompass the emotional health and distress of employees. Most of these programs were internally housed within corporations with mental health counselors as employees. With the advent of managed care and the concomitant downsizing of industry, behavioral health carve-outs began offering EAP services and many corporations chose to outsource mental health and substance abuse assessment and treatment. Such programs are referred to as external EAP programs. Some companies have both internal and external EAPs called a mixed model. Although EAP programs vary, most include health promotion, education, and referral to professional treatment including alcohol and other drug or mental health counseling. Many employers offer EAP services (Roman & Blum, 2002). Many large behavioral healthcare organizations that offer EAP programs could and do deploy their services to communities in the United States affected by disasters such as Columbine, the Oklahoma City bombing, September 11, and Hurricane Katrina, to supplement local and federal resources. There has been a trend for large behavioral carve-outs to further subcontract critical incident response services to specialty vendors. Employee assistance programs and providers, with training in disaster mental health principles, can incorporate disaster mental health education, readiness, and response into existing health promotion and prevention programs because the psychological and behavioral sequelae of disasters involve many of the same issues and disorders that they deal with on a day-to-day basis.

Disaster mental health interventions

Pre-event

Pre-event interventions for managing the consequences of disasters include buy-in from executive and senior management that such activities are worthwhile and cost-effective, and employee receptivity to preparing for disasters. Employer and employee attitudes are shaped by beliefs in the reality and probable realization of such risks. Workplace risks may be industry specific, i.e., plant explosions, location of enterprise, brand or other factors. It is interesting to note that many schools, which are workplaces, practice drills in the event of school shootings due to history. In each case, preparedness is critical to the outcome.

Morgan Stanley's response to September 11 has been widely cited as an example of workforce preparedness for terrorism. Soon after the 1993 World Trade Center bombings, Morgan Stanley launched a preparedness program involving serious evacuation drills directed by its corporate security department. On the morning of September 11, 1 min after the North Tower was struck, Rick Rescorla, security Vice President, instructed Morgan Stanley's employees to evacuate the South Tower immediately, to stay calm and follow their well-practiced drills. This resulted in a loss of only 7 of its 2700 employees (Coutu, 2002).

The example above reinforces the findings of a classic study (Weisaeth, 1989) that identified the concept of "disaster behavior" in the context of a workplace critical incident. The study of the aftermath of a paint factory explosion in Norway found that an individual's level of preparedness was the strongest predictor of an optimal disaster outcome. Employees without prior training did not fare well after a workplace explosion.

Disaster behaviors are of critical importance in the workplace, especially in tall buildings occupied by multiple employers, referred to as vertical communities (Hall et al., 2003; Ursano & Norwood, 2003). During the 1993 World Trade Center explosion, 32% of individuals had not begun to evacuate by over 1 h, 30% decided not to evacuate, and only 36% had participated in a previous emergency evacuation (Aguirre et al., 1998). Large groups (greater than 20 people) took 6.7 min longer to initiate evacuation, a time frame of life or death in many disasters. Large groups often take on the group dynamics of large committees seeking consensus and direction in decision-making. In addition, the higher the location, the greater the delay in initiating evacuation, and the more people were known to one another, the longer the group took to initiate evacuation (Aguirre et al., 1998). Recent studies of the World Trade Center evacuation found nearly 25% of employees believed the roof could be used for evacuation and only 10% had ever entered a stairwell as part of a fire drill (Gershon, 2005).

Adaptive disaster behaviors may include evacuation, shelter-in-place and quarantine. These are often overlooked as important human continuity issues and health interventions in occupational settings, yet they are central to organizational resilience (Fullerton et al., 2003; Hall et al., 2003; Ursano & Norwood, 2003; Ursano et al., 2003). Therefore, preparing people and organizations for terrorism and disaster response and recovery requires understanding such disaster behaviors (Ursano & Vineburgh, 2004, 2005; Ursano et al., 2004b).

Several United States studies indicate that, despite the public's belief there will be more terrorism, the public is generally not knowledgeable about preparedness within their own workplace (National Center for Disaster Preparedness, 2003). One national survey found only 36% of citizens familiar with emergency plans in their workplace, yet citizens reported interest in having their workplace update their plans and practice drills (Council for Excellence in Government, 2004). Another national study found that nearly half of US workers felt their employer was not prepared for a terrorist attack; of those, 9% said it did not matter because they believed their company will never be affected (ComPsych Survey, 2004).

The pre-event role of disaster mental health providers – be they consultants to or employees of industry, or organizations that provide corporate behavioral health services or firms that provide subcontracted crisis management services – is to educate leadership, management, and employees directly about the concept of disaster behaviors. Studies have shown that people are more receptive to changing behaviors when risk is personalized (Tierney *et al.*, 2001). The concept of disaster behavior, unlike an abstract concept such as pre-paredness, can personalize risk, reinforcing an individual's sense of agency and responsibility in response to crisis.

Event

In the face of the actual disaster event, leadership visibility and organizational communication are the two most important interventions to prevent, mitigate, and foster recovery from the event's impact (Gifford & Tyler, 1990; Ingraham, 1989; Tyler & Gifford, 1991). Two recent Harvard Business Review case studies on corporate responses to September 11 (Argenti, 2002; Greenberg, 2002) illustrate the importance of communications and communication strategies in the immediate after-math of workplace disasters, and how such com-munication fosters organizational recovery and resilience. The Chief Executive Officer (CEO) of Marsh and McLennan Companies, a corporation that suffered severe losses (295 employees), emphasizes the importance of CEO visibility in communicating during the immediate aftermath of a disaster (Argenti, 2002; Greenberg, 2002). Improvization and creativity were touted as essential to deal with downed power and telephone lines. Public address systems, a technology often overlooked because it is dated, became central (Greenberg, 2002). The media, often regarded with ambivalence during crises, became partners with corporations to communicate information about

employee whereabouts and safety issues (Argenti, 2002). Communication through leadership visibi-lity that is clear, honest, and compassionate reas-sures employees. Grief leadership, the ability of a CEO or city official to show and model emotion and compassion, is an integral part of leadership visibility (Ingraham, 1989). Reassuring employees helps to re-establish operational continuity, enhancing the resilience of people and business.

Occupational health programs must collaborate with human resources to disseminate the corpor-ate communication message through existing help lines and benefits websites. It is essential that corporate communication is consistent and repetitious to reinforce information on employee safety, workplace resumption and schedules, and employee resources for information and help-seeking. An important role in this phase is provi-sion of Psychological First Aid: promoting personal care, sleep, exercise, and return to normal routine (NIMH, 2002).

Postevent interventions

The goal of postevent disaster interventions is to restore organizational safety, cohesion, and trust through return to work, resumption of routine, and restoration of health and good morale of workers. This requires thoughtful planning in the pre-event stage and execution of plans by numerous functions and collaborative efforts postevent. Security trans-parency is vital to re-establishing a sense of safety. In some corporations directly affected by September 11, security worked side by side with employee assis-tance to walk the halls and talk with employees. Gathering around food available throughout an organization brings people together to talk infor-mally. One corporation used a bomb dog as a ther-apy dog, letting workers pet and befriend this important security tool. Human resources collabor-ates with communications to ensure that there are procedures around employee whereabouts, that contact information is valid and updated, and that there is ongoing communication around the disaster and its effects on return to work and schedules.

Workplace health and productivity professionals must evaluate the impact of the event and provide necessary resources to aid in the recovery. Critical Incident Stress Debriefing (CISD) has become a staple in the employer's arsenal of postevent workplace crisis response (Ursano *et al.*, in press). While its clinical effectiveness is subject to debate (McNally *et al.*, 2003; NIMH, 2002; Raphael, 2003; Rose *et al.*, 1999, 2001; Schouten *et al.*, 2004), a larger issue is that CISD has become an industry in which large behavioral health organizations that provide outsourced employee assistance further subcontract CISD services to private firms. Many employers may not be aware of what kinds of postdisaster interventions they are receiving and who provides them (Benedek *et al.*, 2005).

Long before it was confirmed in epidemiologic studies of combat veterans or survivors of the September 11 terrorist attacks, the idea that traumatic exposure may lead to the development of acute stress disorder (ASD) or PTSD simultaneously in large groups or communities was recognized. Military commanders have long used after-action reviews in an effort to evaluate the effectiveness and damage resulting from combat operations. More recently this process has evolved into a number of techniques applied to groups of law-enforcement personnel, emergency service providers, and civilians, collectively referred to as psychological debriefing. The CISD is a popular form of semi-structured, staged, group psychological debriefing. While there are reports that many who receive debriefing experience the process as beneficial (Boscarino *et al.*, 2005), there is no evidence to suggest that debriefings prevent PTSD and some studies suggest that the process may be harmful (Bryant, 2005). The current American Psychiatric Association practice guidelines do not recommend CISD or other forms of psychological debriefing for the prevention or treatment of ASD or PTSD. The guidelines do call for the development of population-based approaches to exposure to mass violence aimed at the reduction of distress and maladaptive distress behavior in communities and populations as well as the prevention of ASD

and PTSD (American Psychiatric Association, 2004). A longitudinal, population-based survey (Boscarino *et al.*, 2005) that supports the use of postdisaster mental health interventions in the workplace as beneficial to employee mental health status (reducing the risk of binge drinking, alcohol dependence, PTSD symptoms, major depression, somatization, anxiety and global impairment) does not provide a description of what constituted these interventions. Some affected employers in the aftermath of September 11 abandoned CISD in favor of a resilience model made up of educational briefings aimed at restoring safety and work routine (Ursano *et al.*, in press). It is also important to consider the legal implications of not providing postdisaster mental health interventions or providing some that produce negative effects (Tehrani, 2002). At present, Psychological First Aid and use of crisis intervention needs assessment teams are valuable early workplace interventions.

It is important to reach out to vulnerable populations. Gender and predisaster psychiatric history are strong predictors of post-trauma psychiatric difficulties (North, 2003; North *et al.*, 1999). After disasters, women are more likely to experience PTSD and major depression, and men are at greater risk for substance abuse. Individuals with pre-existing mental disorders are more likely to experience renewed difficulties. Because some workplaces are predominantly male or female, such findings can inform pre- and postdisaster interventions.

Specific groups may require special interventions. These include identified cultural groups whose perception of the disaster may be markedly different as a result of past experiences with disasters (i.e., refugee, individuals recently exposed to traumas, ethnic groups). The number of refugees worldwide is growing, and many are relocated in the United States, as well as in workplaces throughout the world. The unique characteristics of refugee groups, including cultural, ethnic, and language considerations, torture or trauma experiences, multiple losses, minimal resources, and an uncertain future need to be considered in developing mental health services (Gerrity & Steinglass, 2003). Workplace disasters can affect their surrounding communities and affect vulnerable populations such as occurred in Enschede, Holland when a plant fire explosion affected a large Turkish population causing extensive mental distress and disorder (Drogendijk *et al.*, 2003).

An important role of human resource professionals is to stay alert to the opening of fault lines from terrorist events. Terrorism opens the fault lines of a society revealing its vulnerabilities and divisive tendencies along racial, ethnic, and religious lines (Ursano, 2002). This can result in scapegoating, discrimination against ethnicities perceived akin to the terrorist agent, as well as fallout around perceived inequities in disaster treatment responses.

The response to the anthrax attacks of 2001 created "the perception of a double standard," that opened the fault lines around race and socioeconomic status (Walsh *et al.*, 2004). The rapid response to workers on Capitol Hill, their evacuation and distribution of ciprofloxacin contrasted sharply against the Brentwood postal workers' ongoing risk of exposure and belated receipt of medication. This resulted in serious and persistent mistrust that undermined the cohesion of the postal service workplace and included legal ramifications (Holloway & Waldrep, 2004; Steury *et al.*, 2004). These behavioral consequences of terrorism have important implications for the human capital and continuity of organizations about which human resource personnel must be knowledgeable.

While resilience is the expected outcome of disaster, attention to the psychological and behavioral implications of trauma are important. Attention to these issues fosters employee and organizational resilience (Coutu & Hyman, 2002; Ursano, 2002; Vineburgh, 2004). Leadership down through management must demonstrate that employees matter. A large corporation affected by September 11 established human continuity by the leadership's assurance of job security to every employee in the enterprise, even those whose offices no longer existed.

Disaster mental health consultation and application to industry

The beginning of the twenty-first century has already witnessed devastating natural and human-made disasters that have dramatically affected, and in a number of instances been targeted at, the workplace. Whether these events happen or culminate *within* workplaces (September 11), *outside of* (Hurricane Katrina) or *on transportation routes* to work (London), employers and employees must be prepared, both in their occupational settings and through family and work communication plans. The impact of workplace disasters on communities and regions, such as the Union Carbide, India, and the Valdez Oil Spill (Ijzermans *et al.*, 2005), can be substantial.

Disaster mental health professionals – consultants as well as those within the workplace – should view the following areas and issues as points of interest and points of access for dissemination of workplace trauma knowledge and interventions (see Table 13.4)

Talking to industry about disaster mental health involves knowledge about an organization's view of business and human continuity, defining events and resilience.

Table 13.4 Workplace disaster preparedness and response

I. **Knowledge of corporate:**
  - Business continuity
  - Human continuity
  - Defining events
  - Resilience
II. **Buy in:**
  - Leadership
  - Corporate security
  - Occupational health
  - Corporate communications and public affairs
III. **Understanding of corporate:**
  - Structure, function, and culture
  - Integration and collaboration
  - Disaster training
  - Community interface

Business continuity and human continuity

The traditional view of business continuity has been focused on the infrastructure of an enterprise, i.e., its facilities and hardware. As a result of September 11, many corporations have recognized that people are the most important asset of organizations. The individual functions of and collaboration between corporate communications, security, human resources, occupational health services, and leadership attitudes are vital in protecting and sustaining the human continuity of a corporation.

Defining events

Many corporations have experienced a defining event or events that become a template for their approach in preparing for and responding to workplace crises and traumatic events. Defining events include industrial accidents, workplace violence, acts of disgruntled employees, natural disasters, and the experience of September 11. A corporation's crisis management philosophy, team, and training are often organized around one or more of these defining events.

Resilience

Defining events act as a benchmark of an organization's resilience. Positive responses to previous corporate disasters set the standard upon which leaders and management base their disaster responses and expectations. Responses that are not positive become lessons learned for future planning and responding.

Talking with industry about disaster mental health involves buy-in from corporate leadership, security, occupational health, communication, and public affairs.

Corporate leadership

Corporate leadership must champion the importance of disaster and terrorism preparedness in order for management to facilitate preparedness activities. A corporation that provides preparedness education sends a message that it cares, and this can counterbalance a corporation's fear that undertaking such activities runs the risk of fear mongering or increasing employee anxiety. Policies and leadership behavior must maximize people's sense that they matter, and be informed by the idea that best practices for training or preparing one subculture within a corporation may not be as effective in other subculture populations.

Corporate security

Corporate security directors are often highly knowledgeable, articulate about disaster and terrorism preparedness, and interested in advancing this knowledge directly to management and employees. Many see their role as going beyond the traditional corporate security functions of "gates, guns, and guards." Security directors may understand that preparedness and response to disaster are about human behavior.

Occupational health

Functions of occupational health, internal and outsourced, include medical, employee assistance, occupational nursing, wellness, and worklife. Participation of the corporate medical director in crisis management highlights planning for normal epidemics (e.g., influenza), and creates opportunities for better response to other health threats, such as the recent SARS outbreak or fears around new pandemics such as Avian flu. Importantly, the medical director can provide information and assessment around product contamination and related issues around bioterrorism (anthrax).

Employee assistance provider (EAP) programs are the locus of health promotion, assessment, and sometimes treatment for a range of employee psychological and behavioral health problems, including workplace stress, substance abuse, mental disorders, and domestic violence. Most companies outsource their EAP services. Corporations must be vigilant and conscientious in setting expectations for outsourced services that relate to employee security or preparedness.

Corporate communications and public affairs

Corporate communications are essential for provision of information, provided on a consistent and reliable basis, in disaster events. Communications focus on information to employees, leadership and then on disseminating the leadership's message to management, employee families, community stakeholders, customers, and the media. This necessitates ongoing employee information updates and having some positive mechanism for ensuring the updates really occur. The latter requires having ways to communicate with employees who are not at the office and means that contact lists must be current. Often these functions reside in human resources or exist separately but work in tandem.

Working with industry to achieve disaster mental health preparedness and response plans necessitates an understanding of an organization's: (1) structure, function, culture; (2) integration and collaboration; (3) disaster training; and (4) the corporate–community interface.

Organizational structure, functional areas, and corporate culture

Organizational structure, functional areas, and corporate culture affect preparedness planning and its position in each corporation. The functional areas that are represented on the crisis management team, and how they interact with one another appears to be extremely important in determining what information is considered in corporate planning. The organization's culture can facilitate or impede a crisis management team's objectives, as well as individual employee behavior before, during, and after a terrorist event. Our interviewees identified several important organizational, functional and cultural factors that enhanced or impaired crisis response.

Integration, collaboration and cross-functionality

Corporations describe effective crisis management as requiring cross-functionality and teamwork. Many functions that formerly operated in silos (e.g. independently) collaborate around crisis management. Collaboration between corporate security, corporate communications, and occupational health services can strengthen employee outreach, education, and training for disaster and terrorism. The collaboration between human resources, EAP, and security is essential to address back-to-work policies and programs following critical incidents. The collaboration between security, medical, and human resources is critical in order to address bioterrorism and pandemic threats.

Disaster training

Discussion with corporations following questions specific to their terrorism preparedness training programs often leads to general discussions about safety, health, leadership, and communication. Each of these areas and topics involves trainable skills, especially in relation to a disaster or terrorist attack. Corporations vary in what exercises they conduct. Some have active programs including table top exercises with senior management; others may participate in exercises with less frequency and with less sophistication. An all-hazards response to anticipated corporate disaster is the norm.

Corporate – community cooperation and the public – private interface

Disaster and terrorism preparedness and response requires coordination and cooperation between the public and private sectors, including a company's community or communities, as well as state and federal agencies. The public – private interface around terrorism preparedness can range from issues of research, to sharing and interpretation of threat information, to the role and resources of a business in response to a major disaster and to the local fire department and law enforcement in responding to corporate needs.

Conclusion

Throughout history, the workplace has been affected by natural and human-made disasters. Natural disasters that affect communities and regions can destroy businesses and disrupt productivity, resulting in economic, social, and health consequences. Human-made disasters in the form of industrial accidents can originate in a workplace and affect communities emotionally and economically (Sago mine disaster); likewise, industrial accidents that originate within a workplace can disrupt and devastate communities as happened in a firework explosion in Enschede, the Netherlands (Drogendijk *et al.*, 2003) and the Exxon Valdez oil spill (Arata *et al.*, 2000). Some human-made disasters such as terrorism have targeted the workplace as a way of spreading fear and disrupting economic stability and growth.

The workplace is an important if not primary social context that provides routine, purpose, and economic and social resources to one's life, all of which can be undermined by exposure to disaster. The workplace has a plethora of resources that can assist in the planning, response and recovery phase of disasters. Many organizations have internal occupational health and mental health resources in the form of medical, employee assistance and wellness programs that have knowledge of a company's culture and health issues. But, occupational health and mental health resources have undergone dramatic transformation in the past quarter of a century. Corporations are increasingly outsourcing their medical and employee assistance services to private health companies and large behavioral health companies who in turn subcontract out crisis management services to specialty firms.

Since September 11, there has been increased interest in the field of disaster mental health – and how its knowledge and practice can be incorporated into the workplace setting. A public health approach to integrating the psychological and behavioral principles of disaster mental health provides a model for pre-event, event, and post-event responses.

Integration of multiple corporate functions can facilitate pre-event planning, event and postevent collaboration between security, human resources, communications, and EAP. EAP is essential to motivate employees to understand and operationalize adaptive disaster behaviors (Gershon, 2005). The voice and visibility of leadership and management are essential to fostering a sense of mattering, which nurtures community cohesion and resilience.

Mental health professionals – psychiatrists, organizational psychologists, social workers who are EAPs – can have an important role. Those employed by the organization must seek integrated participation in crisis planning to educate about and address psychological and behavioral issues involved in disaster consequence management.

Mental health consultants can work with leadership and management to educate them about disaster behaviors and grief leadership. This role of working with leadership and management in consultation and training has a tradition in occupational mental health history.

Importantly, mental health professionals can consult with the EAP and crisis management industry to ensure that providers and subcontractors are providing quality crisis response services – both in the form of pre-event, employee education and evidence-based postdisaster services.

REFERENCES

Aguirre, B.E., Wenger, D. & Vigo, G. (1998). A test of the emergent norm theory of collective behavior. *Sociological Forum*, **13**, 301–320.

American Psychiatric Association. (2004). Practice guideline for the treatment of patients with acute stress disorder and posttraumatic stress disorder. Arlington, Va.: American Psychiatric Association, pp. 1–57.

American Psychological Association Help Center. (2004). The road to resilience: www.apahelpcenter.org, accessed May 11, 2007.

Anderson, V.V. (1944). Psychiatry in industry. *The American Journal of Psychiatry*, **100**, 134–138.

Angell, M. (1997). The ethics of clinical research in the third world. *New England Journal of Medicine*, **337**, 847–849.

Arata, C.M., Picou, J.S., Johnson, G.D. & McNally, T.S. (2000). Coping with technological disaster: an application of the conservation of resources model to the Exxon Valdez oil spill. *Journal of Traumatic Stress*, **13**, 23–39.

Argenti, P. (2002). Crisis communication: lessons from September 11. *Harvard Business Review*. Cambridge, Mass: Harvard Business School of Publishing.

Artiss, K.L. (1963). Human behavior under stress: from combat to social psychiatry. *Military Medicine*, **128**, 1011–1015.

Bender, E. (2003). Employers see value in raising workers' awareness of mental health issues. *Psychiatric News*, **38**, 8–9.

Benedek, D.M., Ursano, R.J. & Holloway, H. (2005). Military and disaster psychiatry. In *Comprehensive Textbook of Psychiatry*, Vol. II, 8th edn., eds. B. Sadock & V. Sadock. New York: Lippincott, Williams & Wilkins.

Birnbaum, H.G., Greenberg, P.E., Barton, M. *et al.* (1999). Workplace burden of depression: a case study in social functioning using employer claims data. *Drug Benefit Trends*, **11**, 6BH–12BH.

Birnbaum, H.G., Cremieux, P.Y., Greenberg, P.E. & Kessler, R.C. (2000). Management of major depression in the workplace: impact on employee work loss. *Disability Management Health Outcomes*, **3**, 3.

Blythe, B.T. (2002). *Blindsided: A manager's Guide to Catastrophic Incidents in the Workplace*. New York: Penguin Group.

Boscarino, J.A., Adams, R.E. & Figley, C.R. (2005). A prospective cohort study of the effectiveness of employer-sponsored crisis interventions after a major disaster. *International Journal of Emergency Mental Health*, **7**, 9–22.

Bowie, V., Fisher, B.S. & Cooper, C.L. (2005). *Workplace Violence: Issues, Trends, Strategies*. Cullompton: Willan Publishing.

Bryant, R.A. (2005). Psychosocial approaches of acute stress reactions. *CNS Spectrum*, **10**, 116–122.

Budd, J.W., Arvey, R.D. & Lawless, P. (2001). Correlates and consequences of workplace violence. *Journal of Occupational Health Psychology*, **6**, 255–269.

ComPsych Survey. (2004). Employees feel sense of inertia around terror warnings. Available at www.compsych.com/jsp/en_us/core/home/press Releases List 2004.jsp? cid=420#, accessed May 14, 2007.

Council for Excellence in Government. (2004). From the home front to the front lines: America speaks out about homeland security. *Hart-Teeter Research*. Available at www.excelgov.org/ index.php? keyword = a432949724f-861, accessed May 14, 2007.

Coutu, D.L. (2002). How resilience works. *Harvard Business Review On Point*. Cambridge, Mass: Harvard Business School Publishing.

Coutu, D.L. & Hyman, S.E. (2002). Managing emotional fallout: parting remarks from America's top psychiatrist. *Harvard Business Review*. Cambridge, Mass.: Harvard Business School Publishing.

De Angelis, C., Drazen, J.M., Frizelle, F.A. *et al.* (2005). Is this clinical trial fully registered? A statement from the International Committee of Journal Editors. *New England Journal of Medicine*, **252**, 2436–2438.

Dhara, V.R. & Dhara, R. (2002). The Union carbide disaster in Bhopal: a review of health effects. *Archives of Environmental Health*, **57**, 391–404.

Drogendijk, A.N., Velden, P.G., Kleber, R.J. *et al.* (2003). Turkish victims of the Enschede firework disaster: a comparative study. *Gedrag and Gezondheid*, **31**, 145–162.

Dutton, J.E., Frost, P.J., Worline, M.C., Lilium, J.M. & Kanov, J.M. (2002). Leading in times of trauma. *Harvard Business Review*, **80**, 54–61, 125.

Fullerton, C.S., Ursano, R.J. & Norwood, A.E. (2003). Workplace interventions following trauma: a review of interventions to prevent or treat psychological and behavioral consequences of occupational or workplace exposure to mass traumatic events. Final Report to NIOSH, Uniformed Services University, Bethesda, Md.

Galea, S., Ahern, J., Resnick, H. *et al.* (2002). Psychological sequelae of the September 11 terrorist attacks in New York City. *New England Journal of Medicine*, **346**, 982–987.

Gerrity, E.T. & Steinglass, P. (2003). Relocation stress following catastrophic events. In *Terrorism and Disaster: Individual and Community Mental Health Interventions*, eds. R.J. Ursano, C.S. Fullerton & A.E. Norwood. Cambridge: Cambridge University Press.

Gershon, R. (2005). RRM WRC Evacuation Study: lessons for high rise building preparedness. Paper presented at the Uniformed Services University, Department of Preventive Medicine and Biometrics, Bethesda, Md. Available at www.mailman.hs.columbia.edu/CPHP/wtc/, accessed may 13, 2007.

Gifford, R.K. & Tyler, M.P. (1990). Consulting in grief leadership: a practical guide. *Disaster Management*, **4**, 218–224.

Gochfeld, M. (2005a). Chronologic history of occupational medicine. *Journal of Occupational Environmental Medicine*, **47**, 96–114.

Gochfeld, M. (2005b). Occupational medicine practice in the United States since the industrial revolution. *Journal of Occupational Environmental Medicine.* **42**, 115–131.

Greenberg, J.W. (2002). September 11, 2001: a CEO's story. *Harvard Business Review*, **80**, 58–64, 128.

Greenberg, P.E., Stiglin, L.E., Finkelstein, S.N. & Berndt, E. R. (1990). The economic burden of depression in 1990. *Journal of Clinical Psychiatry*, **54**, 11.

Grieger, T.A., Fullerton, C.S. & Ursano, R.J. (2003). Post-traumatic stress disorder, alcohol use, and perceived safety after the terrorist attack on the pentagon. *Psychiatric Services*, **54**, 1380–1382.

Grieger, T.A., Waldrep, D.A., Lovasz, M.M. & Ursano, R.J. (2005). Follow-up of Pentagon employees two years after the terrorist attack of September 11, 2001. *Psychiatric Services*, **56**, 1374–1378.

Hall, M.J., Norwood, A.E., Ursano, R.J. & Fullerton, C.S. (2003). The psychological impacts of bioterrorism. *Biosecurity and Bioterrorism: Biodefense Strategy, Practice, & Science*, **1**, 139–144.

Henderson, R. & Bacon, S. (1953). Problem drinking: the Yale plan for business and industry. *Quarterly Journal of Studies on Alcohol*, **14**, 247–262.

Holloway, H.C. & Waldrep, D.A. (2004). Biopsychosocial factors in bioterrorism: consequences for psychiatric care, society and public health. In *Bioterrorism: Psychological and Public Health Interventions*, eds. R.J. Ursano, A.E. Norwood & C.S. Fullerton. Cambridge: Cambridge University Press.

Ijzermans, C.J., Dirkzwager, A.J.E. & Breuning, E. (2005). *Long-Term Health Consequences of Disaster: A Bibliography*. Utrecht: Nivel.

Ingraham, L.H. (1989). Leading through loss: grief leadership in the army. Presented at the Army Leadership Conference, Center for Army Leadership, Kansas City, Mo., April 13, 1989.

Institute of Medicine. (2003). *The Future of the Public's Health in the 21st Century*. Washington, D.C.: The National Academies Press.

Kahn, J.P. & Langlieb, A.M. (2003). *Mental Health and Productivity in the Workplace: A Handbook for Organizations and Clinicians*. San Francisco: Jossey-Bass Publishers.

Kinnane, A. (2002). *Dupont: From the Banks of the Brandywine to Miracles of Science*. E.I. du Pont de Nemours and Company, Baltimore: Johns Hopkins University Press.

LeBlanc, M.M. & Kelloway, E.K. (2002). Predictors and outcomes of workplace violence and aggression. *Journal of Applied Psychology*, **87**, 444–453.

Levinson, H. (1965). The future of health in industry. *Industrial Medicine and Surgery*, **34**, 321–334.

Lott, M.G. (1946). Emotional first aid stations in industry. *Industrial Medicine*, **15**, 419–422.

Mangione, T.W., Howland, J. & Lee, M. (1998). Alcohol and work: results from a corporate drinking study. In *To Improve Health and Healthcare 1998–1999*, eds. S.L. Isaacs & J.R. Knickman. San Francisco: Jossey-Bass Publishers.

Mankin, L.D. & Perry, R.W. (2004). Terrorism challenges for human resource management. *Review of Public Personnel Administration*, **24**, 3–17.

Mayo, E. (1934). *The Human Problems of an Industrial Civilization*. New York: McMillan.

McLean, A.A. (1973). Occupational mental health: review of an emerging art. In *Industrial Mental Health and Employee Counseling*, ed. R.L. Noland. New York: Behavioral Publications.

McNally, R.J., Bryant, R.A. & Ehlers, A. (2003). Does early psychological intervention promote recovery from posttraumatic stress? *Psychological Science in the Public Interest*, **4**, 45–79.

Miguel-Tobal, J.J., Cano-Vindel, A., Gonzalez-Ordi, H. et al. (2006). Madrid March 11 train bombings. *Journal of Traumatic Stress*, **19**, 69–80.

Miller, M.W. (1993). Dark days: the staggering cost of depression. *The Wall Street Journal*, December 2.

National Center for Disaster Preparedness (NCDP). (2003). How Americans feel about terrorism and security: two years after September 11. Presented by the Mailman School of Public Health in collaboration with The Children's Health Fund, Columbia University, New York City.

National Institute of Mental Health. (2002). Mental health and mass violence: evidence-based early Pschological intervention for victims/survivors of mass violence. A Workshop to reach consensus on best practices. NIH Publication No. 02–5138. Washington, D.C.: US Government Printing Office.

North, C.S. (2003). Psychiatric epidemiology of disaster responses. In *Trauma and Disaster: Responses and Management*, eds. R.J. Ursano & A.E. Norwood. Arlington, Va: American Psychiatric Publishing.

North, C.S., Nixon, S.J., Shariat, S. *et al.* (1999). Psychiatric disorders among survivors of the Oklahoma City Bombing. *Journal of the American Medical Association*, **282**, 755–762.

North, C.S., Tivis, L., McMillen, J.C. *et al.* (2002). Coping, functioning, and adjustment of rescue workers after the Oklahoma City bombing. *Journal of Trauma Stress*, **15**, 171–175.

Nundy, S. & Gulhati, C.M. (2005). A new colonialism? Conducting clinical trials in India. *New England Journal of Medicine*, **352**, 1633–1636.

Pfefferbaum, B. & Doughty, D.E. (2001). Increased alcohol use in a treatment sample of oklahoma city bombing victims. *Psychiatry*, **64**, 296–303.

Raphael, B. (2003). *Debriefing*. Cambridge: Cambridge University Press.

Rogers, K.A. & Kelloway, E.K. (1997). Violence at work: personal and organizational outcomes. *Journal of Occupational Health Psychology*, **2**, 63–71.

Roman, P.M. & Blum, T.C. (2002). The workplace and alcohol problem prevention. *Alcohol Research and Health*, **26**, 49–57.

Rose, S., Brewin, C.R., Andrews, B. & Kirk, M.A. (1999). Randomized controlled trial of individual psychological debriefing for victims of violent crime. *Psychological Medicine*, **29**, 793–799.

Rose, S., Bisson, J. & Simon, W. (2001). Psychological debriefing for preventing post traumatic stress disorder. *Cochrane Database System Review*, **4**, 70.

Rosenberg, M. & McCullough, B.C. (1981). Mattering: inferred significance and mental health among adolescents. *Research in Community and Mental Health*, **2**, 163–182.

Rubin, G.J., Brewin, C.R., Greenberg, N., Simpson, J. & Wessely, S. (2005). Psychological and behavioural reactions to the bombings in London 7 July 2005: cross sectional survey of a representative sample of Londoners. *British Medical Journal*, **331**, 606.

Schat, A.C. & Kelloway, E.K. (2000). Effects of perceived control on the outcomes of workplace aggression and violence. *Journal of Occupational Health Psychology*, **5**, 386–402.

Schouten, R., Callahan, M.V. & Bryant, S. (2004). Community response to disaster: the role of the workplace. *Harvard Review of Psychiatry*, **12**, 229–237.

Southard, E.E. (1920). The modern specialist in unrest: a place for the psychiatrist in industry. *Journal of Industrial Hygiene*, **4**, 500.

Steele, P.D. (1989). A history of job-based alcoholism programs: 1955–1972. *Journal of Drug Issues*, **19**, 511–532.

Stein, B.D., Elliott, M.N., Jaycox, L.H. *et al.* (2003). A National Longitudinal Study of the Psychological Consequences of the September 11, 2001 Terrorist Attacks: reactions, impairment, and help-seeking. *Psychiatry*, **667**, 105–117.

Steury, S., Spencer, S. & Parkinson, G.W. (2004). The social context of recovery. *Psychiatry: Interpersonal and Biological Processes*, **67**, 158–163.

Stewart, W.F., Ricci, J.A., Chee, E., Hahn, S.R. & Morganstein, D. (2003). Cost of lost productive time among US workers with depression. *Journal of the American Medical Association*, **289**, 3135–3144.

Stith Butler, A., Panzer, A.M. & Goldfrank, L.R. (2003). *Preparing for the Psychological Consequences of Terrorism: A Public Health Strategy*. Washington, D.C.: National Academies Press.

Tehrani, N. (2002). Workplace trauma and the law. *Journal of Traumatic Stress*, **15**, 473–477.

Tierney, K.J., Lindell, M.K. & Perry, R.W. (2001). *Facing the Unexpected: Disaster Preparedness and Response in the United States*. Washington, D.C.: Joseph Henry Press.

Trice, H. & Schonbrunn, W. (1981). A history of job-based alcoholism programs: 1900–1955. *Journal of Drug Issues*, **11**, 171–198.

Tyler, M.P. & Gifford, R.K. (1991). Fatal training accidents: the military unit as a recovery context. *Journal of Traumatic Stress*, **4**, 233–249.

Ursano, R.J. (2002). Terrorism and mental health: public health and primary care. Status Report: meeting the mental health needs of the country in the wake of September 11, 2001. Presented at the Eighteenth Annual Rosalynn Carter Symposium on Mental Health Policy, The Carter Center, Atlanta, Ga.

Ursano, R.J. & Norwood, A.E. (2003). *Disaster: Responses and Management*. Washington, D.C.: American Psychiatric Publishing, Inc.

Ursano, R.J. & Vineburgh, N.T. (2004). *EAP Leadership for Terrorism Response: A Resiliency Health Promotion Strategy*. Washington, D.C.: US House of Representatives In-Service.

Ursano, R.J. & Vineburgh, N.T. (2005). EAP *Leadership for Terrorism Response: Disaster Behaviors for Resiliency*. Architect of the Capitol In-Service.

Ursano, R.J., Fullerton, C.S. & Norwood, A.E. (2003). *Terrorism and Disaster: Individual and Community Mental Health Interventions*. Cambridge: Cambridge University Press.

Ursano, R.J., Vineburgh, N.T. & Fullerton, C.S. (2004a). Corporate Health and Preparedness: bioterrorism preparedness. Presented at The Imperative for a Public Private Partnership: Sam Nunn Bank of America Policy Forum, Atlanta, Ga.

Ursano, R.J., Hall, M.J. & Gifford, R. (2004b). Psychological impact of transportation terror. Transportation Safety Administration, US Homeland Department of Transportation. Washington, D.C.: RAND corporation.

Ursano, R.J., Vineburgh, N.T., Gifford, R.K., Benedek, D.M. & Fullerton, C.S. (2006). Workplace preparedness for terrorism: Report of findings to Alfred P. Sloan Foundation. www.usuhs.mil/psy/Workplace Preparedness Terrorism.pdf, accessed May 11, 2007.

Vineburgh, N.T. (2004). The power of the pink ribbon: raising awareness of the mental health implications of terrorism. *Psychiatry*, **67**, 137–146.

Vineburgh, N.T. (2006). Book essays and reviews: My name is Bill. *Psychiatry*, in press.

Vineburgh, N.T., Ursano, R.J. & Fullerton, C.S. (2005a). Workplace preparedness and resiliency: an integrated response to terrorism. In *Workplace Violence: Issues, Trends, Strategies*, eds. V. Bowie, B. Fisher & S. Cooper. Collumpton: Willan Publishing.

Vineburgh, N.T., Ursano, R.J. & Fullerton, C.S. (2005b). Disaster consequence management: an integrated approach for fostering human continuity in the workplace. In *The Integration of Employee Assistance, Work/life, and Wellness Services*, eds. M. Attridge, P.A. Herlihy & R.P. Malden. Binghamton, New York: Haworth Press.

Vineburgh, N.T., Ursano, R.J. & Fullerton, C.S. (2005c). Disaster consequence management: an integrated approach for fostering human continuity in the workplace. *Journal of Workplace Behavioral Health*, **20**, 159–181.

Vlahov, D., Galea, S., Resnick, H. *et al.* (2002). Increased use of cigarettes, alcohol, and marijuana among Manhattan, New York residents after the September 11th terrorist attacks. *American Journal of Epidemiology*, **155**, 988–996.

Wallace, M. & Webber, L. (2004). *The Disaster Recovery Handbook*. New York: American Management Association.

Walsh, M.E., Norwood, A.E. & Hall, M.J. (2004). The 2001 anthrax attacks in the media. In *Bioterrorism: Psychological and Public Health Interventions*, eds. R.J. Ursano, C.S. Fullerton & A.E. Norwood. Cambridge: Cambridge University Press.

Weisaeth, L. (1989). The stressors and the post-traumatic stress syndrome after an industrial disaster. *Acta Psychiatrica Scandinavica*, **80** (Suppl. 355), 25–37.

14

Healthcare systems planning

Brian W. Flynn

Introduction

Few things are axiomatic in the field of disaster mental health. The need to plan and value of preparation for extraordinary events are on this short list. This level of consensus probably stems more from the demonstrated value of preparation inherent in seemingly unrelated areas such as national defense, community and personal protection, and the anthropological legacy, at least in the European context, of needing to preserve and store food for winter. Being prepared seems to work better than not being prepared. There is little argument about the value of anticipating what is possible and probable, identifying what needs to be done and who is to do it, and setting about the task of getting ready. Then why is it so difficult to design and implement sound disaster preparedness to address psychosocial issues in general, and in healthcare systems specifically?

This chapter will attempt to identify some of these obstacles to effective planning, describe components of sound approaches to preparedness, and suggest strategies to implement viable and sustainable plans. The chapter concludes with describing implications for public health, clinical care, and research.

The healthcare systems have many diverse components. In addition, across governmental lines, especially across national and regional boundaries, these systems may look quite different.

This chapter assumes a healthcare system that is, at minimum, composed of public health, hospital and community medical services, emergency medical services, and specialty health and medical care. This chapter will include discussion of community components traditionally thought of as outside the healthcare system but which are inextricably linked to healthcare in emergency situations. Examples include schools, law enforcement, and work places to name but a few.

Why is planning for behavioral health consequences important for the healthcare system?

The healthcare system is already in the mental health and disaster preparedness business. More than half of all mental health services are delivered by primary care providers (DeGruy, 1996). Most components of the healthcare system are accustomed to planning and preparing for exceptional events. In the United States, the Joint Commission on the Accreditation of Health Care Organizations (JCAHCO) accredits healthcare organizations on the basis of many factors, including the adequacy of their plans in the event of disasters. JCAHCO provides specific guidance for healthcare organizations in creating and sustaining emergency preparedness systems (JCAHCO, 2003). Most, even small, clinics and provider offices have rudimentary evacuation and emergency plans. Regrettably, few healthcare systems or components of healthcare systems have even minimally prepared for the psychosocial consequences that are visited upon them in times of disaster. Those that have plans have frequently limited their planning to dealing with people presenting with a psychiatric illness and/or coping with disruption caused by highly agitated and acting-out patients and citizens. These contingencies represent only a small portion of the psychosocial needs with which healthcare organizations are faced.

Even as overall emergency preparedness in the healthcare system has improved, many, if not most, components of the healthcare system have failed to accurately anticipate either the type or the magnitude of the psychological and psychosocial consequences. They are ill-prepared for what has repeatedly proven to be the largest health consequence of disaster: those of behavioral health. In situation after situation across the globe, the psychological footprint of large-scale disasters (particularly those with perceived health risk) has far exceeded the medical footprint. Two case examples demonstrate this phenomenon.

Case 1: *The Gulf War* (Karsenty *et al.*, 1991)

In Israel, during the 1991 Gulf War, there was widespread fear that Iraqi missiles carrying poison gas would be launched toward Israel. There were 23 missile attack alerts, 5 false alarms, and, in the end, there were no attacks using poison gas. During these attacks, there were 1059 emergency room visits representing 234 direct medical casualties, and 835 psychological casualties (78% of all casualties). About half of these psychological casualties were suffering from acute anxiety; 230 people had autoinjected atropine without exposure; 40 were injured while running to sealed rooms; 11 people died; 7 suffocated in their gas masks; and there were 4 fatal heart attacks.

In summary, there were more fatalities from fear-driven behaviors than from missile impact and there were more hospital visits resulting from psychological responses than from medical injury.

Case 2: *Sarin gas attack* (Kawana *et al.*, 2001)

In 1995, Sarin gas was released in the subway system of Tokyo, Japan. There were 12 deaths, 17 critical injuries, and 1370 mild to moderate injuries. There were 5510 emergency room visits, yet of that number more than 4000 had no medical effects at all. Many of those seeking care in emergency rooms arrived there within hours of the incident, seriously taxing medical resources. In this case, psychological casualties arrived very quickly and significantly outnumbered medical casualties.

Finally, the integration of behavioral health into the healthcare system has support and foundation well beyond disaster situations. In the first ever *Mental Health: A Report of the Surgeon General* (US Department of Health and Human Services, 1999), the then Surgeon General, David Satcher, MD, made several recommendations germane to the topic of this chapter. He noted that mental health is fundamental to good health. He recommended that mental health should be part of the mainstream of healthcare. He urged that the split between mental and physical health be mended. The field of disaster mental health has an opportunity to help move the nation and the world toward those goals.

The larger context of planning

Although the field of disaster mental health is relatively young, overall planning has evolved significantly over a long period of time. If the healthcare system is to develop usable and sustainable plans, a basic understanding of the larger planning context is important. Specifically, the overall approach to planning used by emergency managers at all governmental levels, overarching plans that are in place, and how incidents are managed are critical.

All-hazards planning

In recent history, many remember a time when planning was conducted on a hazard-specific basis.

For example, a community might have a tornado plan, a flood plan, a plan for widespread fires, and so forth. Because it is impossible to anticipate every eventuality, most emergency planning around the world is currently based on some form of all-hazards model. As an example, this is the model utilized by the United States' national emergency preparedness and response entity, the Federal Emergency Management Agency (FEMA), within the Department of Homeland Defense. They describe (US Department of Homeland Security/ Federal Emergency Management Agency, 1996) an all-hazards plan as one that:

- Assigns responsibility to carry out actions in emergencies
- Sets forth lines of authority and organizational relationships
- Describes how people and property will be protected in emergencies
- Identifies personnel, equipment, facilities, supplies, and other resources available
- Identifies steps to address mitigation.

All-hazards planning recognizes that in most events, irrespective of type, there are roles, relationships, and core activities that remain the same. This planning model then goes on to identify specific types of events (e.g., floods, fires, terrorism, etc.) and describes any specific issues, actions, and relationships necessary to respond effectively.

Clearly, the healthcare system is an extraordinarily important part of community infrastructure and may be called upon to plan central roles in the event of many types of disasters and emergencies. It behooves all healthcare systems to understand and participate in planning within the context of the community beyond health and to integrate mental health into the medical incident management infrastructure (DeMartino & Flynn, 2004; Flynn, 2005).

In the aftermath of September 11, 2001, FEMA placed even more emphasis on preparedness (US Department of Homeland Security/FEMA, 2002) and required that states address special elements on several activities that are related directly to healthcare systems:

- Identification and protection of critical infrastructure
- Inventory of critical response equipment and teams
- Interstate and intrastate mutual aid agreements
- Resource typing
- Resource standards to include interoperability protocols and a common incident command system
- State and local continuity of operations (COOP) and continuity of government (COG)
- Citizen and family preparedness, including Citizen Corps and other volunteer initiatives in responding to an incident.

The National Response Plan

In the United States, there is an overall plan, based on an all-hazards approach, that governs and guides the country in the management of domestic incidents. That document is the National Response Plan (NRP) (US Department of Homeland Security, 2004).

The NRP forms the basis of how the federal government coordinates with state, local, and tribal governments and the private sector during incidents. The goals of the NRP are to:

- Save lives and protect the health and safety of the public, responders, and recovery workers
- Ensure security of the homeland
- Prevent an imminent incident, including acts of terrorism, from occurring
- Protect and restore critical infrastructure and key resources
- Conduct law enforcement investigations to resolve the incident, apprehend the perpetrators, and collect and preserve evidence for prosecution and/or attribution
- Protect property and mitigate damages and impacts to individuals, communities, and the environment

- Facilitate recovery of individuals, families, businesses, governments, and the environment.

The NRP is the foundation of all state and local planning and a document with which planners in the healthcare system should be intimately familiar.

Incident management

Until recently, in the United States there was little uniformity in how the management of the early stages of an incident was organized. The result was sometimes disorganization, delay, and conflict among responders (including health). To reduce the potential of these adverse outcomes, a national program is being put in place called the National Incident Management System (NIMS) (US Department of Homeland Security/FEMA, 2005). The goal of NIMS is to help responders at all levels to work together more effectively to manage domestic incidents no matter what the cause, size or complexity.

The Federal Emergency Management Agency (FEMA) hopes that the national adaptation of this system will result in the following positive benefits:

- Standardized organizational structures, processes and procedures
- Standards for planning, training and exercising, and personnel qualification standards
- Equipment acquisition and certification standards
- Interoperable communications processes, procedures, and systems
- Information management systems
- Supporting technologies – voice and data communications systems, information systems, data display systems, and specialized technologies.

With the exception of those in the emergency medical system, this program to unify command and standardize incident management is probably unfamiliar. All those in the healthcare system who have responsibilities for planning for, and responding to, disasters will be well served by becoming very familiar with this emerging system.

In the early hours of a major incident, the structure of response (including the role of components of the healthcare system) will be based on NIMS. Components of the healthcare system, and individuals within those components, will be required to know the NIMS (and probably have that knowledge certified) and function within it.

The what, if, and with whom of planning

Hazard identification

The first element of sound planning involves determining what is being planned for. This is far easier said than done. How can any element of a healthcare system possibly anticipate every eventuality? They cannot. While careful analysis of potential threats is useful (see Table 14.1), not every eventuality can ever be foreseen.

Hazard potential

Not all hazards are equally likely to occur. Working with knowledgeable experts in the field such as emergency management, public health, and law enforcement, healthcare providers can assess (although not with certainty) the types of events that might be most likely to occur in their communities. No planning effort can anticipate all potential events but careful review with knowledgeable community partners can go a long way toward identifying those types of event that may be most likely. Members of the healthcare community can play an important role in identifying the potential health (including behavioral health) consequences of a wide variety of incidents.

Potential community partners

Planning occurs within a community context. A comprehensive and integrated plan requires the involvement of many formal and informal community partners, each of which will be affected by the function of the others during any incident.

Table 14.1 Potential hazard types and potential causes (adapted from US Department of Health and Human Services, 2003)

Type	Natural	Human-caused (intentional)	Human-caused (unintentional)
Flooding (flash/slow rising) and dam failure	+	+	+
Hazardous materials (including chemicals)		+	+
Hurricane	+		
Fire	+	+	+
Earthquake	+		
Military chemical agents and munitions		+	+
Radiological hazards (medical usage, educational, educational institutions, military, manufacturing companies, transport of nuclear materials)		+	+
Nuclear power plants		+	+
Snow/ice	+		
Tornado	+		
Transportation emergency (aircraft, train, bus, multi-vehicle, boat)		+	+
Tsunami	+		
Civil unrest/community violence		+	
Agricultural disaster/emergencies	+	+	+
Emerging infectious diseases	+	+	+
Immigration emergencies		+	+
Incendiary devices		+	+
Terrorism		+	

The role of disaster behavioral health in planning

Much disaster planning has occurred without significant input from, and the participation of, behavioral health professionals with expertise and experience in disaster preparedness and response. One can speculate as to why this is the case. Reasons may include lack of awareness regarding the scope of behavioral health disaster impact and what behavioral health professionals can contribute, stereotypes about behavioral health issues and providers, and lack of interest, skills, sophistication, and initiative by behavioral health professionals in approaching and informing emergency managers.

The result, in many cases, is a limited, inaccurate, and stereotypical view by emergency managers of the nature and scope of behavioral health consequences. There are often limited opportunities to correct inaccuracies and expand understanding. Participation in the planning process is one of those opportunities.

Several significant documents can provide a broad understanding of the contribution that behavioral health professionals can and should make. Many of the findings and recommendations have a direct bearing on planning.

First, two meetings of disaster experts (Ursano *et al.*, 2001, 2002) produced recommendations about mental health and behavioral planning,

Table 14.2 Potential community planning partners

Health	Government	Agencies	Voluntary	Others
Hospitals	Public health authority	Head Start	Red Cross	Private schools
Specialty care providers (including behavioral health)	Mental health authority	Daycare	Salvation Army	Major business and industry
Nursing homes	Substance abuse authority	Social service agencies	Faith community	Small employers
Private practice providers	Developmental Disability Authority	Vocational rehabilitation providers	Crime victim advocates	Media organizations
Managed behavioral healthcare companies	Public education/ schools		Health advocacy organizations	Unions
Managed care organizations	Emergency management agencies		Behavioral health advocate organizations	
Emergency Medical Services	Homeland security agencies		Service organizations	
	Veterans Affairs		Child/school advocacy organizations	
	Military institutions Vocational rehabilitation agencies Social service agencies Law enforcement			

education and training, public health policy for the psychological consequences of bioterrorism, communication, decision support, and research.

Second, in the fall of 2001, 58 disaster mental health experts met to address the impact of early psychological interventions following mass violence (e.g., school violence, terrorism, work-place violence). After reviewing the evidence, this group made recommendations in the following areas (National Institute of Mental Health, 2002), many of which have planning implications:

- Secure basic needs
- Provide Psychological First Aid
- Conduct needs assessment
- Monitor the rescue and recovery environment for stressors
- Conduct outreach and disseminate information
- Provide technical assistance
- Provide consultation to leadership
- Provide training
- Foster resilience and recovery
- Conduct psychological triage
- Provide treatment.

In addition to providing sound guidance, the products of the above meeting illustrate the very wide variety of contributions that experts in beha-vioral health can provide in the planning, response, and recovery phases of disasters.

Definitions of disaster, how they unfold, and planning challenges

For planning purposes, it may be helpful to think beyond the type of incident to how that event impacts on the capacity of any given community. That impact can be expressed as a function of the relationship between needs and resources. This allows any given community to consider a differential response within a common language and to recognize that different communities have different definitions of "disasters." In the planning process, this taxonomy, or something similar, is important as much of disaster response involves rapid analysis of needs and the prevailing availability and adequacy of resources.

For example, the following definitions are commonly used:

Emergency – a situation that is urgent but can be managed within the resources of the community

Crisis – a situation that can be handled adequately within existing resources but those resources are pressed to their limits

Disaster – a situation where needs exceed resources but where supplemental resources can bring the situation under control and recovery can begin

Catastrophe – a situation in which needs greatly overwhelm resources and the basic infrastructure of the response is either destroyed or unable to remain functional.

Using this schema, consider an apartment house fire that leaves six people alive but critically burned. In a major metropolitan area, with several hospitals containing burns centers, this would probably constitute an emergency in which care was available and accessible. In a medium-sized city, this may be a crisis where local hospitals could absorb these casualties but capacity would be exhausted. In a rural community or on an isolated island, where there were few or no medical services available, such an incident would probably be considered a disaster. If this apartment house fire was caused by a massive earthquake that destroyed roads, bridges, electrical grids, and several hospitals, it might be considered a catastrophe.

Life cycle of a disaster

Sound planning anticipates needs and opportunities in at least three stages in the life cycle of a disaster. Additional differentiations may be helpful. These stages are:

Pre-event – what types of preparedness, training, alliances, threat monitoring/identification strategies can/should occur in advance of any event?

Response (during and immediately following) – who does what, when, where, and to whom while an event is occurring or shortly thereafter?

Recovery (longer term) – when the event has passed, how do individuals, families, organizations and institutions, and communities begin to rebuild and reconstitute.

Changing planning assumptions/challenges

Viable planning must incorporate the notion of a dynamic and ever changing environment and the plan itself must be a living and changing document. The plans for any given healthcare system should include new risks such as expanded transportation patterns, emerging diseases, and changing work, housing, and social patterns. Categories of planning assumptions might include natural disasters, unintentional human-generated events (e.g., accidental chemical spill from a derailed train), and intentional events (e.g., terrorism). In addition, government at all levels continues to produce expectations and requirements (optimally with funding) which all response and recovery organizations must absorb.

Goals of good planning

What are we trying to accomplish by good planning? This question can be answered for both the healthcare system itself and from the perspective of the healthcare system as part of the fabric of the community(ies) which it serves (Shultz *et al.*, 2004).

Healthcare system level

At the healthcare system level, good planning tries to:
- Provide care for disaster victims/survivors
- Maintain care for current existing patients
- Safeguard staff
- Support responders
- Exercise effective leadership before, during, and following a crisis.

Community level

As part of the fabric of the community, the healthcare system strives to:
- Promote community health
- Reduce exposure, illness, and injury
- Reduce mortality
- Promote pro-social behavior
- Reduce fear-driven behavior
- Safeguard the healthcare system.

Elements of good planning

There are many useful sources of information and guidance for healthcare system disaster planning found throughout this chapter. Few address behavioral health issues in a comprehensive manner. *Mental Health All-Hazards Planning Guidance* (US Department of Health and Human Services, 2003) contains considerable guidance regarding both the planning process and the contents of the plans. It should be noted that the intended audience of the *Mental Health All-Hazards Planning Guidance* is mental health planners, not necessarily health system planners. Nonetheless, the process and content recommendations have broad applicability. The following two subsections draw heavily on that document. In addition, the Appendix contains a matrix similar to one found in the *Mental Health All-Hazards Planning Guidance* but slightly adapted for healthcare systems and organizations.

When thinking of goals of planning and preparedness, one should not lose site of the opportunity for primary prevention of adverse medical and psychological consequences. The best plan would be one that prevents disastrous events. While only the ignorant and arrogant would attempt to change patterns of nature there may be opportunities to do a better job of removing ourselves individually and collectively from harm's way. As an example, perhaps primary prevention means the opportunity and responsibility to inform development decisions, such as building on barrier islands or in flood-prone areas.

With respect to the physical and mental health consequences of human-caused events such as terrorism or other mass violence clearly it would be best if those types of events could be prevented from occurring in the first place. It would be wise to commit our expertise to that cause. If these events cannot be prevented, perhaps some of their health consequences can. Health and mental health experts should care a great deal about how buildings are constructed, how glass breaks, and how transportation security is designed and implemented. If we can prevent the exposure, we have prevented the trauma. If we can reduce physical trauma, we can reduce psychological trauma. Sometimes the most basic opportunities are missed.

The planning process

The process of planning is nearly as important as the resulting plan. Even if no incident occurs, many have found that relationships established and strengthened in the disaster planning process have paid dividends in other ways. Who is involved, who leads, who has what roles, how agreement is reached and conflicts resolved are all critical determinants of the quality and success of any plan.

One of the most common and significant errors is the failure in the planning process to include those who are being planned for (Lasker, 2004).

This has resulted in inaccurate assumptions about how people behave, a reduction in compliance, trust, and confidence, and a lack of understanding by planners of the factors that influence the public's comfort with, and confidence in, planning.

There are several foundational elements necessary for sound planning. While they may initially seem obvious and intuitive, planning that proceeds without assuring that these factors are addressed has a high probability of failure. These elements include:

Human resources – are there adequate numbers, skills, and perspectives represented in the planning process?

Time – good planning takes time. Is there adequate time to consider a full range of risks, roles, resources and to bring all factors together in a meaningful plan that can be reviewed and endorsed by all stakeholders?

Sanction – do those doing the planning have the authority to plan and to make commitments for organizations, governmental entities, and diverse community elements?

Funding – planning is not free. In addition to the time of planning participants (often considerable), there are usually expenses related to logistics, special analysis/studies, and duplication and publication. Are there adequate funds to get the job done?

Adaptation – planning is not a single-stage process resulting in a permanent document. Viable plans change continuously over time as a product of many factors including:

- changing risks
- changing community composition and constellation
- changing governmental and community organizations
- changing laws, rules, technology, and science
- lessons learned from drills, exercises, and actual events.

Even during the initial planning process, planners should consider how plans will be changed and updated. The who, how, when, and with what resources questions of plan viability and sustainability should be addressed in the planning process.

A checklist intended to identify key elements of a sound planning process are included in Table 14.3.

Table 14.3 Key elements of the planning process (adapted from US Department of Health and Human Services, 2003)

□ Secure support/sanction for planning	□ Involve representatives who can make decisions for their organizations
□ Know the "culture" of the city, county, state, etc.	□ Keep expectations and timelines realistic
□ Anticipate problems from the start	□ Optimize use of existing data/information/experience
□ Err on the side of over inclusion of interested parties	□ Define populations at risk/to be served
□ Have a leader	□ Assure attention to cultural factors and cultural competence in the process
□ Keep reminding participants of the benefits of the effort	□ Include representation of the interests of special populations
□ Appreciate and acknowledge the concerns/constraints/expertise of all	□ Even at the start, assure a plan for adapting the plan over time
□ Assure adequate human resources to get the job done	□ Assure adequate funding to complete the planning process and assure sustainability
□ Assure that those who are being planned *for* are involved in the public planning process	□ Other considerations

Plan content

The content of a plan will be the product of many factors including who is involved in the plans development, licensing and accreditation requirements, state and local laws and regulations, and the particular needs of the healthcare system. The content of the plan will also obviously be a product of the nature of the agency or organization doing the planning.

A template intended to provide an example of potential elements of an all-hazards plan can be found in the Appendix. Not all elements of the template will apply to all organizations. The template is included to serve as a guide intended to be modified and adapted to the particular needs of the organization and location.

Roles of the healthcare system

In disaster situations, the healthcare system serves at least three major functions (Shultz *et al.*, 2004). Sound planning in each of these functional areas, in all three stages discussed earlier, can provide a solid template for planning (Table 14.4).

Patient care providers

Healthcare organizations exist to treat patients. In the event of a disaster, patient care may involve caring for existing patients; managing a surge of new patients who have been, believe they are, and fear they are, injured and/or exposed; screening and triaging large numbers of people seeking care;

Table 14.4 Model for phase roles of healthcare provider organizations

Phases	Roles patient care provide	Work place	Community partner
Pre-event			
During event			
Postevent			

and assisting people attempting to find loved ones, people. For most of these individuals and families fear and anxiety will be a significant part of their presentation.

Work places

All parts of the healthcare system are operated by people. In the well intentioned rush to provide good patient care, the needs of workers of all types, and the responsibilities of healthcare organizations to support and care for workers and their families are all too often overlooked. Overwork, potential exposure and illness, exposure to large-scale death, injury, and mutilation, and concern for family welfare and safety are more common than not in many types of disaster situations. Planning elements should include making provision for assuring staff safety and security, staff and family support; reducing and managing staff stress; and assuring a range of psychosocial interventions for staff when necessary.

Healthcare organizations can assist their workers by encouraging them to develop personal and family disaster plans. Staff who have taken planning seriously in their own lives are more likely to be able to play their occupational roles in times of disaster. Several guides to personal disaster preparedness are available (American Red Cross, 2005; Federal Emergency Management Agency, 2005; US Department of Homeland Security/ FEMA, 2004).

Community partners

The importance of community partnerships was noted earlier in this chapter. All elements of the healthcare system exist in the context of the communities in which they reside and operate. At the same time, individual elements of the healthcare system, including hospitals, public health, primary and specialty care community providers, and specialty facilities, relate to each other and those outside the healthcare system in unique ways.

These relationships are often missing, strained, or unclear even at the best of times. It is not difficult so see why operating partnerships are difficult to manage during a disaster. Planning before an event is the best way to ensure that things will go well during an event. It is frequently said that during an event is not the time to be meeting and exchanging business cards for the first time!

The context of communities includes their characteristics and the individual and organizational roles of its members. Planning should be sensitive to such factors as current and historic stresses, resilience, rivalries, vulnerabilities, and formal and informal leadership.

Critical linkages for the healthcare system

In recent years (in the United States especially since the attacks of September 11, 2001) there has been much more emphasis on preparing for extraordinary events. There has been increased activity at governmental, organizational, community, family, and individual levels. In fact, this motivation to prepare for adversity may be one of the few positive consequences of these traumatic events.

On the other hand however, it appears that much planning and preparedness continue to occur primarily inside organizational silos and the integration of organization and systems preparedness necessary for a viable response is not as common as it needs to be.

For example, hospital disaster planning is common (even though the behavioral health components of planning may be seriously underdeveloped). However, little hospital planning is focused on integration with other key elements of the community such as schools. Many hospital staff have children in schools. If schools are closed or evacuated, it is highly likely that hospital staff may not come to work, may leave work, or be so distracted from their hospital roles that performance and safety are compromised. Much work is needed in horizontally integrating the expanded effort that has gone into improved vertical integration.

Overall relationships in the disaster response environment should be guided and informed by the requirements of the NRP discussed earlier in this chapter. While describing an overall all-hazards approach, the plan also identifies specialized support functions (Emergency Support Functions or ESFs) and identifies key governmental departments and agencies to carry out these support functions. Primary and secondary responsibilities are prescribed. While the NRP addresses federal agencies, all states closely follow the format of the NRP for regional, state, and local planning. Members of the healthcare community will want to pay special attention to no. 8 – Public Health and Medical Services. To illustrate the scope of health-related activities identified under the NRP, Table 14.5 lists the various ESFs and identifies those in which governmental health agencies have primary and secondary responsibilities.

While Table 14.5 is helpful in identifying and illustrating the wide variety of roles in which the healthcare system may be important during a disaster, it provides little in the way of identifying important behavioral health opportunities and responsibilities. However, it is very useful in providing a framework in which to explore opportunities to provide assistance and leadership. It is not a difficult leap to review the various ESFs and identify ways in which experts in the behavioral sciences can help evaluate needs, provide critical psychosocial information and education, provide consultation and training to leadership, and so forth.

There are also opportunities to be helpful even in areas where no health role is identified in the NRP. For example:

- Psychosocial support to firefighters (ESF no. 4)
- Helping the public deal with the fear and distress caused by energy failures (ESF no. 12)
- Providing stress support to veterinarians who face the task of killing large numbers of apparently healthy animals (ESF no. 11).

Each healthcare system should assess the requirements and opportunities to link with key community partners. The following are a few examples of critical linkages.

Table 14.5 Health roles in the National Response Plan

ESF[a]	P/S	Description
ESF no. 1 – Transportation		
ESF no. 2 – Communications		
ESF no. 3 – Public works and engineering	S[b]	Environmental health, water supply, wastewater
ESF no. 4 – Firefighting		
ESF no. 5 – Emergency management	S	Expert advice
ESF no. 6 – Mass care, housing & human services	S	Shelter operations, medical care, medical supplies, technical expertise on food, water supply
ESF no. 7 – Resource support		
ESF no. 8 – Public health & medical services	P[c]	Public health surveillance, health needs assessment, medical supplies and personnel, information & education, expert advice, patient evacuation, worker safety, drugs and biologicals, food safety and security, behavioral health care, protection of animal health, public health and medical information, vector control, victim identification/mortuary services
ESF no. 9 – Urban search & rescue	S	Support for medical teams
ESF no. 10 – Oil & hazardous material	S	Assess health hazards, worker safety, establish disease registries, health information and education, disposal of contaminated food
ESF no. 11 – Agriculture & natural resources	S	Protect food supply, surveillance for zoonotic diseases, lab & diagnostic support, field investigators for tracing, investigation and eradicating disease
ESF no. 12 – Energy		
ESF no. 13 – Public safety & security		
ESF no. 14 – Long-term community recovery & mitigation	P/S	Provide expertise in long-term health and medical concerns and mental health services
ESF no. 15 – External affairs	S	

[a] ESF = Emergency Support Function.
[b] S = Secondary role/responsibility.
[c] P = Primary role/responsibility.

Emergency management

In natural disasters local, regional, and national government emergency management organizations have primary authority and responsibility for planning and response. It is critical that all elements of the healthcare system be part of that planning to ensure that accurate assumptions regarding the healthcare system are being made and that elements of the healthcare systems understand their roles and the relationship of their roles to others.

Increasingly, emergency managers are recognizing the importance of understanding and incorporating psychosocial considerations in their work. Assistance in the form of expertise, information, consultation, and training is often welcomed.

Education

Many of any community's children spend considerable portions of their days in schools. In addition, schools and school systems are typically significant employers of adults in the community. In many cases, schools are part of the healthcare system. Schools have nurses, crisis teams and can benefit from participating with the larger healthcare system in realistic drills and simulations (Shaw & Shaw, 2004). The integration and coordination of healthcare and school plans are critical.

Because of the pervasiveness of all-hazards approaches in schools as well as other community elements, schools have special planning challenges to deal not only with emergencies and disasters outside schools but also emergencies (e.g., violence within schools) that have significant impact on the healthcare system.

Law enforcement

In disaster situations, law enforcement agencies have many responsibilities. At minimum, they will have significant roles in access to, egress from, and movement within the disaster zone. In significant public health emergencies, law enforcement will have major roles in enforcing movement restrictions (e.g., quarantine or shelter in place). For healthcare systems, even this single law enforcement function will have implications for staff and patient movement to and from healthcare providers. In situations involving terrorism, the disaster scene is also a crime scene and the injured are both crime victims and witnesses. There may be conflicting priorities of medical response and recovery and the preservation of evidence and crime documentation. While no amount of planning can eliminate all potential problems, good planning can help reduce conflicts and thereby enhance the function of both healthcare systems and law enforcement.

Clearly pre-event planning involving the healthcare system and law enforcement can help address many behavioral health elements. These areas include managing disruptive behavior, factors influencing collective behavior, dispelling myths about panic, stress management approaches, to name a few.

Transportation

Every aspect of transportation impacts the healthcare system. A transportation accident may be the disaster itself (e.g., plane crash or multi-vehicle accidents). The degree to which the transportation system is intact or compromised following a disaster will have significant impact on all elements of the healthcare system. For example, if critical roads are closed, hospitals may receive only a small proportion of the injured patients they might otherwise receive. At the same time, they may experience a surge of patients who might normally be seen elsewhere. Healthcare system plans should be fully integrated with transportation planning. The intactness of transportation systems will be a factor in family reunification following a disaster – a major source of fear and distress.

Business and industry

Much disaster planning is focused on public sector organizations. Too little attention is paid to the centrality of business and industry to the life and fabric of a community and the importance of economic (heavily influenced by the resilience of business and industry following a disaster) issues in mental health outcomes. In a disaster, the artificial and often only theoretical membrane that separates family and personal life from work life is often torn.

Following September 11, 2001 in New York, the walls between the public and private sectors literally came down. For individuals and communities to recover from disaster, planning must forge and sustain partnerships with business and industry so that unique roles, needs, and resources can be identified.

Critical challenges for healthcare system planning

Education of funders/leaders

Perhaps the greatest impediment to optimal preparedness is the lack of appreciation of the

are axiomatic in the field. What are the beliefs that underlie this perspective? They are twofold:

1. Planning results in a more rapid response, a more appropriate response, and a more efficient response.
2. Planning results in responses that reduce and also prevent adverse psychosocial effects.

Unfortunately, these beliefs have little evidentiary support. They simply have not been tested to the point where we can say with confidence what types of planning, in what contexts, involving who, and implemented in what ways have what types of effects.

In addition, and just as importantly, there are at least four areas that beg for more evidence and data, and that lack consensus among leaders in the field. These are:

1. Planning to do what? What are we fundamentally trying to accomplish as a result of the interventions we are planning for? Treat a disorder? Prevent a disorder? Provide comfort and support? Change the trajectory of psychosocial response? Promote mental health, positive coping, resilience? Until we are clear on what we are trying to accomplish, it is difficult to plan with precision.
2. Services provided by whom? What we are trying to do will have a major influence upon deciding who is best qualified to do it. There is significant divergence of views on what can best be done by mental health professionals, trained paraprofessionals, clergy/chaplains, teachers, and others. Within healthcare organizations there is discussion about what can and should be done by most staff (such as Psychological First Aid), what can be done by a variety of health professionals, and what should be done by licensed mental health professionals. Even if there is consensus on using resources outside healthcare organizations, these issues must be arranged during the planning process to ensure that legal issues are addressed.
3. Programming using what strategies? What interventions work best for whom, when, and under what circumstances? For example, when is Psychological First Aid, or cognitive-behavioral therapy, or crisis counseling indicated? Should approaches be population based or based on risk? What is the role of activities such as training, consultation to leadership, risk and crisis communication?
4. Strategies based on what? What are the criteria for evaluating the efficacy of different interventions? Should they be evidence based/informed? What about field experience? Belief? Consensus?

Conclusion

It may seem that the planning process, the content of plans, and the as yet unanswered questions about intervention are overwhelming. They are but we must not be overwhelmed to the point of inaction. In spite of the difficulty and gaps, planning within the healthcare system to respond capably to the wide variety of behavioral health needs is imperative. If we are honest, many elements of healthcare are implemented with incomplete and sometimes controversial foundations.

Victims and survivors deserve the best we can do, yet they cannot wait for us to have all the answers to all the questions. Involving a wide variety of stakeholders in a demanding and unending process is no small task … yet it must be done. Disasters do not wait.

Acknowledgments

Much of the content regarding healthcare in this chapter draws heavily upon training curricula developed for public health and healthcare organizations by the Disaster and Extreme Event Preparedness (DEEP) Center at the Miller School of Medicine, University of Miami. The development of these curricula was supported by the Florida Department of Health using funds from the Centers for Disease Control and Prevention and the Health Services and Resources Administration. I have worked closely with DEEP Center in the development

Appendix 14.6 Example of a template for an all-hazards disaster planning guide

	NA	Assigned	Time	Comment
1. Introductory material A. Signature page B. Dated title page C. Record of changes D. Record of distribution E. Table of contents	NA	Assigned	Time	Comment
2. Executive Summary Summary describing basic plan	NA	Assigned	Time	Comment
3. Purpose General statement of plan's purpose	NA	Assigned	Time	Comment
4. Situation and assumptions – general A. Assumptions (limits of organization, highest probability scenarios, etc.) B. Situation (probable impact, vulnerable/special facilities & populations, include low-probability/ high-impact events, etc.) C. Include matrix of events if desired	NA	Assigned	Time	Comment
5. Concept of operations – general (sequence and scope of response) A. Overview of approach (what should happen, when, at whose direction) B. Division of responsibility (state, federal, regional, etc.) C. General sequence of actions before, during, after event Who is D. authorized to request aid in what situations	NA	Assigned	Time	Comment
6. Authorities and references Citation of legal authorities and reference documents as appropriate	NA	Assigned	Time	Comment
7. Organization and assignment of responsibilities A. Listing, by position and organization, of what types of tasks are to be performed (matrix of primary/secondary/ shared responsibilities?) B. Documents tasks in FEMA format: definition of objective, characterization of the situation, general plan of action, delegation of responsibilities, information on resources and administrative support necessary to accomplish tasks. Include description of treatment responsibilities (internal/external) C. Describes health tasks in an emergency that are outside organization's normal role D. Tasks related to other governmental units and organizations (e.g., Red Cross, faith organizations, DHS, FEMA, adjoining jurisdictions, etc.)	NA	Assigned	Time	Comment Included in several places but incomplete. Review all to assure consistence

Appendix 14.6 (cont.)

E. Describes coordination with components of
   government such as Mental Health Authority, Criminal
   Justice, Law Enforcement, Fire and Rescue, Parks and
   Recreation, Animal Care and Control, Victims Services,
   Social Services, Education
F. Relationship/coordination with governmental
   emergency plans ensured, complete, and described

8. Administration, logistics, legal	NA	Assigned	Time	Comment

A. Admin: recording and reporting program activities
B. Admin: recording and reporting expenditures &
   obligations
C. Admin: recording and reporting human resources
   utilization
D. Admin: expectations of situation reports
   (format & frequency)
E. Admin: recording and reporting of services
   provided by volunteer agencies
F. Admin: management of volunteer offers/services
G. Logistics: arrangements for support needs
   (food, water, fuel, etc.)
H. Logistics: provision for self support for at least 72 h
 I. Logistics: replacement/repair of damaged/destroyed
   essential equipment
J. Logistics: access of personnel to impacted area
   (badging, transportation)
K. Logistics: availability, transport, administration,
   safeguarding, recording medications
L. Logistics: existence and scope of mutual aid
   agreements
M. Legal: issues including licensing, informed
   consent, confidentiality, providers licensed in other
   jurisdictions, personal, professional, and organizational
   liability, management of patients records

9. Plan development and maintenance	NA	Assigned	Time	Comment

A. Describes who is responsible for modifications and
   updating, assuring coordination with other emergency
   planning elements

10. Communications	NA	Assigned	Time	Comment

A. Situation assumptions (types of situations likely to
   occur – should relate to earlier assumptions, types of
   communications necessary such as telephone, data, etc.)
B. Methods of communication among medical and
   psychiatric hospitals, community-based treatment

Appendix 14.6 (cont.)

		NA	Assigned	Time	Comment

facilities, EMA, Regional or Field Offices, emergency
medical services, hospitals and clinics, shelter facilities.
Assure organization is on notification list when
emergencies occur
  C. Alternatives in the event of failed
     communication capacity
  D. Availability of technical expertise

11. Public information   NA   Assigned   Time   Comment
  A. Identification of responsibility
  B. Policies for public information (who can speak on
     what with what authority)
  C. Existence of PI materials (fact sheets, guides,
     multiple languages, access to services, distribution
     of materials, etc.)
  D. Relationship with other PIOs
  E. Identified means of disseminating information
  F. Identification of experts/resources outside
  G. Pre-event relationships with media

12. Warning/mobilization (internal/external)   NA   Assigned   Time   Comment
  A. Internal: links with emergency management
     warning activities
  B. Internal: describe methods and procedures for
     notifying staff, facilities, service providers, other as
     appropriate (link to organizations risk management
     as appropriate)
  C. Internal: policies and procedures for offices and
     facilities (e.g., sending staff home, holding staff in
     place, recall of essential staff, facilities evacuation, etc.)
  D. External: identifies groups with special warning
     needs (e.g., deaf, blind, etc.)
  E. External: notify public healthcare
     system (providers, etc.)
  F. External: notification of private sector
     health resources

13. Evacuation   NA   Assigned   Time   Comment
  A. Plan for evacuation of organizations' offices
     and facilities
  B. Plan for alternative sites (hot, warm,
     cold sites as appropriate)
  C. Clear linkage with emergency management's
     evacuation plans and operations
  D. Plan for services at shelters/mass care facilities

Appendix 14.6 (cont.)

14. Mass care	NA	Assigned	Time	Comment

A. Documentation of coordination with emergency
   management mass care plan
B. Linkage with Red Cross facilities and other
   VOAD Agencies

15. Special health and medical considerations	NA	Assigned	Time	Comment

A. Health plans document coordination with
   emergency management
B. Health plan documents responsibilities under ESF-8
C. Roles identified in areas of services/consultation to
   primary victims, secondary victims, response and
   recovery workers, incident command, public
   information, body identification and recovery,
   mortuary services, other Agencies and
   Departments (e.g., education, social services, etc.)
D. Health plan documents roles and responsibilities
   of Agencies and Departments with secondary
   responsibilities
E. Documentation of coordination with Red Cross Services
F. Initial Epi activities (human resources, material
   resources, information collection/analysis and
   utilization plans clear)
G. Movement restriction plans
H. Strategic National Stockpile (SNS)
 I. Mortuary Services/ME's Office
 J. Documents relationships with support agencies
   consistent with disaster response plan

16. Resource management	NA	Assigned	Time	Comment

A. Purpose: document means, organization, and
   process by which organization will find, obtain,
   allocate, and distribute of necessary resources
B. Personnel
C. Transportation for staff
D. Emergency equipment as necessary
E. Mass care supplies for organization's resources
F. Regional mutual aid
G. Management of offers of assistance and
   invited/uninvited volunteers
H. Availability of aid from other States and Federal
   government
 I. Plan for maintaining financial and legal
   accountability
 J. Resources for needs assessment

Appendix 14.6 (cont.)

	NA	Assigned	Time	Comment
17. All-hazards specific planning materials (natural and accidental)				

   A. Plan allows for accommodation of unique aspects of hazards
   B. Identifies nature of hazard
   C. Identifies areas of high risk
   D. Flooding (flash and slow rising) and dam failure
   E. Hazardous materials (including chemicals)
   F. Hurricane
   G. Fire
   H. Earthquake
   I. Military chemical agents and munitions
   J. Radiological hazards (medical usage, educational institutions, military, manufacturing companies, transport of nuclear material)
   K. Nuclear power plant(s)
   L. Nuclear conflict (War)
   M. Snow/Ice
   N. Tornado
   O. Civil unrest/community violence
   P. Immigration emergencies
   Q. Other(s) (specify)

	NA	Assigned	Time	Comment
18. Terrorism				

   A. Describes nature of potential hazards (chemical, biological, nuclear/radiological, explosive, cyber, combined)
   B. Potential targets are identified and/or reflective of disaster response plan
   C. Describes incident management for organization
   D. Describes and/or reflects disaster response plan, situational assumptions (environment, populations, infrastructure, transport patterns, airports, trains/subways, government facilities, recreation facilities, military installations, HazMat facilities, other high-risk targets such as financial institutions, national landmarks, embassies, universities, hospitals, research institutes, schools, day care centers)
   E. Reflects coordination with disaster response plan's modeling of potential release areas
   F. Incident management reflects roles of other organization and government roles and resources
   G. Consequence management reflects involvement of various external components
   H. Health plan reflects knowledge of and integration with disaster response plan with respect

Appendix 14.6 (cont.)

to warning, communication, emergency public
information, protective actions, mass care,
behavioral health, resource management
I. Describes plan and procedures for medical
screening of potential victims and includes mental
disorders and psychogenic symptomatology,
functional impairment, substance abuse, etc.
J. Describes health structure for surveillance,
screening, consultation, intervention planning,
risk communication
K. Describes health role in risk communication
planning and response

19. Continuity of operations   NA   Assigned   Time   Comment
A. Contains overview of goals of continuity of
operations plan (e.g., to maintain/re-establish vital
functions of organization during the first 72 h
following an event that would seriously
compromise or halt normal operations)
B. Documents coordination with overall government
continuity of operations plans
C. Identifies vital functions to be maintained
within first 72 h
D. Identifies vital records/data necessary to
function within first 72 h
E. Describes plans related to human resources
(e.g., essential staff, staff notification, family support)
F. Describes alternative locations of essential operations
G. Describes transportation and staff support
H. Describes alternative vital record/document
sites (e.g., assurance of access to disaster plan,
staff rosters, patient vital medical records if
existing sites are destroyed or inaccessible)
I. Describes plan and procedures for medical
screening of potential victims and includes
mental disorders and psychogenic symptomatology,
functional impairment, substance abuse, etc.
J. Describes health structure for surveillance,
screening, consultation, intervention planning,
risk communication
K. Describes health role in risk communication
planning and response

20. Other special planning concerns   NA   Assigned   Time   Comment
A. Description of health's presence and role
in emergency management structure

Appendix 14.6 (cont.)

    B. Documentation of regional planning
       and coordination

    C. Describes various issues around licensing
       within jurisdiction, out-of-state providers,
       scope of practice, etc.

    D. Documentation of plans to prepare and
       support organization's staff during and following
       deployment under the plan (physical, health,
       special medical needs, family support, psychological)

    E. Documentation of public sector linkage with
       private health and medical resources

    F. Documentation of coordination with business
       and corporations and other private sector interests
       in planning for health response and consequences

    G. Documentation of appropriate planning
       linkages with institutions of higher learning
       (academic departments, student health services, etc.)

    H. Provides assurance that all health providers
       and facilities meet JCAHCO or other appropriate
       standards for disaster and emergency preparedness

    I. Health's role in risk communication

    J. Training and exercises

    K. Coordination of research

    L. Data collection/evaluation

21. Standard operating procedures and checklists   NA   Assigned   Time   Comment
    A. Contains applicable SOPs
    B. Contains applicable check lists (e.g., emergency
       contact numbers, lists of facilities, etc.)

22. Glossary of terms   NA   Assigned   Time   Comment
    A. Organization's specific terms
    B. Emergency Management terms
    C. Public health terms

---

and delivery of these materials over the past 2 years, especially with its Director, James M. Shultz, Ph.D, and Zelde Espinel, MD, MPH. The collaboration has been so synergistic and complete that it is often difficult to recall who contributed what content…the mark of a truly successful collaboration.

During my many years in the field of disaster behavioral health, I have been honored and privileged to be with individuals and communities in their darkest hours. Their pain, suffering, loss, and resilience have informed, inspired, and motivated me and positively changed my life and work forever. It has also been a privilege to work alongside so many fine colleagues across the globe. Their big brains and even bigger hearts cast a great shadow in which I gratefully and humbly stand.

I dedicate this chapter to my grandson, Matthew Edward Flynn, Jr. Each time I see him, I am reminded why this work must be done.

REFERENCES

American Red Cross. (2005). *Be Prepared: American Red Cross Preparedness Information*. Available at www.red-cross.org/services/disaster/0,1082,0_500_,00.html, accessed May 13, 2007.

DeGruy, F. (1996). Mental health in the primary care setting. In *Primary Care: America's Health in a New Era*, eds. M.S. Donaldson, K.D. Yordy, K.N. Lohr & N.A. Vanselow. Washington, D.C.: Institute of Medicine, National Academy Press.

DeMartino, R. & Flynn, B.W. (2004). Bioterrorism: a strategy for preparedness, response, and recovery. In *Bioterrorism: Psychological and Public Health Interventions*, eds. R.J. Ursano, A.E. Norwood & C.S. Fullerton. Cambridge: Cambridge University Press.

Federal Emergency Management Agency. (2005). *Your Family Disaster Plan*. Available at: www.fema.gov/plan/index.shtm, accessed May 13, 2007.

Flynn, B.W. (2005). Mental health response to terrorism in the United States: an adolescent field in an adolescent nation. In *The Trauma of Terrorism: Sharing Knowledge and Shared Caring – an International Handbook*, eds. Y. Danieli, D. Brom & J. Sills. Binghampton, NY: The Haworth Maltreatment and Trauma Press.

Institute of Medicine. (2003). *Preparing for the Psychological Consequences of Terrorism: A Public Health Strategy*. Washington, D.C.: The National Academies Press.

Joint Commission on Accreditation of Health Care Organizations. (2003). *Health Care at the Crossroads: Strategies for Creating and Sustaining Community-wide Emergency Preparedness Systems*. Available online at www.ncsl.org/programs/health/ep3–12–03.pdf, accessed May 12, 2007.

Karsenty, E., Shemer, J., Alshech, I. *et al.* (1991). Medical aspects of the missile attacks on Israel. *Israeli Journal of Medical Science*, **27**, 603–607.

Kawana, N., Ishimatsu, S. & Kanda, K. (2001). Psychophysiological effects of the sarin attack on the Tokyo subway system. *Military Medicine*, **166**, 23–26.

Lasker, R.D. (2004). *Redefining Readiness: Terrorism Planning Through the Eyes of the Public*. New York: The New York Academy of Medicine.

National Institute of Mental Health. (2002). *Mental Health and Mass Violence: Evidence-Based early Intervention for Victims/Survivors of Mass Violence: A Workshop to Reach Consensus on Best Practices*. NIH Publication No. 02–5138. Washington, D.C.: US Government Printing Office.

Reissman, D.R., Spencer, S., Tanielian, T.L. & Stein, B.D. (2005). Integrating behavioral aspects into community preparedness and response systems. In *The Trauma of Terrorism: Sharing Knowledge and Shared Caring – An International Handbook*, eds. Y. Danieli, D. Brom & J. Sills. Binghampton, NY: The Haworth Maltreatment and Trauma Press.

Shaw, J.A. & Shaw, S. (2004). The psychological effect of a community-wide disaster on children: planning for bioterrorism. In *Bioterrorism: Psychological and Public Health Interventions*, eds. R.J. Ursano, A.E. Norwood & C. S. Fullerton. Cambridge: Cambridge University Press.

Shultz, J.M., Espinel, Z., Cohen, R.E. *et al.* (2004). *Disaster Behavioral Health Training for Health Care Professionals*. Miami, Fla.: Disaster Epidemiology and Emergency Preparedness Center, Miller School of Medicine, University of Miami.

Ursano, R.J., Norwood, A.E. & Fullerton, C.S. (2001). *Planning for Bioterrorism: Behavioral and Mental Health Responses to Weapons of Mass Destruction and Mass Disruption*. Bethesda, Md.: Uniformed Services University of the Health Sciences.

Ursano, R.J., Norwood, A.E. & Fullerton, C.S. (2002). *Responding to Bioterrorism: Individual and Community Needs*. Bethesda, Md: Uniformed Services University of the Health Sciences.

US Department of Health and Human Services, Substance Abuse and Mental Health Services Administration, Center for Mental Health Services, National Institute of Mental Health. (1999). *Mental Health: A Report of the Surgeon General*. Rockville, Md.: US Department of Health and Human Services.

US Department of Health and Human Services. (2003). *Mental Health All-Hazards Disaster Planning Guidance*. DHHS Pub. No. SMA 3829. Rockville, Md.: Center for Mental Health Services, Substance Abuse and Mental Health Services Administration.

US Department of Homeland Security. (2004). *The National Response Plan*. Available at: www.dhs.gov/nrp, accessed May 13, 2007.

US Department of Homeland Security/FEMA. (1996). *Guide for All-Hazard Emergency Operations Planning, State and Local Guide (SLG)*. Washington, D.C.: US Department of Homeland Security/FEMA.

US Department of Homeland Security/FEMA. (2002). *State and Local EOP Planning Guidance*. Available at www.fema.gov/plan/gaheop.shtm, accessed May 13, 2007.

US Department of Homeland Security/FEMA. (2004). *Are You Ready? An In-depth Guide to Citizen Preparedness* (IS-22). Available at: www.fema.gov/areyouready/, accessed May 13, 2007.

US Department of Homeland Security/FEMA. (2005). *National Incident Management System*. Available at: www.fema.gov/nims.

PART V

Public health and disaster psychiatry

15

Public health and disaster mental health: preparing, responding, and recovering

Robert J. Ursano, Carol S. Fullerton, Lars Weisaeth, & Beverly Raphael

Mental health experts are an essential part of planning for and responding to disasters. However, across nations, public mental health planning and care vary greatly from systems in which all healthcare is national and resources are substantial, to those in which no mental healthcare is available or the public resources are greatly limited. Regardless of resources, disasters challenge mental health systems in nearly all nations and communities.

In the United States, prior to the 1960s the mental health component of the public health system generally meant public mental hospitals. Beginning in the 1960s and continuing to the early 1970s, the public health-mental health system was the community mental health center. The early 1970s saw the start of a continuous erosion in the comprehensive mission originally included as part of community mental health. Today, with rare exception, the public health component of the United States mental health system refers to community based services for people with serious and persistent mental illness, not to a comprehensive public health approach to the entire mental health and behavioral needs of the community (Institute of Medicine, 2003). There is not a systematic approach to the provision of public medical care for mental health problems across the entire range of primary, secondary, and tertiary prevention including health behaviors and traditional mental health – from community-based prevention pro-

grams to outpatient clinics, inpatient hospital care, and care in the primary care setting where most mental health problems present. In times of disaster, this lack of a comprehensive system is particularly evident.

Disasters require that we respond not only to those who need direct care but also to populations that may need support, assistance, guidance, and psychological and health-related information. Emergency care providers must discriminate between physical and anxiety symptoms to assure the integrity of the medical system (see Chapter 8). Mental health providers must respond to a range of emotional and behavioral demands, e.g., anger, fear, depression, increased substance use, and in some disasters such as epidemics or bioterrorism, the special stresses of quarantine, shelter in place and altered travel behaviors that may threaten the economic stability of a nation. The public health system must address mental healthcare across all of its dimensions. Mental health and behavior are critically important elements of our healthcare system for responses to disasters. Mental health and behavioral preparedness are one step in the process.

Preparing for disasters including terrorism is a focused, yet often forgotten, need of disaster communities. A study conducted by The Marist Institute for Public Opinion for Columbia's Mailman School of Public Health (National Center for Disaster Preparedness, 2003) found 76% of

Americans were concerned about terrorism in the United States 2 years after September 11. A majority, however, lack confidence in the United States' health system's capacity to respond effectively to a biological, chemical or nuclear attack, and many Americans are unaware of emergency plans at their workplace or in their children's schools. Despite the fact that the most prevalent concern of Americans (66%) was the need to account for the whereabouts and safety of family members, the study found that fewer than one in four families (23%) actually have a basic emergency plan. Nationally, only 58% of parents are aware of the emergency or evacuation plans at their child's school, and only 19% are familiar with the details of their children's school plan. The Asian tsunami of 2004 and Hurricanes Katrina and Rita in the United States are powerful reminders of the critical need to include mental health services in the primary care setting before disaster strikes (Davidson, 2006; Weisler *et al.*, 2006).

The psychological and behavioral consequences of disasters include behavior change, distress symptoms and, for some, psychiatric illness (for review, see Norris *et al.*, 2002a, 2002b; North *et al.*, 1999) (see Figure 15.1). In the immediate aftermath of a disaster, individuals and communities may respond in adaptive, effective ways or they may make fear-based decisions, resulting in unhelpful behaviors. The adaptive capacities of individuals and groups within a community are variable, and need to be understood before a crisis in order to effectively identify postevent needs (Ursano & Norwood, 2003). Interventions to sustain psychological function and alleviate psychiatric disease as well as distress are dependent upon the rapid, effective, and sustained mobilization of resources. Knowledge of a community's risk and protective factors before a disaster or terrorist event, as well as understanding the psychological responses to such an event enables leaders and medical experts to talk to the public, promoting resilient healthy behaviors, sustaining the social fabric of the community, and facilitating recovery (Institute of Medicine, 2003).

Psychological casualties present a significant challenge to medical and health providers in the aftermath of disaster. Traditional natural disaster or transportation accident models of providing health services after a disaster must be altered for terrorist events. Effective, consistent health responses to the psychological, behavioral, and mental health needs after disaster require that preparedness and response activities fit within the framework of all-hazards disaster planning (Flynn, 2003).

New models of monitoring shifting community healthcare needs in realtime (i.e., mental health surveillance) as well as innovative models for delivering care are required (Bryant, 2006). A disaster mental healthcare response requires the collaborative efforts of the public health system, medical care system, and emergency response systems (see Figure 15.2). The mental healthcare system, as part of the medical care system, must join with the public health and emergency response systems to address needs for triage, surge capacity, and health surveillance in order to best provide care for communities exposed to disasters (Raphael, 2006). This invariably involves public health, health and mental health authorities, state and local emergency planners, disaster relief organizations, healthcare institutions and

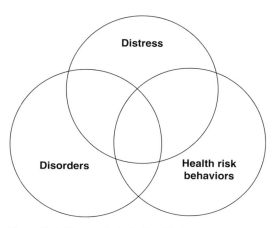

Figure 15.1 The psychological and behavioral consequences of disasters

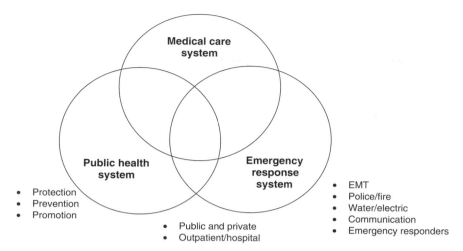

Figure 15.2 The disaster mental health response

providers and representatives of critical infrastructure entities (Ursano *et al.*, 2004). The knowledge base for the interventions draws from a variety of disciplines including sociology, risk communication, education, and disaster mental health. This knowledge can provide guidance to community leaders, local emergency planners, health and mental health planners, and healthcare providers to develop integrated plans and linked preparations for psychological and behavioral consequences of disasters (Litz *et al.*, 2002; National Institute of Mental Health, 2002). Scientists, healthcare responders, and national leaders must work together to assure health, order, and continuity of government and societal function.

For terrorism in particular it has been said that the mental health and behavioral consequences are the most significant, long-term, and most costly effects of a terrorist attack. The development of specific recommendations for the integration of mental health and public health is critical [Institute of Medicine (IOM), 2003; Joint Commission on Accreditation of Healthcare Organizations (JCAHO), 2003; Ursano *et al.*, 2001, 2002]. Preparedness planning is the first of the mental health and behavioral planning needs.

Preparing for the consequences of disasters and terrorism

Although exposure to disasters and other trauma is associated with debility that can persist for decades, resilience is by far the most common finding. For some people, trauma and loss may even facilitate a move toward health (Bonanno, 2004; Bonanno *et al.*, 2006; Card, 1983; Foa *et al.*, 2000; Kessler, 2006; Ursano, 1981; Wessely, 2005).

Disasters overwhelm local resources, and threaten the function and safety of the community. With the advent of instantaneous communication and media coverage, word of a disaster is disseminated quickly and often is witnessed in real time around the globe. The disaster community is soon flooded with outsiders: people offering assistance, curiosity seekers, and the media. This sudden influx of strangers affects the community in many ways. The presence of large numbers of media representatives can be experienced as intrusive and insensitive. Hotel rooms have no vacancies, restaurants are crowded with unfamiliar faces, and the normal routine of the community is altered. At a time when, traditionally, communities turn inward to grieve and assist affected families, the normal social supports are strained and disrupted by outsiders.

Disasters and terrorism strike at the fault lines of our society, increasing the chances of the rupture of society across ethnic, religious, racial, and socioeconomic differences. For example, following Hurricane Katrina, rumors circulated that the government had intentionally blown up the levees to flood the poor minority sections of New Orleans rather than the economically well off and primarily White parts of the town. Similarly in Washington, D.C. after the anthrax attacks the decision to provide ciprofloxacin to those on Capitol Hill and dicloxacillin to those in the post office in Washington, D.C. was interpreted as discriminatory (in fact the Supreme Court also received dicloxacillin). Both were appropriate medications. Avoidance and stigmatization of Arabs was widely reported after the London bombings as well as the World Trade Center attack in the United States.

Disaster behaviors and preparedness behaviors such as decisions about when and how to evacuate, and response to alerts and alarms are a relatively new focus of attention and intervention for mental health and behavior specialists. In addition, in any new infectious outbreak by a new agent – such as severe acute respiratory syndrome (SARS) or Avian influenza – the only available responses are adherence to behavioral interventions such as quarantine and protective behaviors until new vaccination and treatments can be developed. Disaster behaviors are critical to health and morbidity. For example, what determined the decision to evacuate in the face of disasters such as Hurricane Katrina (see Elliott & Pais, 2006)? A large percentage of the population of New Orleans (about one third) did not evacuate despite warnings of an impending hurricane (Kessler, 2006). Studies of the first World Trade Center disaster in New York City, the bombing in 1993, showed that nearly 32% of people had not begun to evacuate over 1 h after the bombing. (Only 36% of those in the tower had participated in a *previous* emergency evacuation.) The higher up one was in the building, the longer it took to decide to evacuate, and 30%

decided *not* to evacuate at all (Aguirre *et al.*, 1998). In addition, people in groups of greater than 20 took over 6 min longer to decide to evacuate. In addition, the more people knew each other in the group, the longer the group took to initiate evacuation (Aguirre *et al.*, 1998). Individual barriers to evacuation of the World Trade Center on September 11 delayed evacuation: doing last-minute work-related tasks, taking personal items, making calls, waiting for instructions/direction. Also, poor familiarity with World Trade Center building, fear of negative impact on job, disabilities and poor physical condition and footwear were associated with problems in evacuation (Gershon *et al.*, 2004).

After a disaster, particularly those that include risk or concerns about toxic exposures, traditional mental health problems may appear as physical health problems (Rundell, 2003). In the face of fears of contamination, multiple unexplained physical symptoms (MUPS) may be the presentation of distress in the outpatient and emergency setting (Engel, 2004; Engel *et al.*, 2003). Health education and risk communication can minimize the numbers seeking healthcare and strengthen the public health response in both the medical and mental health arena (Tucker, 1997).

Bereavement is an inevitable component of disasters (Prigerson *et al.*, 1999; Raphael & Minkov, 1999; Raphael & Wooding, 2004; Raphael *et al.*, 2004; Shear *et al.*, 2005). Both individuals and communities must grieve the loss of loved ones and the hoped-for future. Bereavement begins early, continues for months, and then becomes less of a community focus, often before the individuals themselves are recovered. Bereavement is complicated by ongoing identification of additional remains, the complex interaction of the financial remuneration for victims, and, in the eyes of many victims, the circuitous and puzzling track frequently taken by the criminal justice system.

Post-traumatic responses (not only illness) such as hypervigilance and difficulty sleeping are prominent early on and show rapid recovery for most. For some people symptoms of distress may persist for months. Individuals exposed to terrorism and other disasters have been found to increase their use of alcohol, tobacco, and other drugs, especially those with pre-existing alcohol abuse or other psychiatric difficulties (Galea *et al.*, 2002; North *et al.*, 1999; Pfefferbaum & Doughty, 2001; Ursano & Norwood, 2003; Vlahov *et al.*, 2002). We do not know the course of these behavioral changes. In Manhattan, 1–2 months after September 11, residents south of 110th Street reported increased substance use (alcohol, cigarettes or marijuana), that remained the same 6 months later: 24.6% reported increased alcohol use; 9.7% showed increased cigarette smoking; and 3.2% increased use of marijuana (Vlahov *et al.*, 2002).

Increased cohesion of communities is also common early after a disaster. The period of cohesion is the time in which communities mobilize and natural support groups contribute to the recovery of the community. During this phase, the media serves as a vector for both knowledge and potentially for distress in how it transmits pictures of injury and fear or information and aid. Inevitably, after any major trauma, there are rumors circulated within the community about the circumstances leading up to the traumatic event and the government's response. Sometimes there is a heightened state of fear. For example, a study of a school shooting in Illinois noted that a high level of anxiety continued for a week after the event, even after it was known that the perpetrator had committed suicide (Schwarz & Kowalski, 1991).

Locating loved ones is the first and paramount concern after a disaster. The questions "Where is my loved one?", "Can I find them?", "Can I communicate with them?" comprise the first preoccupation of both individuals and communities. Outpourings of sympathy for the injured, dead, and their friends and families are common and expected. Impromptu memorials of flowers, photographs, and memorabilia are frequently erected. Churches and synagogues play an important role in assisting communities to search for meaning from such tragedy, and in assisting in the grieving process.

Over time, anger often emerges in the community as disillusionment sets in. Typically, there is a focus on accountability, a search for someone who was responsible for a lack of preparation or an inadequate response. Mayors, police, and fire chiefs, and other community leaders are often targets of these strong feelings. A community becomes angry about why things were not done, why it happened, and why things couldn't have been done better. Scapegoating can be an especially destructive process when leveled at those who already hold themselves responsible, even if, in reality, there was nothing they could have done to prevent adverse outcomes. In addition, nations and communities experience ongoing hypervigilance and a sense of lost safety while trying to establish a new norm in their lives.

First responders following a disaster include the traditional firefighters, police, and military, but also healthcare providers. Because the medical community is a "first responder," particularly true in an epidemic or bioterrorist attack, a broad-based educational plan for healthcare providers and organizations is essential. Hospital response plans must incorporate mental health and behavioral interventions at all levels. Medical care for infected/injured people as well as for those people who fear they were infected must be based on proven psychological and behavioral principles (Joint Commission on Accreditation of Healthcare Organizations, 2003). One notable concern is healthcare worker compliance with recommended infection preparedness (e.g., pre-vaccination against smallpox), and the relationship of health-related fears and concerns with absenteeism and other activities at work (e.g., SARS, Avian influenza, anthrax).

The culture of a nation and of its communities influences both responses and possible interventions after a terrorist attack. The recent SARS epidemic is instructive in understanding some of the issues of importance to a bioterrorist attack. Responses to the SARS virus in Canada, Singapore, and China were quite different. In some nations it was possible to immediately mobilize everyone to accept quarantine or shelter in place or to use masks. However, obtaining cooperation will vary in different cultures where control is experienced differently and in nations with different expectations of equitable treatment.

There are many milestones of a disaster that affect the community and may offer opportunities for recovery. There are the normal rituals associated with burying the dead. And later, energy is poured into creating memorials for those who died or performed heroic acts. Memorialization carries the potential to cause harm as well as to do good. There can be heated disagreement about what a monument should look like, and where it should be placed. If a monument is situated too prominently so that community members cannot avoid encountering it, the memorial may heighten intrusive recollections and interfere with the resolution of grief reactions. Anniversaries of an event (1 week, 1 month, 1 year) stimulate renewed grief and offer an opportunity to acknowledge community recovery and resilience.

Public health planning

Responding to the psychological consequences of terrorism

Public health planning for the psychological consequences of disasters must address the range of psychological and behavioral responses. Psychological function and psychiatric disease as well as the distress of individuals and communities are dependent upon the rapid, effective, and sustained mobilization of healthcare and community resources (Ursano & Norwood, 2003). Knowledge of a community's resilience and vulnerability before a disaster or terrorist event, as well as understanding the psychological responses to such an event enable leaders and medical experts to distribute resources, talk to the public, and thus promote healthy behaviors, sustaining the social fabric of the community and facilitating recovery (Joint Commission on Accreditation of Healthcare Organizations, 2003; Ursano et al., 2001, 2002).

Preventive medicine, a familiar organizing structure for conceptualizing infectious outbreaks, can organize models and interventions for behavioral and psychological responses to disasters (Institute of Medicine, 2003; Pfefferbaum & Pfefferbaum, 1998). From the preventive medicine perspective, one identifies the pathogen, its source and vectors of propagation, and those exposed. For the psychiatric consequences of disasters, the stressful psychological, physiological, and social events of the disaster are the pathogens. Terrorist attacks differ from other disasters in the prominence of terror as another agent of disease and disruption.

Prevention can be primary (preparation before the event, sometimes thought of as "inoculation"), secondary (early identification and treatment to limit disability), or tertiary (rehabilitation to prevent chronic social disability) (Ursano et al., 1996). Interventions may be universal (for all individuals regardless of exposure) or selective (meant for particular at-risk populations). Primary (pre-event), secondary (event) and tertiary (postevent) interventions can decrease the risk of maladaptive behaviors, distress, mental disorder, and disrupted functioning (Sorenson, 2002). Importantly, pre-event interventions to decrease exposure to the traumatic event (e.g., evacuation planning, practice drills) or its severity (e.g., seat belts) are an important and often overlooked component of mental health disaster planning (Aguirre et al., 1998; Institute of Medicine, 2003; Ursano, 2002). Identifying the groups of people that are most highly exposed to these stressors is the critical second step in determining the community consequences of a disaster or terrorist attack. Public health strategies to prevent and mitigate the effects of disaster include interventions that can occur before, during, and after a disaster event. (see Figure 15.3). Life-protecting preparedness behaviors, disaster behaviors, and recovery behaviors of individuals and communities are fostered. Such behaviors that increase morbidity or mortality require planning, training, and system interventions to minimize their likelihood.

	Agent: Terror/Injury	Vector: Terrorist	Population: Person

Pre	• Modify building
	  design
	• Educate public to
	  decrease terror
		• Screening of
		  employees
			Preparedness behaviors:
			• Risk assessment
			• Information/plan

During	• Sprinkler system	• Training police • Early detection of intrusion	**Disaster behaviors:** • Active coping • Evacuation
Post	• Emergency response system	• Justice system	**Response/recovery behaviors:** • Psychotherapy • Medication

Figure 15.3 Intervention matrix. Interventions to prevent, mitigate and manage psychological and behavioral consequences of a workplace terrorist explosion

Fostering community and workplace resilience

Prevention of disease is not the only goal of preventive interventions. Increasing resilience and positive outcomes are an important but often forgotten goal of prevention strategies. Thus community resilience is a primary goal of preparation for disaster. Resilience in this case means both decreased adverse responses and more rapid recovery. Community leadership, community resources and functions, and the healthcare system in particular are central to this response. For example, town meetings prior to critical events can foster community efficacy and enable communities to develop neighborhood watch or neighborhood assistance programs, and plan for who will watch the children on the block if mom or dad is not home. If a child needs to be picked up from school, this becomes both a family and a school system responsibility. Around such efforts community cohesion can develop, as can community efficacy (Sampson, 2003; Sampson et al., 1997). Fear may then have a channel in which to flow, constructive action, rather than increase community chaos. There are many decisions communities can make in neighborhoods which are usually defined by schools, churches, public services such as police or fire departments or even grocery/food marts.

The community and workplace serve as physical and emotional support systems. [For children the school system is a major part of this support.] The larger the scale of a disaster, the greater the potential disruption of the community and workplace. Planning for resource distributions is important to preparing for the mental health consequences. Although the airplane crash survivor may experience and witness gruesome sights, for the tornado victim and the natural disaster victim, the recovery environment is also markedly different: home and work site may have been destroyed, and relatives, friends, and coworkers may be dead, injured, or displaced.

Following terrorism, there is the additional burden of continuing altered threat perception and safety experiences for the entire community. The impact of a terrorist event on psychiatric and behavioral morbidity is mediated in part by the effects on individual and community safety and threat perception (Grieger et al., 2003a, 2003b). Before, during, and after a terrorist attack community leaders can foster community resilience through interventions that may directly aid recovery as well as promote hope for the future and the expectation that "we will prevail" (see Table 15.1).

Early intervention

Much work is needed for early mental health and behavioral intervention for disaster-exposed individuals and populations (see Ursano & Blumenfield, 2006). Interventions to sustain the mental health

Table 15.1 Public health approaches to fostering community and workplace resilience

Early intervention
Planning for economic behaviors
Leadership
Mental health surveillance and community preparedness
Workplace preparedness

and performance of community first responders are a pressing need. Evidence-based selective and universal interventions to sustain population and group wellness and operational function are needed. These should build resilience, provide individual care, and foster recovery for communities and individuals. Although there will most likely never be randomized controlled trials of early mental health disaster interventions, specific interventions can be developed using proven mechanisms of change and recovery demonstrated in studies of risk factors, protective factors, and individual interventions.

The community mental health infrastructure is a critical part of a nation's health protection strategy and key to the rapid early intervention. Disaster communities require: (1) ongoing assessment and monitoring of mental health and behavioral needs of disaster communities; and (2) a range of population and individual interventions to foster useful and sustaining actions of the citizenry, reduce social and emotional deterioration, and support key personnel in critical infrastructure.

Psychological First Aid (PFA) (see Chapter 7) is the evolving first-line intervention for the large majority of individuals following disaster. However, PFA requires evaluation. People unlikely to benefit from PFA will require additional clinical assessment and appropriate intervention including pharmacological and psychological treatments.

Culturally informed interventions are a part of recognizing the diversity of every community. Emergent mental healthcare needs, not previously evident, also occur after disaster, such as those with previously untreated or under-treated illness

seeking care after disaster. Responding to this care-needing population is part of the disaster response. Since most mental health problems do not present to specialist care, primary care – the delivery of healthcare through routine primary care providers – is a fundamental component of early intervention for the mental and behavioral healthcare needs after disaster.

Planning for economic behaviors

Certain economic behaviors and decisions are affected directly by a disaster, and by the psychological and behavioral responses to the disaster. For example, after a terrorist attack, decisions and behaviors related to travel, home purchase, food consumption, and medical care visits are altered by changes in availability, but also by changes in perceived safety, optimism about the future, and belief in exposure to toxic agents. Similarly, work productivity and attendance are influenced by whether transportation routes have been destroyed, but also by pre- and post-disaster distress and nonadherence and noncompliance with preparedness and public health interventions such as vaccination, premedication, postmedication, or evacuation planning (e.g., childcare planning). For example, is there a dip in consumer confidence after a bombing or a hurricane? If so, how large and what is its duration? Did the decrease get worse as the crisis continued? Similarly the postdisaster period can bring large inflows of money to areas for construction, creating jobs, economic growth, and changed opportunities – perhaps not for the populations that were victims, but for those who were less affected. Did economic revival bring an economic boom or bust? Was it local, regional or national? Was it in the upper or middle class people or among people of all economic backgrounds?

The fact that warnings of disaster as well as threats and hoaxes of terrorism carry with them economic costs and consequences perhaps best illustrates the importance of psychological and behavioral effects on economic decisions and behaviors and their associated economic costs

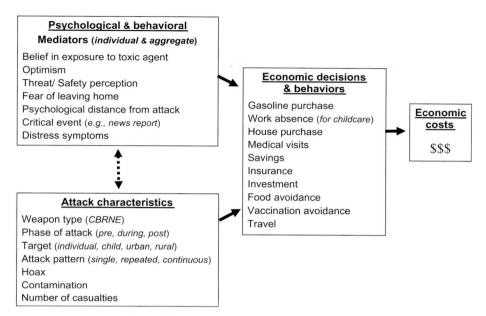

Figure 15.4 Model of economic decisions and behaviors

(see Figure 15.4). The spread of fear or hope via the media and social networks also affects economic decisions and behaviors. The impact of these economic decisions and behaviors on the local or national economy ranges from altered food consumption, savings, insurance, and investment, to changes in work attendance and productivity and broader national or industry-specific consequences such as altered financial and insurance markets or disrupted transportation, communication, and energy networks. Previous disaster and terrorist attack scenarios used in training and tabletop exercises have often failed to consider the effects of psychological and behavioral (individual and aggregate) variables on economic behaviors. The elaboration of the resulting economic cost and consequence models and their derivative response decisions have been inadequate and require new models.

Leadership

A major part of the skill of a leader is his or her sensitivity to the community and the ability to speak the right phrase at the right time to enable the community to speak as well. "Grief leadership" – how to lead a community through loss, mourning, and recovery–is of particular concern. Knowing when to change from rescue of survivors to body recovery is often the first and very delicate step in moving a community to recovery. A leader who says out loud that, "we need help." may allow others to say, "I need help." A leader who scorns the need for care can prohibit others in the community from being able to say they need care.

The stigma associated with psychiatric illness can be decreased by community leaders' acknowledgment of care needs and addressing of barriers to care. Acknowledging that all psychiatric illnesses (i.e., all mental disorders) are not "cancer," that treatment is available, and recovery is expected can be a step in this process. This includes public education by leaders that individuals can be expected to recover from "event-related disorders" (i.e., disorders related to life events) such as acute stress disorder and acute post-traumatic stress disorder. These may be the mental disease equivalent of the sore throat: some may become pneumonia, but most people will recover through their normal healing processes.

Mental health surveillance and community preparedness

Mental health surveillance and adaptation monitoring (Flynn, 2003) have not yet been included in general public health planning. In the United States, Hurricane Katrina has had one of the few postdisaster systematic mental health surveillance programs (Kessler, 2006). Knowledge of an individual's and community's resilience and vulnerability before a disaster or terrorist event as well as understanding in real time the psychological responses to such an event can enable leaders and medical experts to talk to the public, promote healthy behaviors, sustain the social fabric of the community, and facilitate recovery and resource distribution. The adaptive capacities of individuals and groups within a community are variable, and should be understood before a crisis, as well as after, through ongoing mental health surveillance in order to target needs effectively.

Safety is an important and not well studied construct that appears to be related to, but not the same as, risk perception. Community and individual experiences of safety influence behaviors, hope, and family distress. Safety relates to feeling vulnerable, and to feeling protected. Optimism of a community is also an important determinate of emotional and cognitive responses. Optimism bias predicts that people believe they are less at risk for a number of hazards than they are. Optimism may be linked to feelings of controllability through which individuals believe they are safer than they are (e.g., the safety of driving is often rated higher than that of flying although that is not always true). Distance from an event, and the more random an event, the greater the sense of vulnerability and perhaps lower safety. The risk perception of a community is influenced by numerous cognitive and emotional factors. Cognitive (probability-based) and emotional-based risk contribute separately to anticipated changes in behavior (e.g., whether

you will travel) (see Fischhoff *et al.*, 2005). Anger (self-reported or as a result of a manipulation) tends to be associated with decreased risk perception (increased optimism), and fear with increased risk perception (emotion-based judgement) (Lerner *et al.*, 2003). More recent exposure to a threat increases risk perception (availability-based judgement). In contrast, hindsight bias is a well-known effect in which one tends to see past risk as colored by most recent beliefs (Fischhoff *et al.*, 2005).

An enhanced public health infrastructure for mental health requires the means to quickly detect, track, and monitor disaster- and terrorist-caused psychological and behavioral casualties. This entails enhancing the medical incident management infrastructure through standardizing and expanding the manner in which certain illnesses and symptoms are described, recorded, and tracked. In addition, the system requires improved ability to share this information quickly and efficiently, locally and across a nation.

As well as traditional mental health disorders and substance use and abuse, health risk behaviors and distress require community surveillance postdisaster. Additionally important are assessments of: (1) community risk perception; (2) safety perception; (3) changes in behavior, e.g., avoiding air transportation or subways, and purchase behaviors, such as deciding to buy or postpone travel or a major purchase and; (4) preparedness behaviors, e.g., family preparedness plans, evacuation plans (see Table 15.2).

Workplace preparedness

The workplace is a relatively newly recognized environment in which to address public health planning for the psychological consequences of disaster and terrorism (Institute of Medicine, 2003). Because most acts of terrorism in the United States have occurred where and when people work, it is essential that interventions for preparedness, response, and recovery occur in occupational settings. Sustaining the workforce, its

Table 15.2 Postdisaster community
mental health surveillance

Distress
Psychiatric illness/symptoms
Health risk behaviors
Risk perception
Safety perception
Changes in behavior
Preparedness behaviors

organizational health, and the well-being of workers sustains communities and important national resources and services. The prevention of environmental effects on health is a traditional role of public health in the workplace. Following terrorism, the direct effects of threats to life as well as the propagation of terror, such as an agent infecting the workplace, require new and important attention to be paid to the mental health needs of occupational populations.

The behavioral and psychological health and well-being of occupational groups are critical to sustaining workplace health, capabilities, and infrastructure. Disasters including epidemics can result in altered workplace performance, absenteeism, presenteeism and disability. Interventions to prevent, mitigate, and foster recovery from mass trauma in the workplace are needed. Preparedness behaviors, disaster behaviors, and response/recovery behaviors are important targets for a healthy workplace. Workplace interventions include those to: (1) alleviate or mitigate mental health outcomes; (2) provide specific effective treatments in the workplace; and (3) carry out workplace mental health surveillance.

Workplace providers–employee assistance providers (EAPs), corporate medical directors, occupational health and wellness professionals, and human resource personnel – play an important role in disaster preparedness and response because their work includes prevention, health promotion, and treatment (or referral to treatment). In addition, they establish policies for personnel management.

Security directors are also an important part of the behavioral team as they affect many behaviors that decrease exposure to physically and psychologically traumatic events. Worksite health promotion is an integral part of internal EAPs, wellness, occupational health, and corporate medical programs, as are external behavioral care organizations, who view their role as providing health education as well as mental health services for client companies. Workplace health and mental health programs are ideal venues in which to incorporate education around workplace disaster preparedness for managers and supervisors, employees, and employees' families (Ursano, 2005).

Workplace health programs can educate the workforce about disaster-related mental health and behavioral disorders, as well as how to distinguish between normal responses and those that require further evaluation and treatment. This pre-event education can help individuals to self-identify conditions postdisaster requiring further evaluation and treatment, using confidential, interactive screening resources, and/or the in-person assessment and referral that many employers offer.

What we need to know to respond and recover

In order to develop public health approaches to disaster mental health needs, a number of areas must be addressed (see Table 15.3). Early intervention for populations and individuals requires research, planning, and evaluation. A well-supported community mental health system is required as part of the public health infrastructure. Primary medical care sites are important to the delivery of disaster mental healthcare. This requires a systematic approach to education of providers, patient education and assessment, and the availability of referral for specialty care. Adherence/compliance to medical recommendations (e.g., medication, quarantine, shelter in place) is not well understood or taught to healthcare providers. Yet management of these behaviors is as important as

Table 15.3 Public health needs for disaster mental health

- Integration of mental health care into primary care
- Individual – and population-level early interventions
- Interventions to foster adherence to medical recommendations
- Mental health surveillance integrated into public health surveillance
- Inclusion of mental health in training exercises
- Knowledge of community, family, and cultural responses to disaster
- Interventions to foster workplace preparedness and recovery

prescribing or delivering the correct interventions. Mental health and behavioral surveillance should be an integral part of ongoing public health surveillance to facilitate identifying resource needs postevent. This requires substantial rethinking of past paradigms to initiate and establish the utility of both ongoing and potentially real-time surveillance of mental health and behavioral and distress-related symptoms and behaviors.

Models of emergency screening to enable triage of those needing rapid decontamination or hospitalization from those with anxiety and somatic symptoms of distress are needed for our healthcare systems, which may need to respond to real or perceived toxic exposure events. Inclusion of mental and behavioral experts in the training and exercises can facilitate this process. Understanding and modeling economic behaviors postdisaster can facilitate planning for both public education and economic interventions to sustain the function of communities and nations.

Because of the central importance of public education, increased knowledge of public education's limits and possibilities to prepare, educate, motivate, and foster resilient responses is needed. Understanding the behaviors, emotions, and cognitions that affect family and community function (e.g., anticipatory fear, threat perception, risk, and safety perception, threat generalization, and social spread of fear) across the neurobiological and interpersonal perspectives will enable effective interventions. To limit morbidity and mortality, public health planners will need increased knowledge of attachment behaviors in high stress environments that may increase health risk, and at other times decrease health risk (e.g., evacuation effects, warning effects, social supports, separation fears).

Developing better ways to prepare the workplace–business and industrial communities–to embrace the challenges of human continuity as part of their efforts to assure business continuity is a major challenge. An integrated approach that includes security, human resources, occupational health, and leadership may be most effective. Assuring continuity of human capital is as important as assuring the continuity of buildings and information systems, and requires consideration of integrated leadership, medical, employee, and human resource planning.

Overall, the public health challenges of disaster mental health span health services planning, intervention, treatment, training, education, and research into the neurobiological, psychological and sociocultural aspects of disaster behaviors, preparedness behaviors, and response behaviors of individuals and groups. The all-hazards approach can integrate these efforts and find common ground.

REFERENCES

Aguirre, B.E., Wenger, D. & Vigo, G. (1998). A test of the emergent norm theory of collective behavior. *Sociological Forum*, **13**, 301–320.

Bonanno, G.A. (2004). Loss, trauma, and human resilience: have we underestimated the human capacity to thrive after extremely aversive events? *The American Psychologist*, **59**, 20–28.

Bonanno, G.A., Galea, S., Bucciarelli, A. & Vlahov, D. (2006). Psychological resilience after disaster: New York city in the aftermath of the September 11th terrorist attack. *Psychological Science: A Journal of the American Psychological Society*, **17**, 181–186.

Bryant, R. (2006). Early intervention and treatment of acute stress disorder. Presented at conference *Early psychological intervention following mass trauma: the present and future directions*. Valhalla, New York: New York Medical College, School of Public Health.

Card, J.J. (1983). *Lives after Viet Nam*. Lexington, Mass.: Lexington Books.

Davidson, J.R.T. (2006). After the tsunami: mental health challenges to the community for today and tomorrow. *Journal of Clinical Psychiatry*, **67**, 3–8.

Elliott, J.R. & Pais, J. (2006). Race, class, and Hurricane Katrina: social differences in human responses to disaster. *Social Science Research*, **35**, 295–321.

Engel, C.C. (2004). Somatization and multiple idiopathic physical symptoms: relationship to traumatic events and posttraumatic stress disorder. In *Trauma and Health: Physical Health Consequences of Exposure to Extreme Stress*, eds. P.P. Schnurr & B.L. Green, pp.191–215. Washington, D.C.: American Psychological Association.

Engel, C.C., Jaffer, A., Adkins, J. *et al.* (2003). Population-based health care: a model for restoring community health and productivity following terrorist attack. In *Terrorism and Disaster: Individual and Community Mental Health Interventions*, eds. R.J. Ursano, C.S. Fullerton & A.E. Norwood, pp.287–307. Cambridge: Cambridge University Press.

Fischhoff, B., Gonzalez, R.M., Lerner, J.S. & Small, D.A. (2005). Evolving judgments of terror risks: foresight, hindsight, and emotion. *Journal of Experimental Psychology Applied*, **11**, 124–139.

Flynn, B.W. (2003). Promoting psychosocial resilience in the face of terrorism. Briefing for members of the United States House of Representatives. Washington, D.C.

Foa, E.B., Keane, T.M. & Friedman, M.J., eds. (2000). *Effective Treatments for PTSD: Practice Guidelines from the International Society for Traumatic Stress Studies*. New York: Guilford Press.

Galea, S., Ahern, J., Resnick, H. *et al.* (2002). Psychological sequelae of the September 11 terrorist attacks in New York City. *New England Journal of Medicine*, **346**, 982–987.

Gershon, R., Hogan, E., Qureshi, K.A. & Doll, L. (2004). Preliminary results from the world trade center evacuation study–New York City. *MMWR Morbidity and Mortality Weekly Report*, **53**, 815–817.

Grieger, T.A., Fullerton, C.S. & Ursano, R.J. (2003a). Acute stress disorder, alcohol use, and perception of safety among hospital staff after sniper attacks. *Psychiatric Services*, **54**, 1383–1387.

Grieger, T.A., Fullerton, C.S. & Ursano, R.J. (2003b). Posttraumatic stress disorder, alcohol use, and perceived safety after the terrorist attack on the pentagon. *Psychiatric Services*, **54**, 1380–1382.

Institute of Medicine (IOM). (2003). *Preparing for the Psychological Consequences of Terrorism: A Public Health Strategy*. National Academies of Science, Washington D.C.: National Academies Press.

Joint Commission on Accreditation of Healthcare Organizations (JCAHO). (2003). Health care at the crossroads. Strategies for creating and sustaining community-wide emergency preparedness systems. Washington, D.C.: Joint Commission on Accreditation of Healthcare Organizations.

Kessler, R. (2006). Overview of baseline survey results: Hurricane Katrina community advisory group. Available at: www.hurricanekatrina.med.harvard.edu, accessed May 13, 2007.

Lerner, J.S., Gonzalez, R.M., Small, D.A. & Fischhoff, B. (2003). Effects of fear and anger on perceived risks of terrorism: a national field experiment. *Psychological Science*, **14**, 144–150.

Litz, B.T., Gray, M.J., Bryant, R.A. & Adler, A.B. (2002). Early intervention for trauma:current status and future directions. *Clinical Psychology: Science and Practice*, **9**, 112–134.

National Center for Disaster Preparedness (NCDP). (2003). *How Americans Feel about Terrorism and Security: Two Years after 9/11*. New York: Columbia University Mailman School of Public Health in collaboration with The Children's Health Fund.

National Institute of Mental Health. (2002). Mental health and mass violence: evidence-based early psychological intervention for victims/survivors of mass violence. A workshop to reach consensus on best practices. Available at: www.nimh.nih.gov/publicat/massviolence.pdf, accessed May 13, 2007. NIH Publication No. 02-5138, Washington, D.C.: US Government Printing Office.

Norris, F.H., Friedman, M.J. & Watson, P.J. (2002a). 60,000 disaster victims speak. Part II: Summary and implications of the disaster mental health research. *Psychiatry*, **65**, 240–260.

Norris, F.H., Friedman, M.J., Watson, P.J. *et al.* (2002b). 60,000 disaster victims speak. Part I: An empirical review of the empirical literature: 1981–2001. *Psychiatry*, **65**, 207–239.

North, C.S., Nixon, S.J., Shariat, S. *et al.* (1999). Psychiatric disorders among survivors of the Oklahoma City bombing. *Journal of the American Medical Association*, **282**, 755–762.

Pfefferbaum, B. & Doughty, D.E. (2001). Increased alcohol use in a treatment sample of Oklahoma City bombing victims. *Psychiatry*, **64**, 296–303.

Pfefferbaum, B. & Pfefferbaum, R.L. (1998). Contagion in stress: an infectious disease model for posttraumatic stress in children. *Child and Adolescent Psychiatric Clinics of North America*, **7**, 183–194.

Prigerson, H.G., Shear, M.K., Jacobs, S.C. *et al.* (1999). Consensus criteria for traumatic grief: a preliminary empirical test. *British Journal of Psychiatry*, **174**, 67–73.

Raphael, B. (2006). Systems, science and populations: effective early intervention following mass trauma: the roles of government, clinicians and communities. Presented at conference Early psychological intervention following mass trauma: the present and future directions. Valhalla, NY: New York Medical College, School of Public Health.

Raphael, B. & Minkov, C. (1999). Abnormal grief. *Current Opinion in Psychiatry*, **12**, 99–102.

Raphael, B. & Wooding, S. (2004). Early mental health interventions for traumatic loss in adults. In *Early Intervention for Trauma and Traumatic Loss*, ed. B.T. Litz, pp.147–178. New York: Guilford Press.

Raphael, B. Martinek, N. & Wooding, S. (2004). Assessing traumatic bereavement. In *Assessing Psychological Trauma and PTSD*, 2nd edn., eds. J.P. Wilson & T.M. Keane, pp.492–510. New York: Guilford Press.

Rundell, J.R. (2003). A consultation-liaison psychiatry approach to disaster/terrorism victim assessment and management. In *Terrorism and Disaster: Individual and Community Mental Health Interventions*, eds. R.J. Ursano, C.F. Fullerton & A.E. Norwood, pp.107–120. Cambridge: Cambridge University Press.

Sampson, R.J. (2003). The neighborhood context of well-being. *Perspectives in Biology and Medicine*, **46** (3 Suppl), S53–S64.

Sampson, R.J., Raudenbush, S.W. & Earls, F. (1997). Neighborhoods and violent crime: a multilevel study of collective efficacy. *Science*, **277**, 918–924.

Schwarz, E.D. & Kowalski, J.M. (1991). Malignant memories: PTSD in children and adults after a school shooting. *Journal of the American Academy of Child and Adolescent Psychiatry*, **30**, 936–944.

Shear, K., Frank, E., Houck, P.R. & Reynolds, C.F. (2005). Treatment of complicated grief. A randomized controlled trial. *Journal of the American Medical Association*, **293**, 2601–2608.

Sorenson, S.B. (2002). Preventing traumatic stress: public health approaches. *Journal of Traumatic Stress*, **15**, 3–7.

Tucker, J.B. (1997). National health and medical services response to incidents of chemical and biological terrorism. *Journal of the American Medical Association*, **278**, 362–368.

Ursano, R.J. (1981). The Vietnam era prisoner of war: precaptivity personality and development of psychiatric illness. *American Journal of Psychiatry*, **138**, 315–318.

Ursano, R.J. (2002). Post-traumatic stress disorder. *New England Journal of Medicine*, **34**, 130–131.

Ursano, R.J. (2005). Workplace preparedness for terrorism: report of findings to Alfred P. Sloan Foundation. Available at: www.usuhs.mil/psy/WorkplacePrepared nessTerrorism.pdf, accessed May 13, 2007.

Ursano, R.J. & Blumenfield, M. (2006). Concluding remarks. Presented at conference *Early psychological intervention following mass trauma: present and future directions*. Valhalla, NY: New York Medical College, School of Public Health.

Ursano, R.J. & Norwood, A.E., eds. (2003). *Trauma and Disaster: Responses and Management*. Washington, D.C.: American Psychiatric Publishing.

Ursano, R.J., Grieger T.A. & McCarroll, J.E. (1996). Prevention of posttraumatic stress: consultation, training, and early treatment. In *Traumatic Stress: The Effects of Overwhelming Experience on Mind, Body and Society*, eds. B.A. vander Kolk, A.C. McFarlane & L. Weisaeth, pp.441–462. New York: Guilford Press.

Ursano, R.J., Fullerton, C.S. & Norwood, A.E. (2001). Planning for terrorism: behavioral and mental health responses to weapons of mass destruction and mass disruption (DTIC: A392688: 189 pages). Bethesda, Md.: Uniformed Services University of the Health Sciences.

Ursano, R.J., Fullerton, C.S. & Norwood, A.E. (2002). Responding to terrorism: individuals and community needs (DTIC: A406540: 186 pages). Bethesda, Md.: Uniformed Services University of the Health Sciences.

Ursano, R.J., Norwood, A.E. & Fullerton, C.S. (2004). Behavioral and mental health responses to bioterrorism: needs for the public's health. In *Bioterrorism: Psychological and Public Health Interventions*, eds. R.J. Ursano,

A. E. Norwood & C. S. Fullerton, pp. 332–348. Cambridge: Cambridge University Press.

Vlahov, D., Galea, S., Resnick, H. *et al.* (2002). Increased use of cigarettes, alcohol, and marijuana among Manhattan, New York, residents after the September 11th terrorist attacks. *American Journal of Epidemiology*, **155**, 988–996.

Weisler, R. H., Barbee, J. G. & Townsend, M. H. (2006). Mental health and recovery in the Gulf Coast after Hurricanes Katrina and Rita. *Journal of the American Medical Association*, **296**, 585–588.

Wessely, S. (2005). Victimhood and resilience. *New England Journal of Medicine*, **353**, 548–550.

Index